Michael Paddock · Amaka C. Offiah

Paediatric Radiology Rapid Reporting for FRCR Part 2B

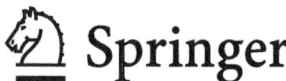

Springer

Michael Paddock
Sheffield Teaching Hospitals
Sheffield
UK

Amaka C. Offiah
Academic Unit of Child Health
Department of Oncology and Metabolism
University of Sheffield
Sheffield
UK

ISBN 978-3-030-01964-8   ISBN 978-3-030-01965-5   (eBook)
https://doi.org/10.1007/978-3-030-01965-5

Library of Congress Control Number: 2018967447

This Springer imprint is published by the registered company Springer Nature Switzerland AG
The registered company address is: Gewerbestrasse 11, 6330 Cham, Switzerland

*To Vaughan—for your unwavering faith,
support and unconditional love*

MP

To my husband and children—you know why

ACO

Foreword

I was delighted to be asked to prepare a foreword for this book written by my colleagues, Dr M Paddock and Dr AC Offiah. As the Training Programme Director for South Yorkshire, it is wonderful to see an enthusiastic radiology trainee producing high-quality teaching material, supported by an established consultant expert in their field of interest. Passing down knowledge continues the important cycle of learning and teaching with benefit to future generations of radiologists.

Reading this book is a must for any specialist trainee in radiology preparing for the final FRCR examination. Paediatric radiology is often an area that is neglected during revision when the RCR curriculum requires a very wide breadth of knowledge. Many trainees have limited exposure to paediatric radiology during their training, and there may have been an interval between a paediatric attachment and preparing for the FRCR 2B examination. Paediatric imaging does however form part of all FRCR examinations, and you will be assessed in this area. I have been an examiner at the Royal College of Radiologists for many years and there is a recognised reduced performance in questions related to paediatric imaging.

This book consists of cases set out in the style of the FRCR 2B Rapid Reporting examination. The high-quality images and attached notes are beautifully presented in a format that is easy to read. Your knowledge will be enhanced with what I think you will find to be an enjoyable learning experience. The carefully selected cases are either commonly seen in daily practice or are important to be aware of. This book will help you prepare for all components of the FRCR 2B examination (not just the Rapid Reporting element) and your future career as an independent practitioner.

Happy reading and good luck!

Ruth Batty
The Royal Hallamshire Hospital/Sheffield Children's Hospital
Sheffield, UK

Preface

Firstly, congratulations on passing the FRCR Part 2A—well done! Now to the FRCR 2B examination where the fun can really begin…

All three components of the 2B examination may contain a significant proportion of paediatric imaging. Candidates 'struggle with interpretation of paediatric imaging—even for common paediatric pathologies' as identified in the Royal College of Radiologists Examiners' report. Better preparation in this component will also help you when faced with paediatric cases in the long case reporting and viva sections, and you will definitely get some!

The amount of paediatric radiology training up and down the country is variable, and some candidates may not feel adequately prepared to tackle paediatric imaging in the Rapid Reporting section of the examination. The reality is that the majority of radiologists will go on to work in District General Hospitals (DGHs) where paediatric imaging can feature prominently in the day-to-day workload of the department. Most children will initially present to and be imaged in DGHs, given that most do not live next to a dedicated paediatric tertiary centre.

The examiners need to make sure that you are a safe radiologist and that you are able to provide a sound radiological opinion which may contribute to effective patient management and care. This is what the 2B examination is assessing—your ability to use your knowledge and skills effectively and your preparedness to practise radiology safely as an independent practitioner.

We felt that there was a lack of dedicated paediatric radiology revision resources for the 2B examination, and we wrote this book to address that need. All radiographs are from standard day-to-day practice and have been collected over a 3-year period by one of the authors: the images range from the obvious buckle fracture to the subtle metaphyseal fracture (specific to physical child abuse) which is easily missed.

Following the answer key for each test, we have expanded on certain abnormal findings or normal variants to further enhance your learning. We have purposefully not used arrows or line diagrams to show you where or what the abnormality is—abnormal radiographs do not come with this in the examination or in real life. As clinical radiologists, we have described the abnormality, and where subtle, it has been magnified as you would do in the examination and in clinical practice. Being a text comprising of paediatric radiographs, the image quality is dependent on the limited dose used to acquire the images. Thus, the quality of some of the magnified images in the explanations may be degraded but still remain adequate to sufficiently demonstrate the pathology. Where relevant, we have included tips for the viva examination. The references also include excellent pictorial reviews and links to educational websites so that you can get the most out of your revision.

We emphasise that the best practice for the Rapid Reporting section of the examination is to report paediatric radiographs and get them checked by your local paediatric radiologists. This book can be used to supplement your learning during normal working hours.

We are extremely grateful to Dr. Jonathan M. Smith and Dr. Robin Dale, specialty trainees on the Sheffield radiology training scheme, for their insight and feedback throughout the preparation of this book.

Finally, we wish you the best of luck in all components of the examination and your future careers. We hope that you will use this book as a future reference text, even after the examination. We welcome any comments, suggestions or feedback, and if you have any queries, please email us on paedsradrapidreporting@gmail.com.

Good luck!

Sheffield, UK   Michael Paddock
                                                                                     Amaka C. Offiah

Testimonies

I used this book in the run up to sitting the Final FRCR Part B examination in autumn 2018 and I believe it played an important role in obtaining a high score in the Rapid Reporting element. Most practice exam sets include a few paediatric radiographs, but no other resource on the market provides a concentrated bank of paediatric radiographs with which you can hone your skills. This makes it particularly useful for candidates like me, who had completed their paediatric rotation a long time before sitting the exam, or for those candidates who are not very confident in paediatric reporting. The explanations are thorough and provide some useful tips for the viva component of the exam, also.

Dr. Jonathan M. Smith

Unlike the online rapids packets I used, this book offers explanations which are really helpful for confidently identifying abnormalities and discounting normal findings unique to paediatric radiology. The discussions are also great for viva preparation. It definitely helped me to pass the FRCR 2B examination.

Dr. Robin Dale

Contents

Abbreviations

ABC	Aneurysmal bone cyst
AFP	Alpha-fetoprotein
AIIS	Anterior inferior iliac spine
ALTE	Apparent life-threatening event
AP	Anteroposterior
ARPKD	Autosomal recessive polycystic kidney disease
ASIS	Anterior superior iliac spine
AVN	Avascular necrosis
β hCG	Beta human chorionic gonadotropin
BBI	Button battery ingestion
BRUE	Brief resolved unexplained event
CLE	Congenital lobar emphysema
CLO	Congenital lobar overinflation
CML	Classic metaphyseal lesion
CMV	Cytomegalovirus
CPAM	Congenital pulmonary airway malformation
CT	Computed tomography
CTPA	Computed tomography pulmonary angiogram
DDH	Developmental dysplasia of the hip
DGH	District General Hospital
DJ	Duodenojejunal
ED	Emergency Department
ETT	Endotracheal tube
FCD	Fibrous cortical defect(s)
FOOSH	Fall onto an outstretched hand
FRCR	Fellowship of the Royal College of Radiologists
GI	Gastrointestinal
GP	General Practitioner
HIV	Human immunodeficiency virus
HME	Hereditary multiple exostoses
ITU	Intensive therapy unit
LCH	Langerhans cell histiocytosis
MCDK	Multicystic dysplastic kidney
MIBG	Metaiodobenzylguanidine

MRI	Magnetic resonance imaging
NAI	Non-accidental injury
NEC	Necrotising enterocolitis
NGT	Nasogastric tube
NICE	National Institute for Health and Care Excellence
NOF	Non-ossifying fibroma
NRSTS	Non-rhabdomyosarcoma soft-tissue sarcoma
NSAID	Non-steroidal anti-inflammatory drug
OCD	Osteochondritis dissecans
OI	Osteogenesis imperfecta
ORIF	Open reduction and internal fixation
PDA	Patent ductus arteriosus
PET-CT	Positron emission tomography-computed tomography
PSIS	Posterior superior iliac spine
RCR	Royal College of Radiologists
RTA	Road traffic accident
SCFE	Slipped capital femoral epiphysis
SLE	Systemic lupus erythematosus
SUFE	Slipped upper femoral epiphysis
TOF	Tracheo-oesophageal fistula
VSD	Ventricular septal defect

About the Authors

Michael Paddock is a final year specialty registrar on the Sheffield radiology training programme, training in general and paediatric radiology.

He completed an EPSRC-funded Biomedical Imaging MSc during his undergraduate medical training at Guy's, King's and St Thomas's School of Medicine at King's College London. After graduating, he undertook foundation training in Dorset followed by clinical paediatric training on the North-West London rotation, including a post at Great Ormond Street Hospital for Children. This led onto an NIHR Academic Clinical Fellowship in clinical radiology at the University of Sheffield which he completed alongside his core clinical radiology training, in addition to completing a Postgraduate Certificate in Clinical Research, whilst successfully attaining the FRCR.

He led a prospective clinical research study assessing fetal brain development using *in utero* magnetic resonance imaging, in addition to conducting research in the imaging of suspected physical child abuse. He has numerous first-author publications and has won national and international research awards for his work.

Amaka C. Offiah is a reader in Paediatric Musculoskeletal Imaging at the Academic Unit of Child Health, the University of Sheffield, and an honorary consultant paediatric radiologist at Sheffield Children's Hospital.

After completing radiology training in Sheffield, she moved to London to Great Ormond Street Hospital for Children and the Institute of Child Health, where she obtained her PhD in the imaging of suspected inflicted injury. She returned to Sheffield as an HEFCE-funded clinical senior lecturer in the Academic Unit of Child Health. She was promoted to reader in January 2015 and is a Fellow of the Higher Education Academy (FHEA).

In addition to over 80 original scientific publications, over 20 peer-reviewed review articles and 10 book chapters, she has co-authored two 'highly commended' textbooks: *A Radiological Atlas of Child Abuse* and *Fetal and Perinatal Skeletal Dysplasias: An Atlas of Multimodality Imaging*. She is chairperson of the European Society of Paediatric Radiologists' (ESPR) Child Abuse Taskforce and the Skeletal Dysplasia Group for Teaching and Research. She has been an expert witness in over 200 cases of suspected child abuse and was the first female and first paediatric radiologist to be appointed the Royal College of Radiologists Roentgen Professor.

Introduction

Purpose of the Rapid Reporting Component of the 2B FRCR Examination

Emergency Department (ED) imaging constitutes a significant proportion of most radiologists' workload. The Rapid Reporting component of the examination assesses candidates' ability to decide rapidly if an image is normal or abnormal and to provide a diagnosis if the image is abnormal. It is important to be able to confidently state when an abnormality is present and exclude it when it is not.

The examination contains 30 radiographs to be reported. The majority of the images are musculoskeletal/extremity radiographs in addition to some chest and abdominal radiographs, as would be expected in a typical ED reporting session. We have replicated this brief, except that all the radiographs are paediatric, ranging from neonates to adolescents.

Structure

Candidates will have 35 min to report all 30 images and denote each image as either normal or abnormal. Each image contains one significant diagnosable abnormality which is *not* complex; as such, differential diagnoses should not be offered. Any anatomical variants (and minor age-related degenerative change in adults) should be recorded as normal. Images will be viewed on a single monitor.

For those radiographs that demonstrate a well-recognised fracture pattern in which two fractures would be expected to occur together, you will be expected to identify and write down *both* fractures to get the mark. This is stated in the Royal College of Radiologists (RCR) Part 2B Spring 2016 Examiners' Report, available at https://www.rcr.ac.uk/sites/default/files/spring2016_cr2b_examiners_report.pdf.

Scoring

Candidates have the opportunity to attain 1 mark per image and thus a maximum of 30 marks. The scoring system used is outlined below and is taken directly from the RCR website:

Image type	Candidate response	Mark
Normal image	Correctly classified	+1
	Incorrectly classified (**appropriate** false positive)	+½
	No answer given	0
Abnormal image	Correctly classified and correctly identified	+1
	Correctly classified but incorrectly identified	0
	Incorrectly classified (false negative)	0
	No answer given	0

What is an **appropriate** false positive? Consider a radiograph designated as 'normal' by the examiners. The candidate denotes the image as 'abnormal' and writes the diagnosis of 'metaphyseal spur', for example. As stated above, whilst normal variants should be categorised as 'normal', the examiners *may* review the radiograph in question and *may* award the candidate half a mark if they agree—however, this will be at the discretion of the examiners.

Subsequently, the total marks attained in the Rapid Reporting component are converted into an overall mark between 4 and 8 as outlined in the table below:

Total marks	Overall mark
00–24	4
24½	4½
25–25½	5
26–26½	5½
27	6
27½–28	6½
28½–29	7
29½	7½
30	8

This score is combined with the scores from the long reporting and the viva examination (two stations are taken over 1 h). Candidates will be given a score of 4–8 in each of the four sections, of which the pass mark in each section is 6, giving an overall pass mark of 24. Additionally, candidates must obtain a mark of 6 (or above) in *at least* two of the four sections to pass the FRCR 2B examination overall.

All candidates should aim for a minimum score of 27/30 (90%) in the Rapid Reporting component to achieve a converted overall mark of 6. Whilst this component is thought of as the most difficult, it is possible for candidates to score full marks and receive a converted overall mark of 8. This can contribute significantly to the final overall score when combined with the scores from the long reporting and viva examination and emphasises the importance of scoring highly in this component.

We encourage all candidates to read all the available Examiners Reports in preparation for their upcoming examination sitting. The latest information pertaining to all components of the examination, the format, the scoring system of each component and the overall scoring allocation, along with guidance for candidates, particularly in light of the recently introduced image-based examination delivered on a digital platform, can be found on the RCR website which should be checked regularly for updates—please see the references.

Hints and Tips

Revising for the Part 2B examination seems like a daunting task, but, as with anything, organisation and preparation are key.

Below are a few hints and tips to help prepare you for your up-and-coming examination sitting:

- Treat the examination as if you were at work and report the radiographs as you would in daily practice.
- Before the exam, report as many radiographs as possible and get them checked by consultant radiologists: this is the only way to receive feedback on your practice and to identify areas for development. Where areas for improvement have been identified, report more of these radiographs and get them checked.
- Best practice, both in the examination and in clinical practice, is to state the side of the abnormality. Given the time limitations in the examination, (L) and (R) can be written in place of 'left' and 'right', respectively. Additionally, writing # in place of 'fracture' is acceptable and will also save time.
- Develop review areas for each body part: there are a number of resources and 'checklists' available online.
- If unsure, denote the radiograph as 'normal'.
- Completing each test in this book within the allotted 35 min (be strict with the timing) will give you the realistic practice needed to succeed in this component of the examination.

Further Reading

The Royal College of Radiologists (2018) Accessed April 2018:

- Final FRCR Part B Examination – Purpose of Assessment Statement. https://www.rcr.ac.uk/sites/default/files/cr2b_purpose_of_assessment_statement.pdf
- Final Examination for the Fellowship in Clinical Radiology (Part B) – Scoring System. https://www.rcr.ac.uk/sites/default/files/docs/radiology/pdf/CR2B_scoring_system.pdf
- Final FRCR Part B Examination. https://www.rcr.ac.uk/clinical-radiology/examinations/final-frcr-part-b-examination-0

- Examiners Reports. https://www.rcr.ac.uk/clinical-radiology/examinations/final-frcr-part-b-examination/examiners-reports
- Final Examination for the Fellowship in Clinical Radiology (Part B) – Guidance Notes for Candidates. https://www.rcr.ac.uk/sites/default/files/cr2b_candidate_guidance_notes_0.pdf

1.1   Images

Image 1

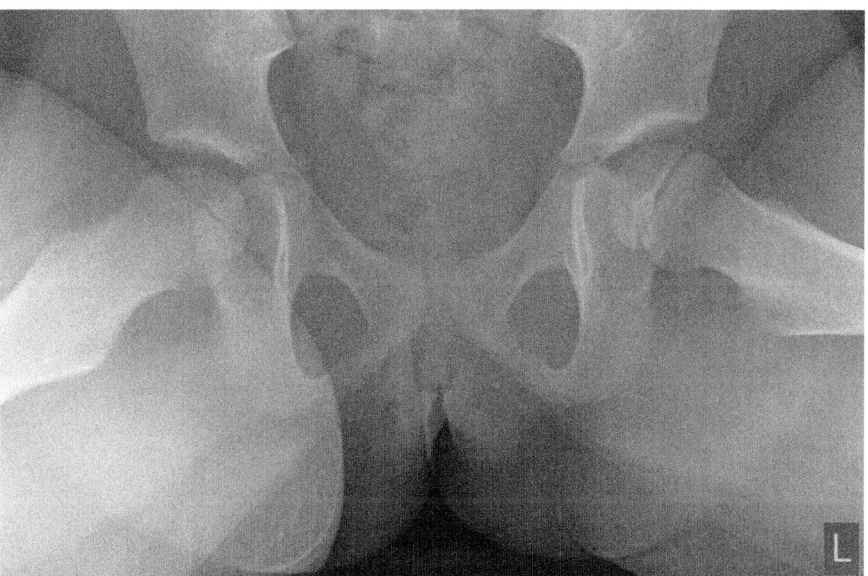

Normal	Abnormal	Diagnosis/Abnormality (only if abnormal)

Image 2

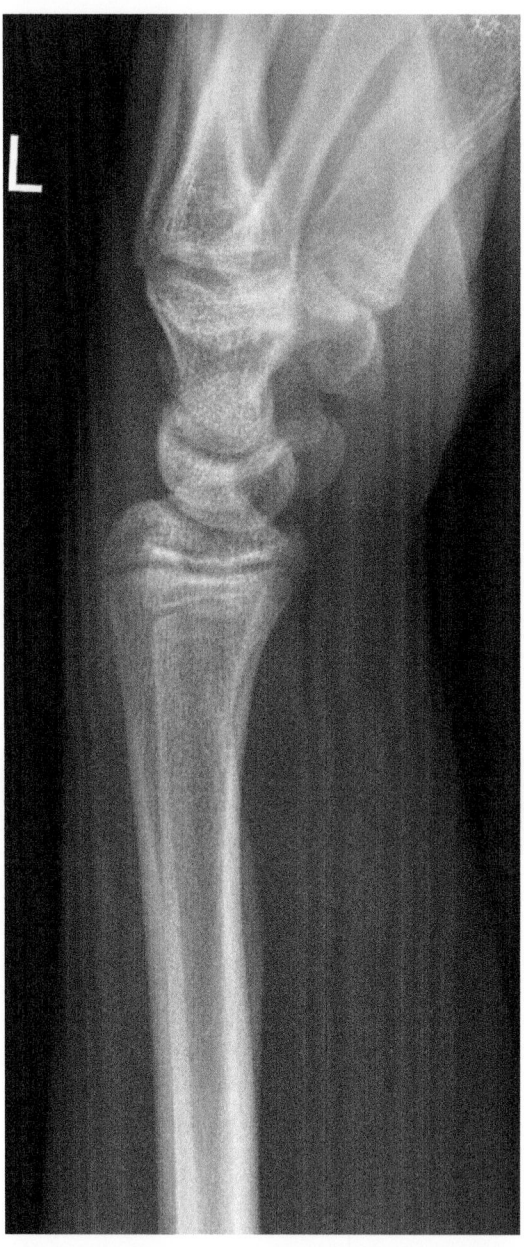

Normal	Abnormal	Diagnosis/Abnormality (only if abnormal)

Image 3

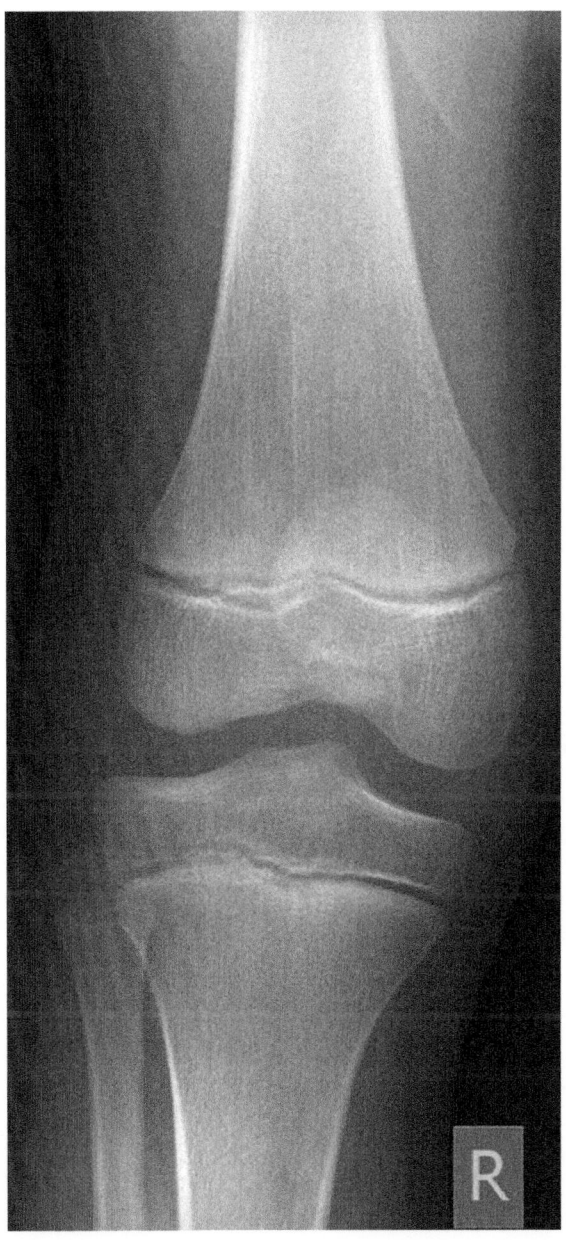

Normal	Abnormal	Diagnosis/Abnormality (only if abnormal)

Image 4

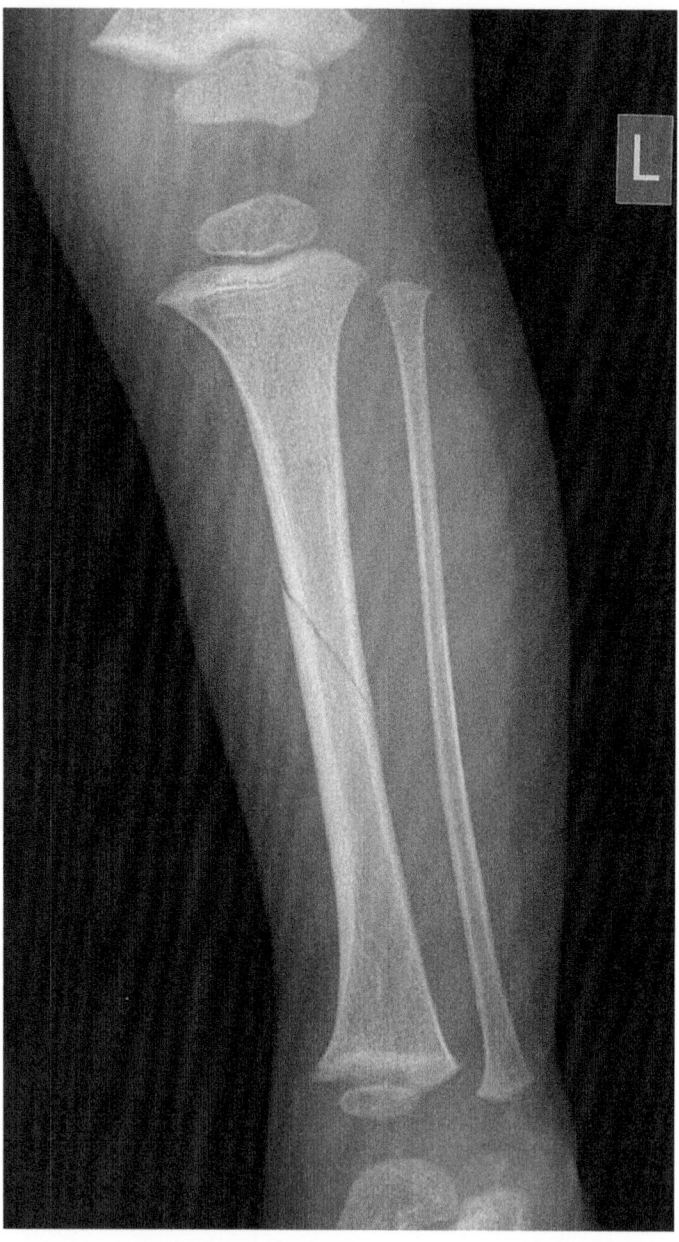

Normal	Abnormal	Diagnosis/Abnormality (only if abnormal)

Image 5

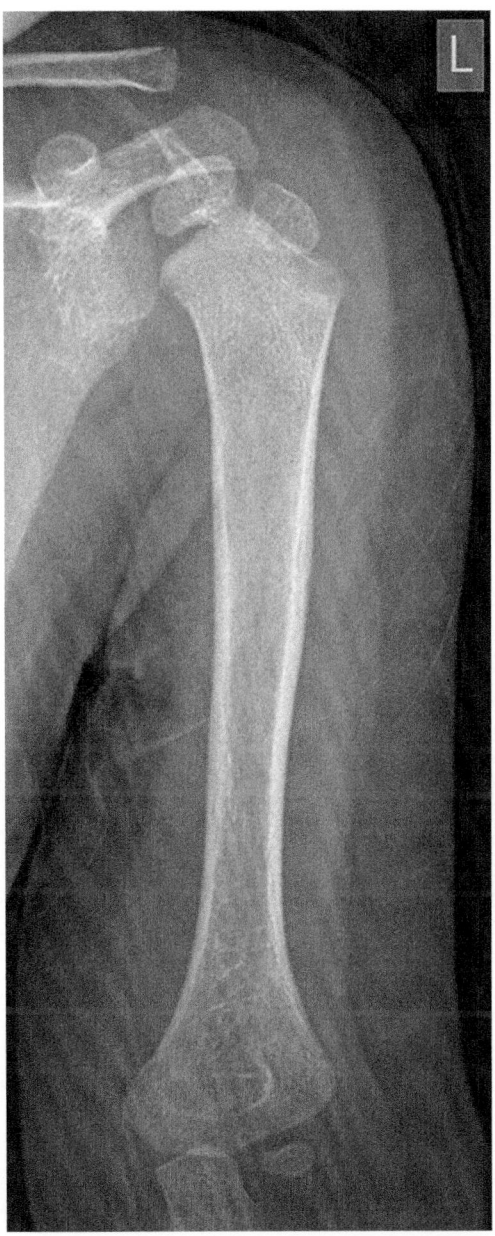

Normal	Abnormal	Diagnosis/Abnormality (only if abnormal)

Image 6

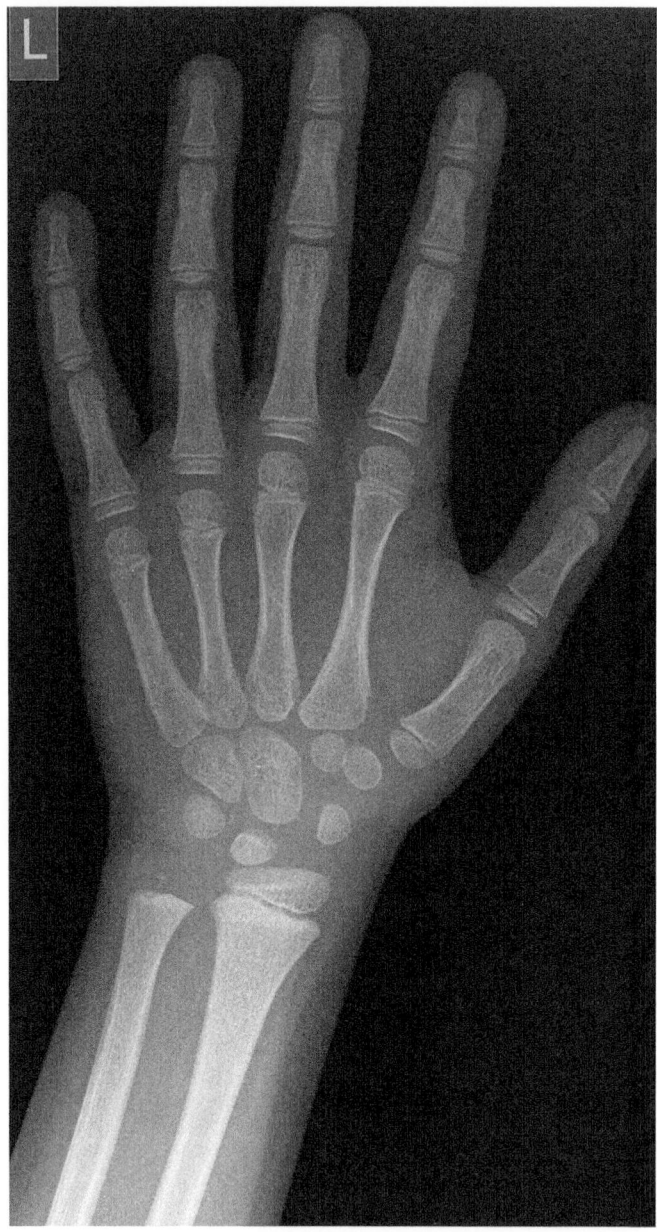

Normal	Abnormal	Diagnosis/Abnormality (only if abnormal)

Image 7

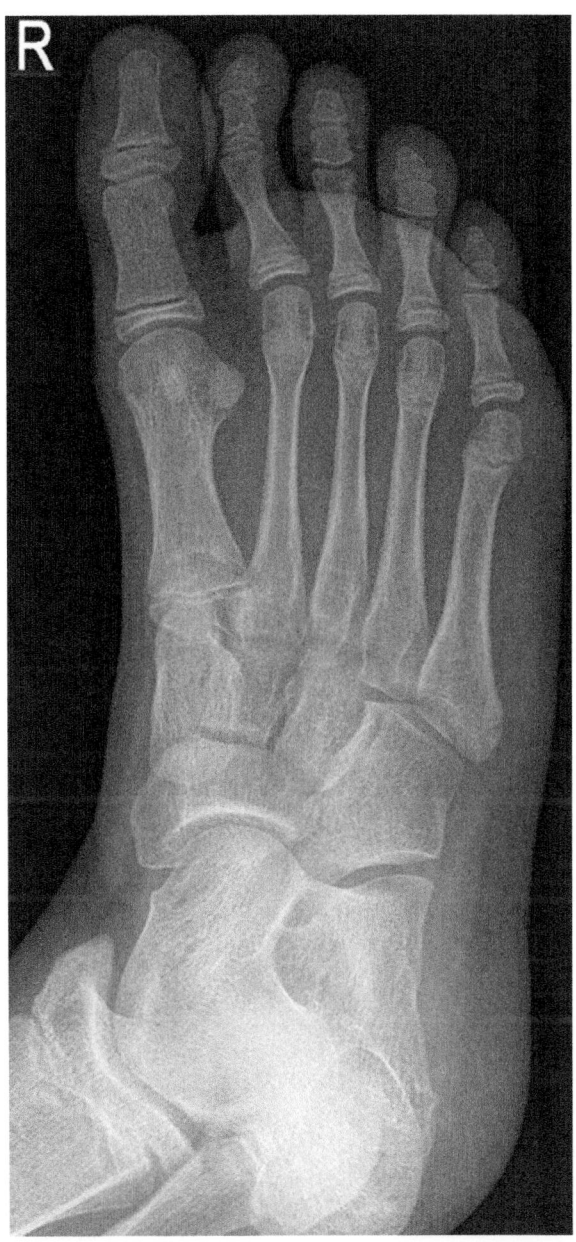

Normal	Abnormal	Diagnosis/Abnormality (only if abnormal)

Image 8

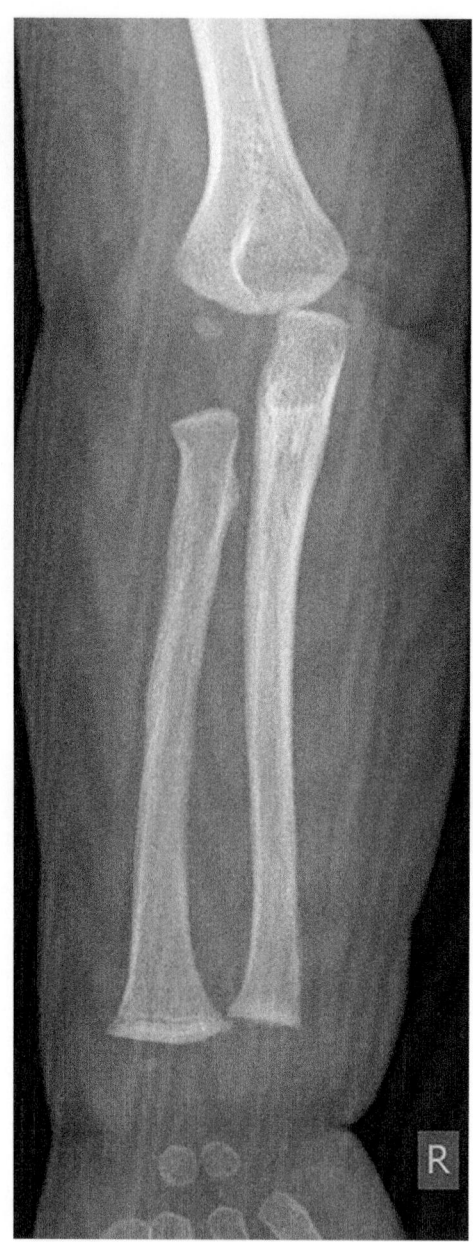

Normal	Abnormal	Diagnosis/Abnormality (only if abnormal)

Image 9

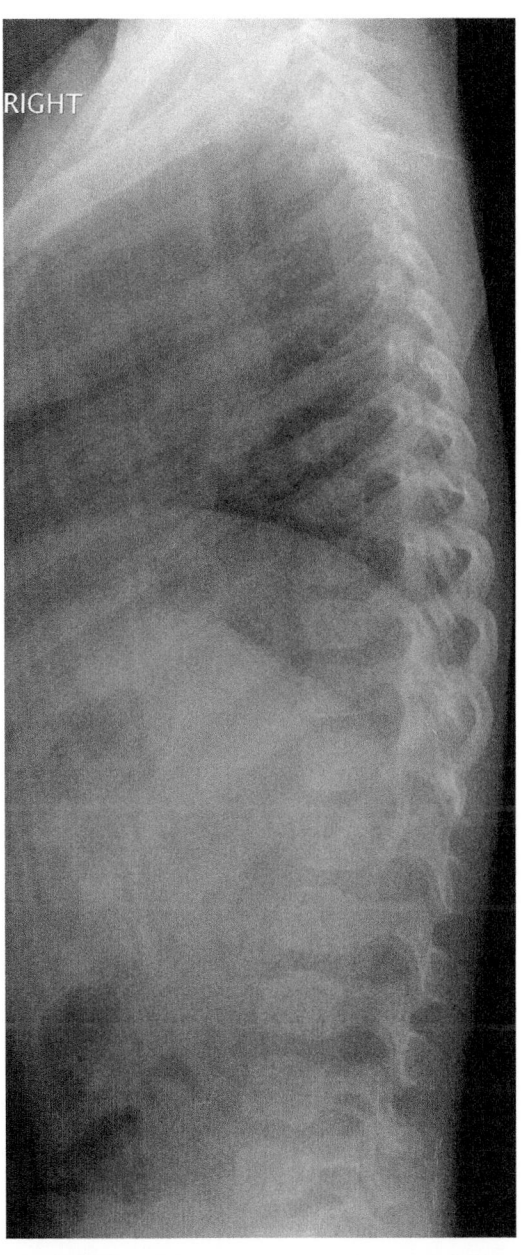

Normal	Abnormal	Diagnosis/Abnormality (only if abnormal)

Image 10

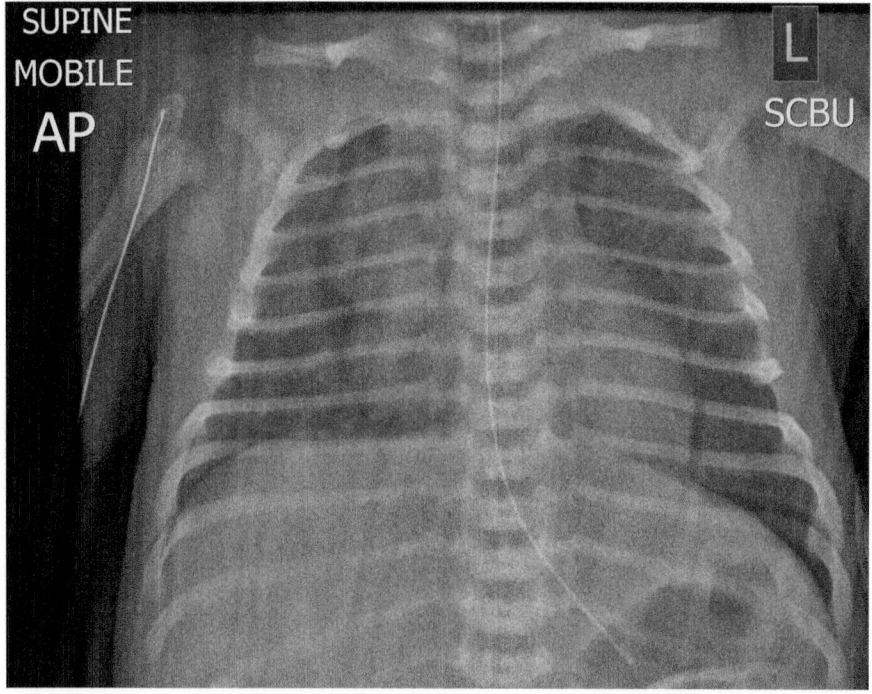

Normal	Abnormal	Diagnosis/Abnormality (only if abnormal)

Image 11

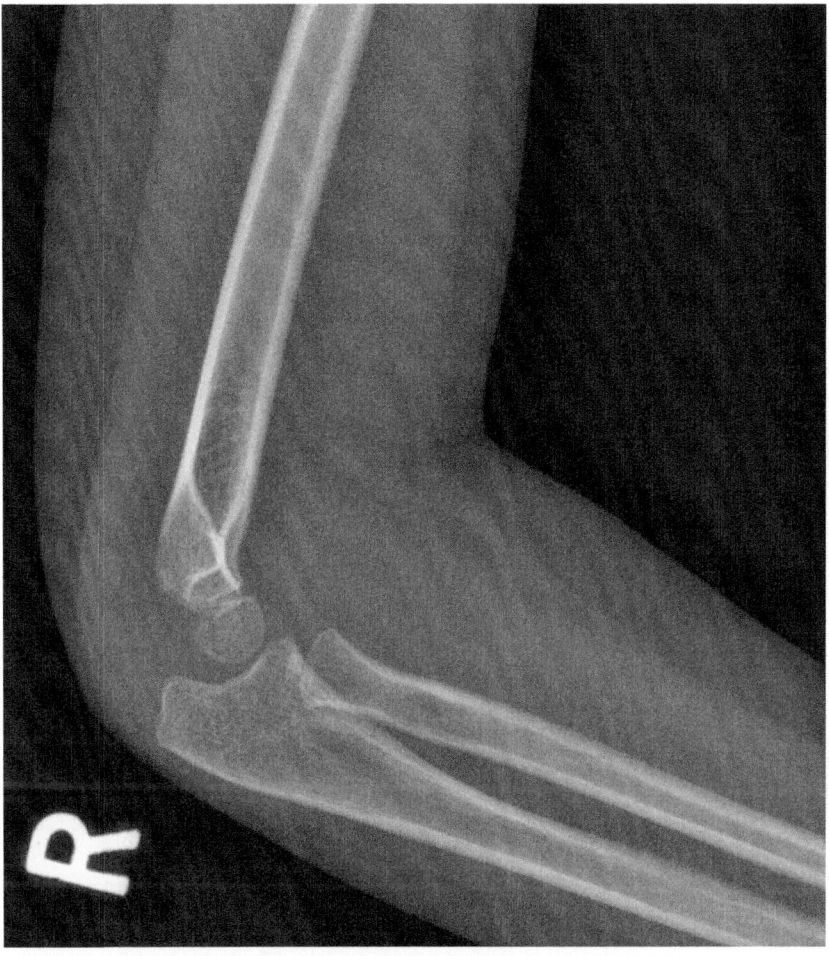

Normal	Abnormal	Diagnosis/Abnormality (only if abnormal)

Image 12

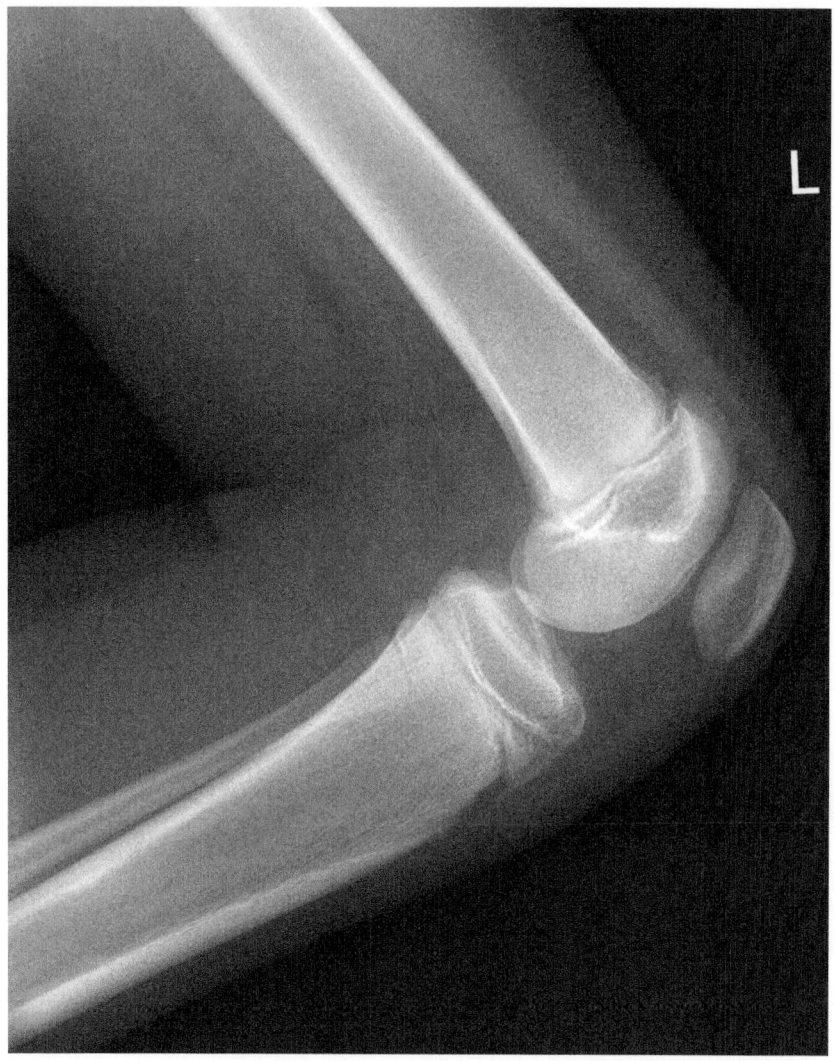

Normal	Abnormal	Diagnosis/Abnormality (only if abnormal)

Image 13

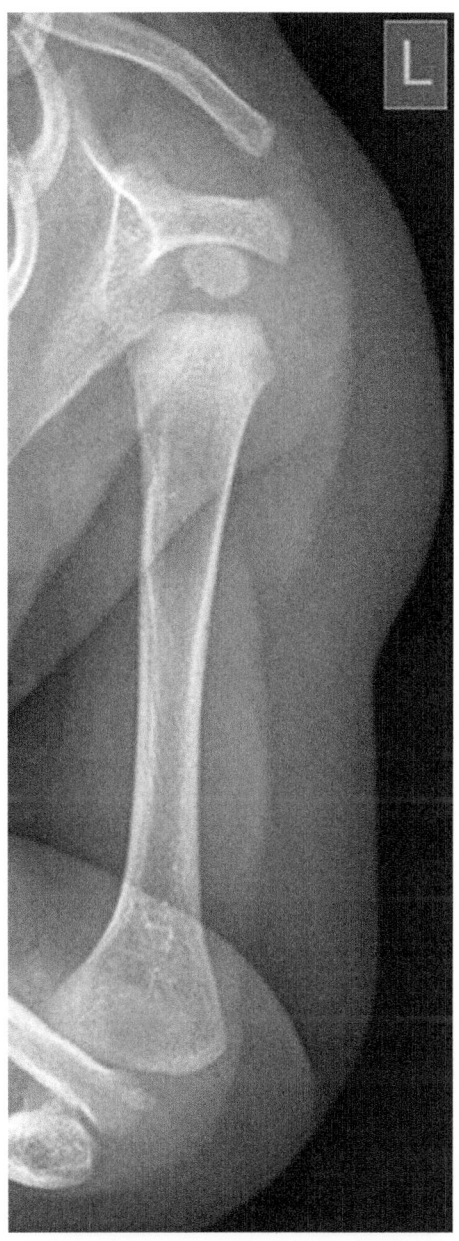

Normal	Abnormal	Diagnosis/Abnormality (only if abnormal)

Image 14

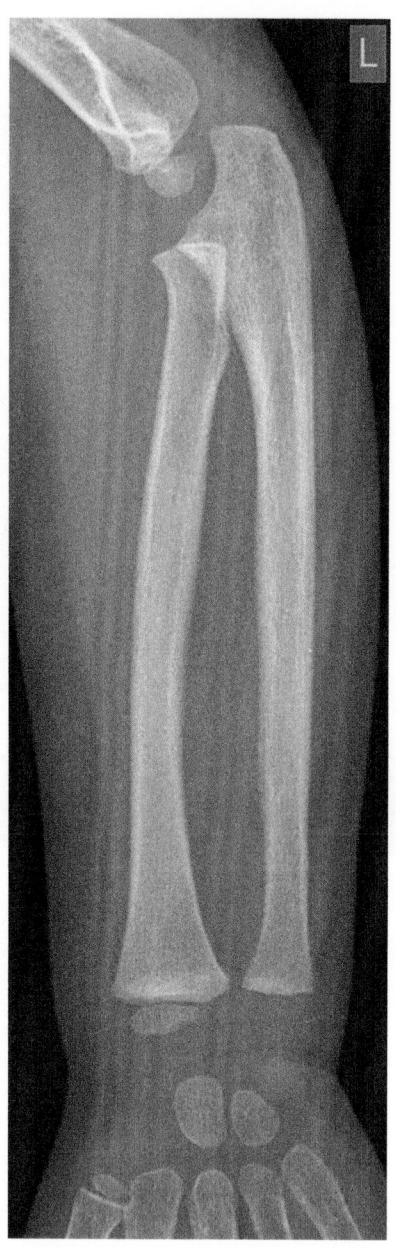

Normal	Abnormal	Diagnosis/Abnormality (only if abnormal)

Image 15

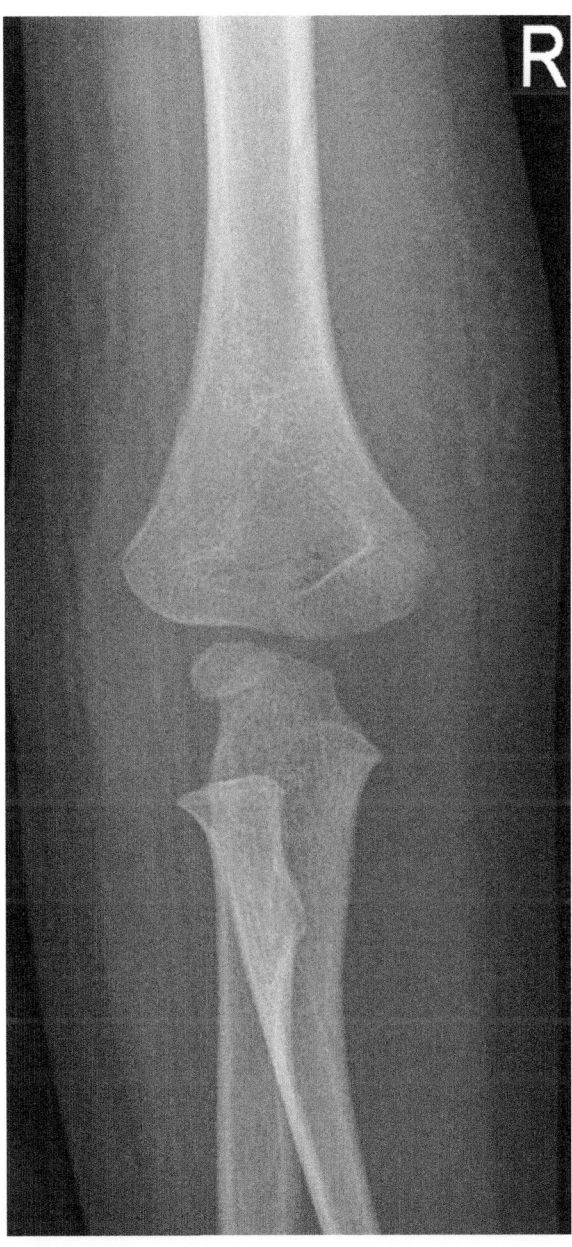

Normal	Abnormal	Diagnosis/Abnormality (only if abnormal)

Image 16

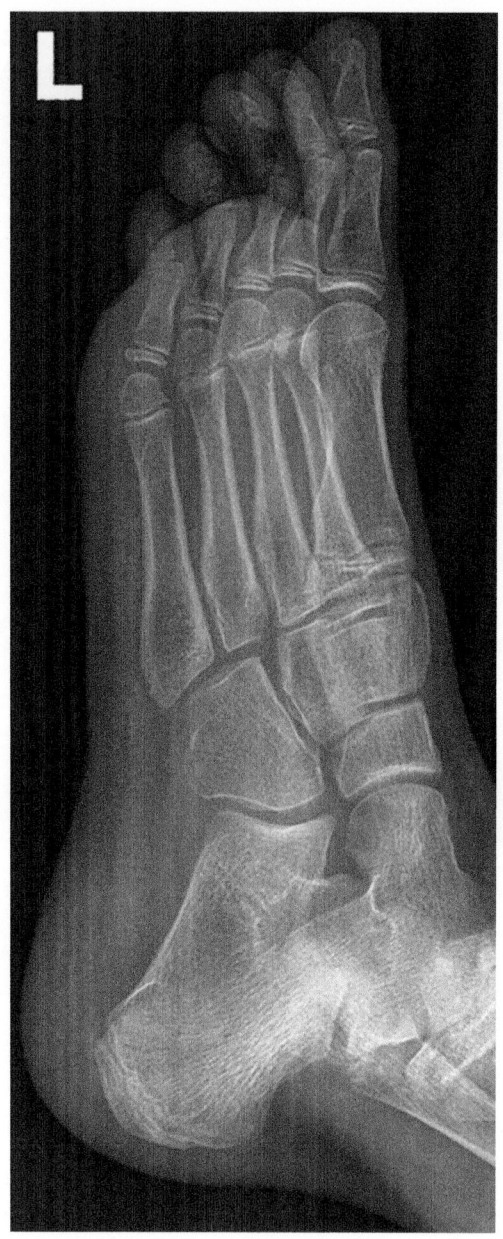

Normal	Abnormal	Diagnosis/Abnormality (only if abnormal)

Image 17

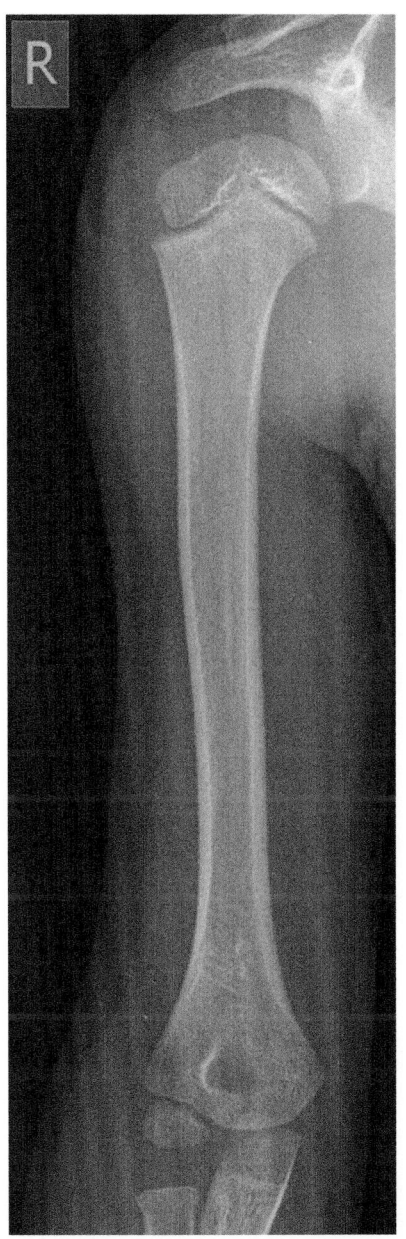

Normal	Abnormal	Diagnosis/Abnormality (only if abnormal)

Image 18

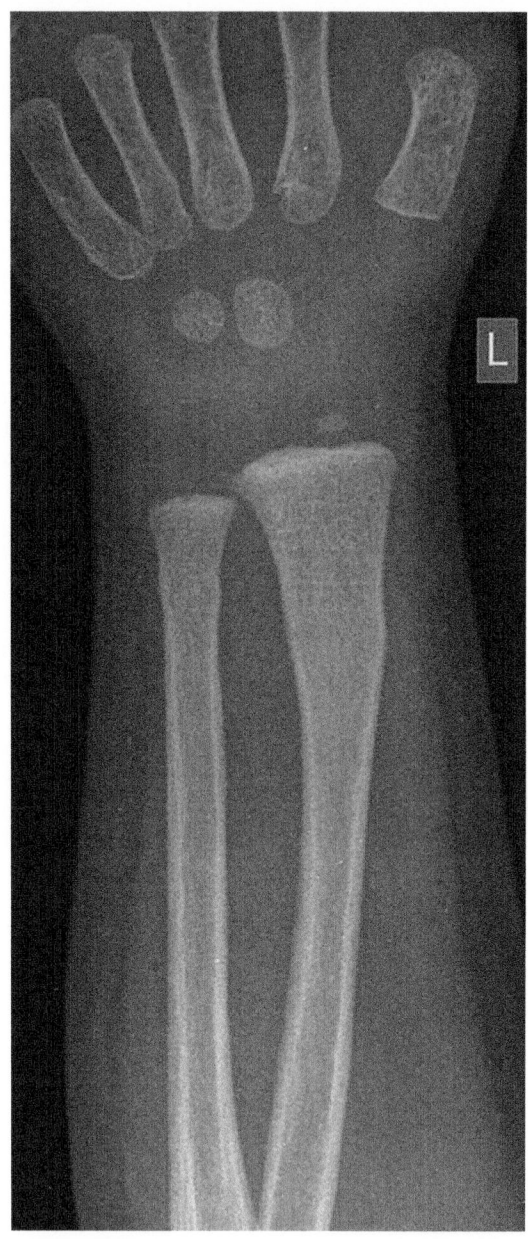

Normal	Abnormal	Diagnosis/Abnormality (only if abnormal)

Image 19

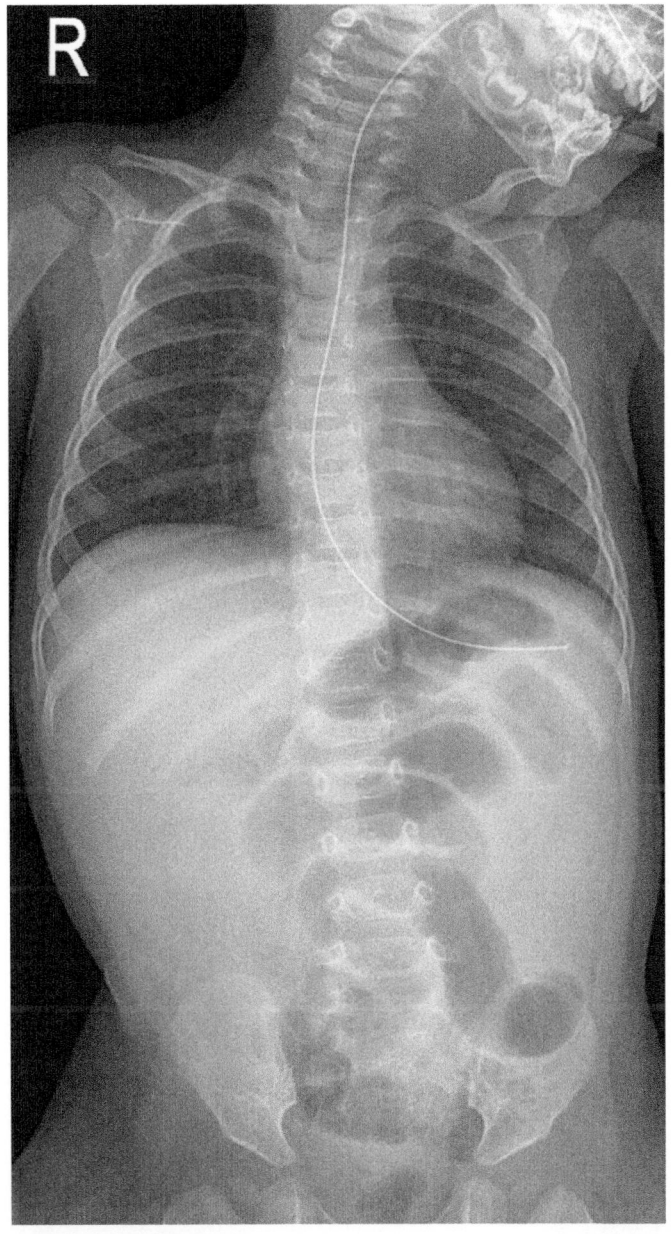

Normal	Abnormal	Diagnosis/Abnormality (only if abnormal)

Image 20

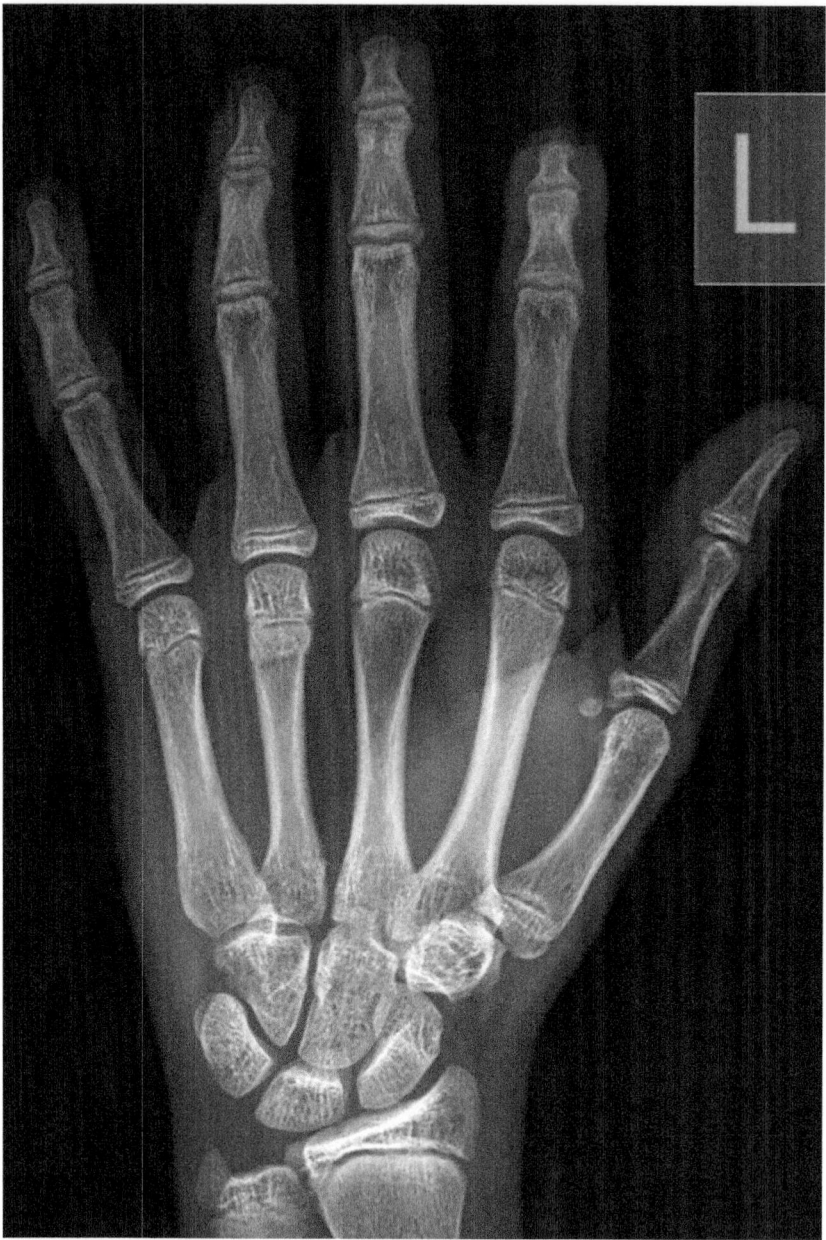

Normal	Abnormal	Diagnosis/Abnormality (only if abnormal)

Image 21

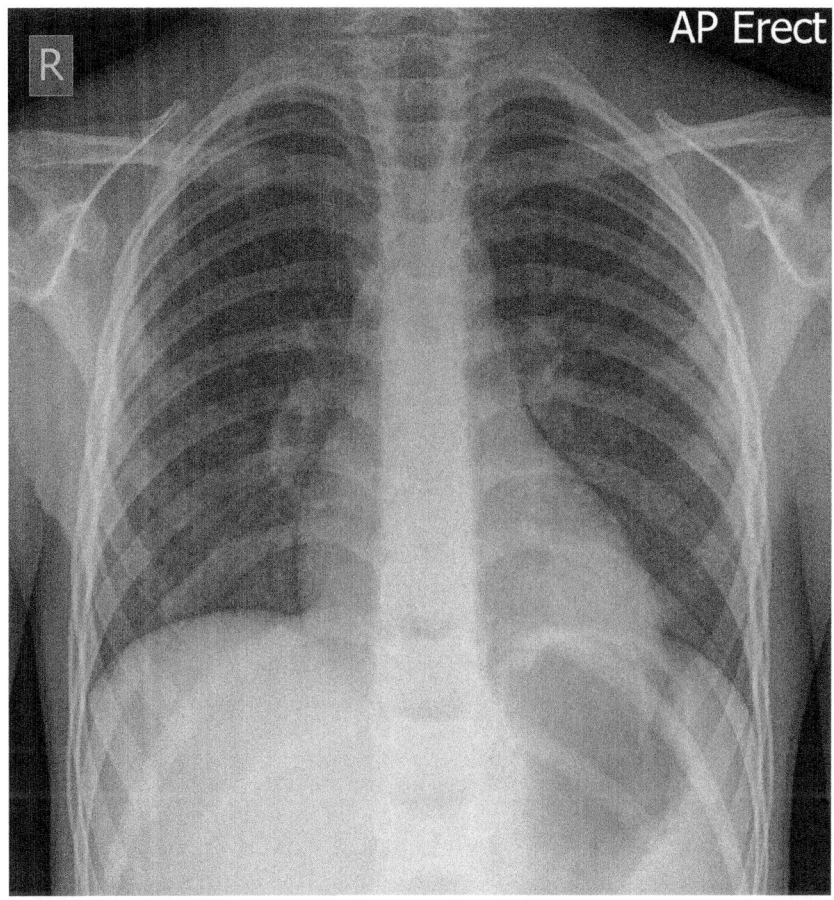

Normal	Abnormal	Diagnosis/Abnormality (only if abnormal)

Image 22

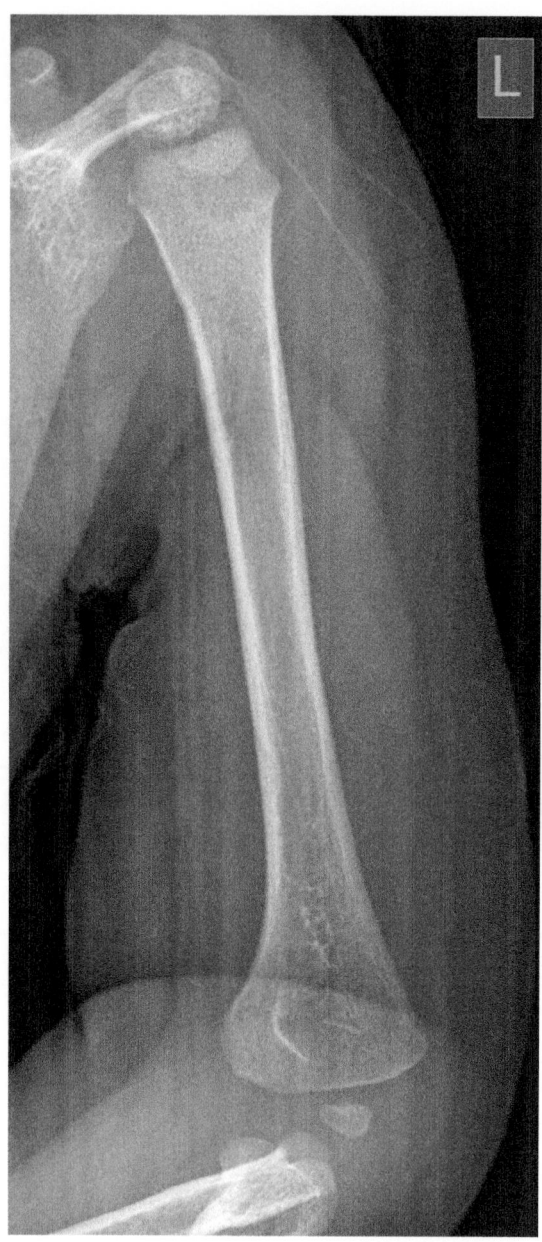

Normal	Abnormal	Diagnosis/Abnormality (only if abnormal)

Image 23

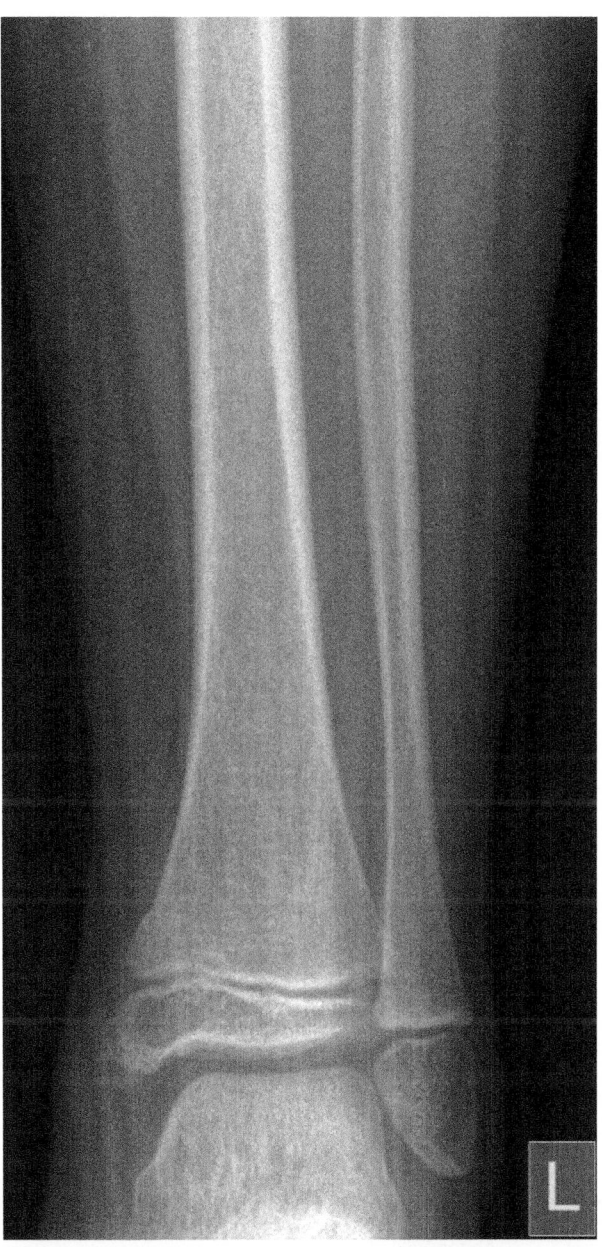

Normal	Abnormal	Diagnosis/Abnormality (only if abnormal)

Image 24

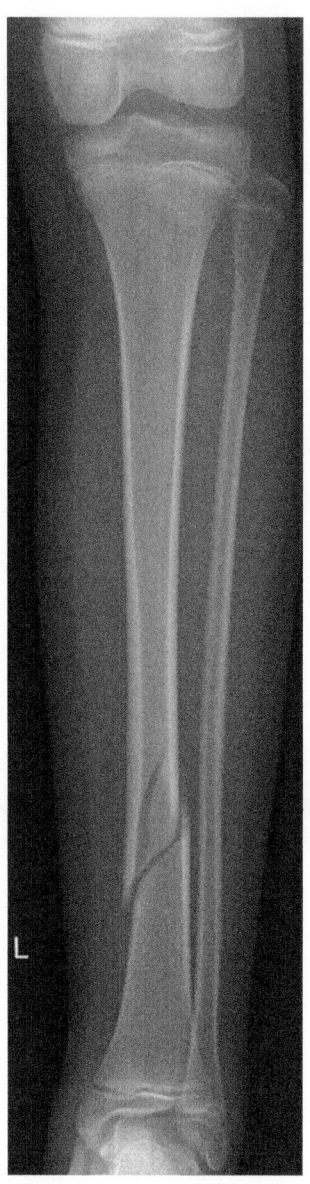

Normal	Abnormal	Diagnosis/Abnormality (only if abnormal)

Image 25

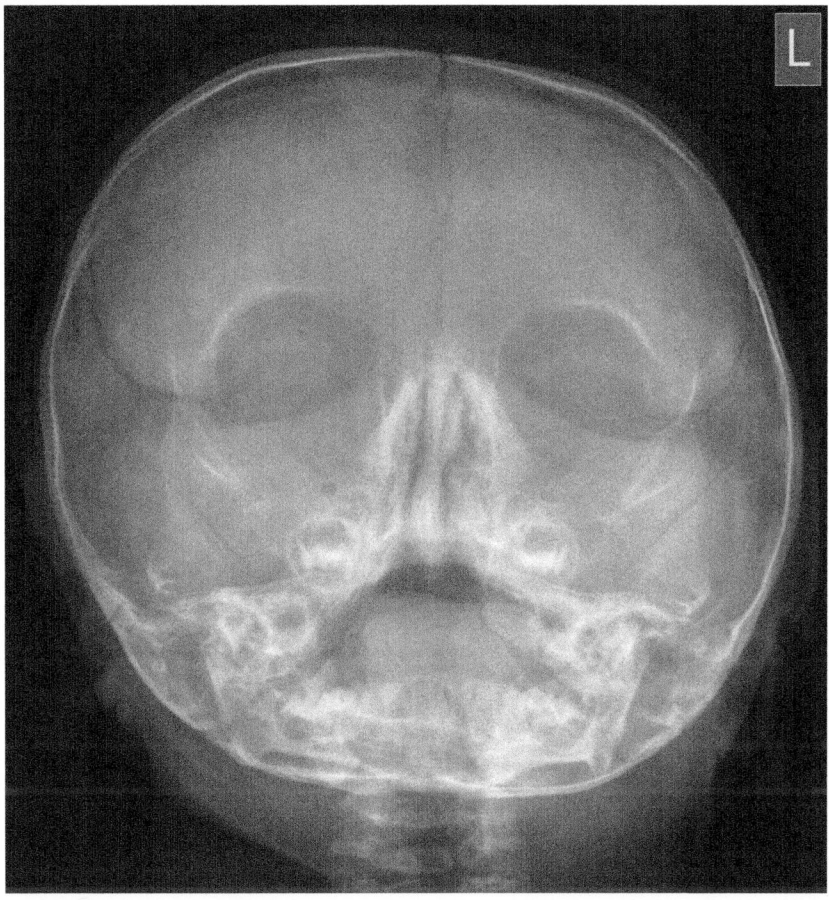

Normal	Abnormal	Diagnosis/Abnormality (only if abnormal)

Image 26

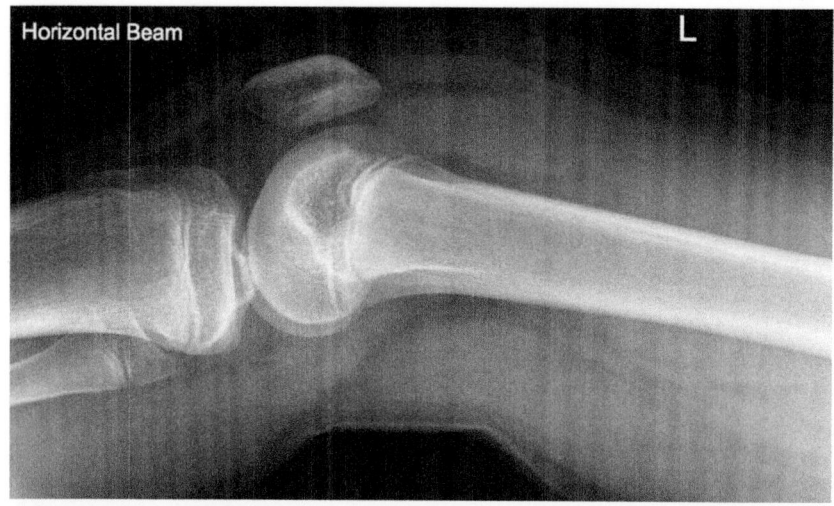

Normal	Abnormal	Diagnosis/Abnormality (only if abnormal)

Image 27

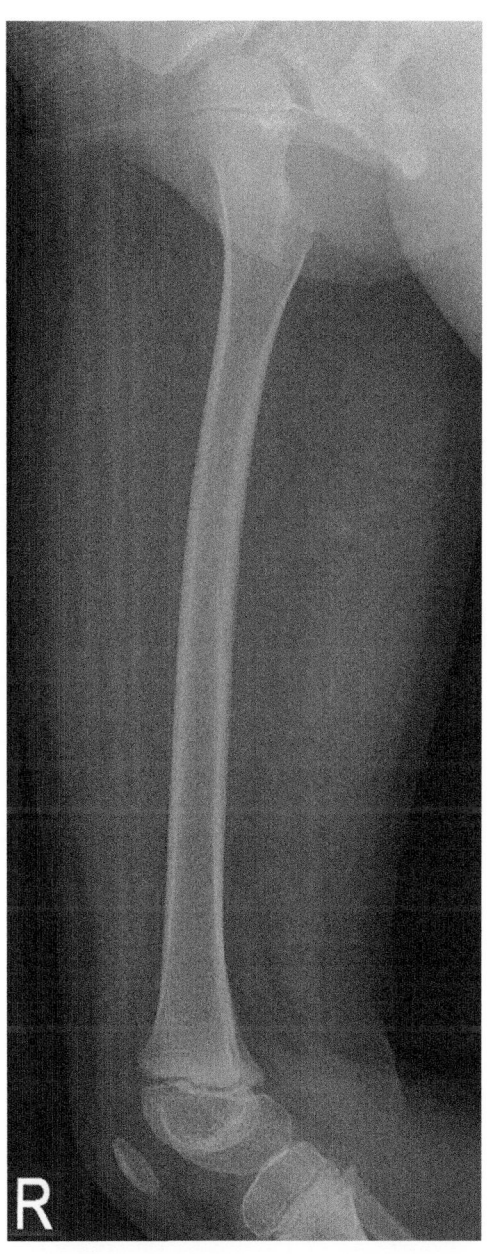

Normal	Abnormal	Diagnosis/Abnormality (only if abnormal)

Image 28

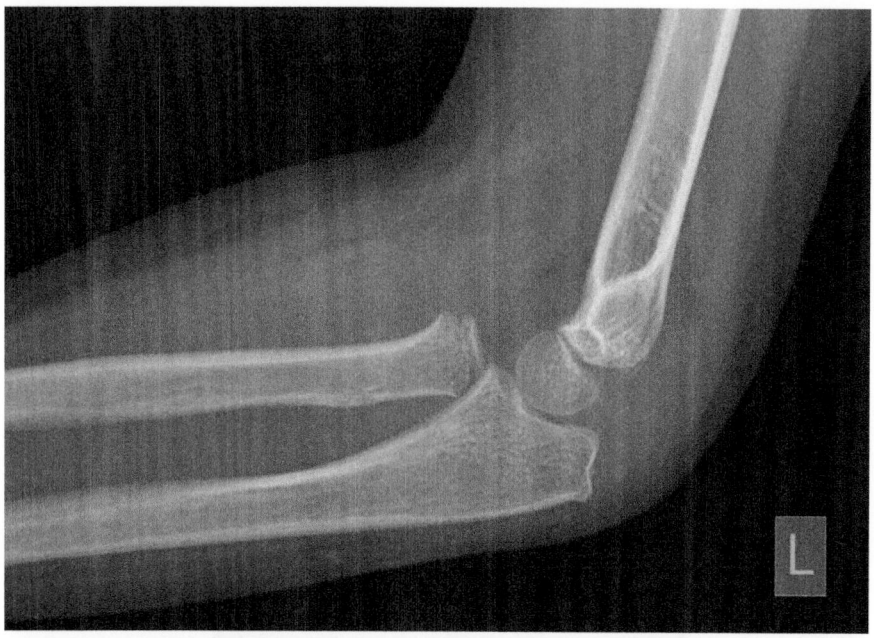

Normal	Abnormal	Diagnosis/Abnormality (only if abnormal)

Image 29

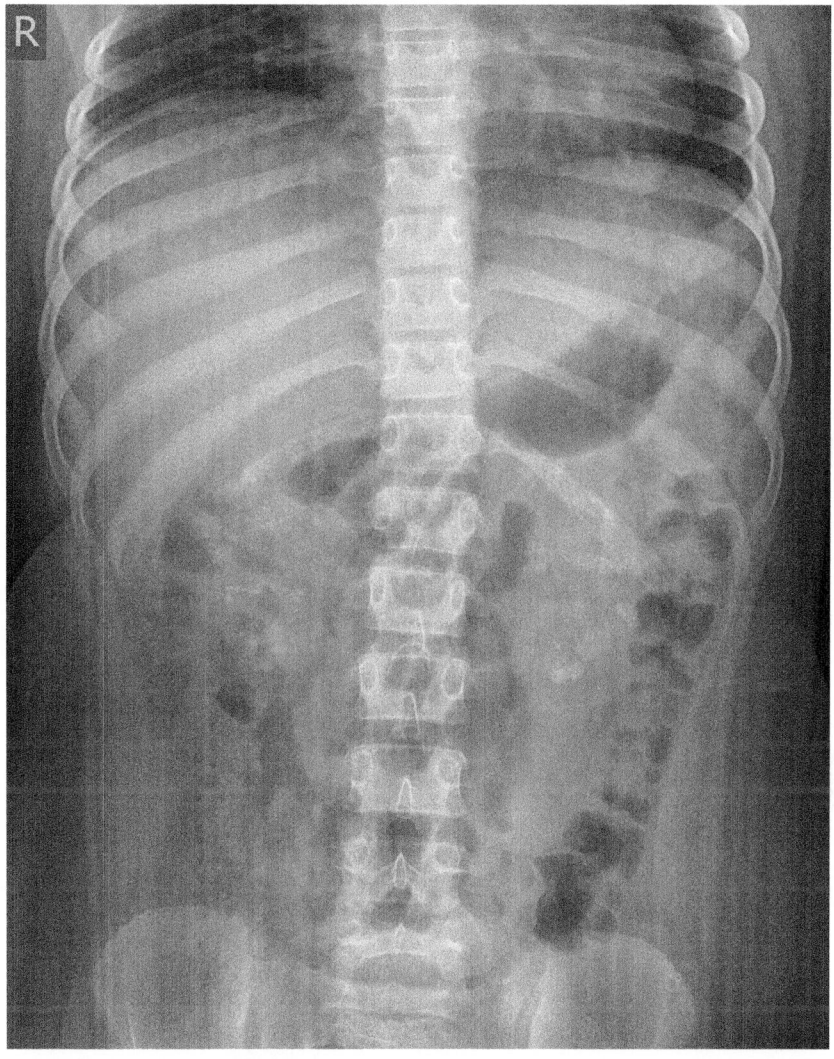

Normal	Abnormal	Diagnosis/Abnormality (only if abnormal)

Image 30

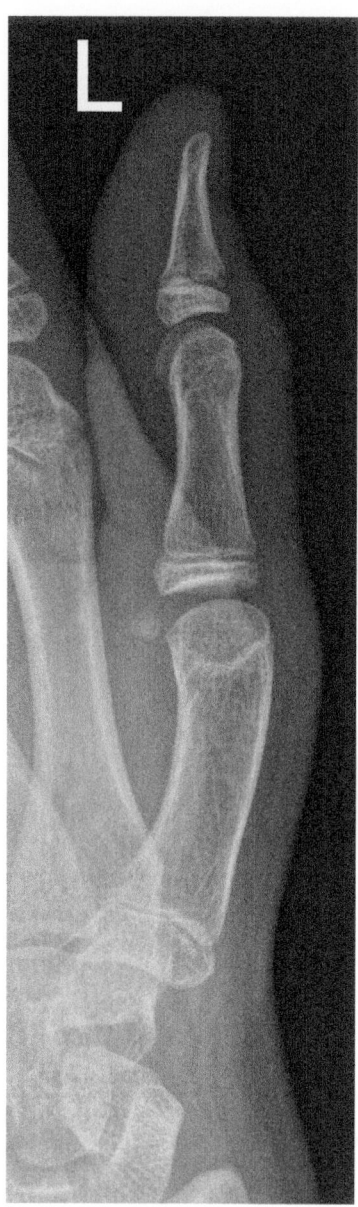

Normal	Abnormal	Diagnosis/Abnormality (only if abnormal)

1.2   Answers

Number	Normal	Abnormal	Diagnosis/abnormality (only required if abnormal column ticked)
1		✓	Avascular necrosis right proximal femoral epiphysis
2	✓		
3	✓		
4		✓	Oblique # left tibial diaphysis
5	✓		
6	✓		
7		✓	# base right fifth metatarsal
8	✓		
9	✓		
10		✓	Bilateral pneumothoraces
11		✓	Joint effusion right elbow
12	✓		
13	✓		
14	✓		
15		✓	Right supracondylar #
16	✓		
17	✓		
18		✓	Buckle #s left distal radius and ulna
19		✓	Bowel obstruction
20		✓	Transverse # left ring finger metacarpal
21		✓	Left lower lobe round pneumonia
22	✓		
23		✓	Buckle # left distal tibia
24		✓	Spiral # left tibial diaphysis and buckle # left proximal fibula
25	✓		
26		✓	Lipohaemarthrosis
27	✓		
28		✓	Left radial head dislocation
29		✓	Bilateral nephrocalcinosis
30		✓	Salter-Harris 2 # distal phalanx left thumb

1.3   Explanations

1. **Avascular necrosis right proximal femoral epiphysis**
   The imaging differential diagnosis of avascular necrosis (AVN) is wide and is summarised by the mnemonic **PLASTIC RAGS**:
   - **P**ancreatitis; **P**regnancy
   - **L**upus (Systemic lupus erythematosus, SLE)
   - **A**lcohol
   - **S**teroids
   - **T**rauma
   - **I**diopathic; **I**nfection
   - **C**aisson disease: also known as decompression illness/syndrome or 'the bends'. The rapid or uncontrolled ascension from a high-pressure environment or deep-sea depth can result in the formation of intravascular nitrogen gas bubbles leading to arterial occlusion and osteonecrosis; **C**ollagen vascular disease.
   - **R**adiation; **R**heumatoid arthritis
   - **A**myloid arthropathy
   - **G**aucher disease: an autosomal recessive lysosomal storage disorder arising from a deficiency of glucocerebrosidase resulting in an accumulation of glucocerebroside within the lysosomes of macrophages in the bone marrow, spleen, and liver. As such, its most common form (type 1) presents with hepatosplenomegaly and skeletal symptoms such as pain, pathological fractures, and osteonecrosis. Consider this as a cause of AVN in the context of hepatosplenomegaly: remember to look for the Erlenmeyer flask deformity in the femur (relative constriction of the diaphysis and flaring of the metaphysis).
   - **S**ickle cell disease

   The cause was idiopathic in this case and is more commonly known as Perthes (or Legg-Calvé-Perthes) disease, the eponymous name for idiopathic AVN of the proximal femoral epiphysis. In the examination, it would be more accurate to write 'avascular necrosis right proximal femoral epiphysis' rather than 'Perthes disease' because you will not know the underlying aetiology in the absence of clinical history.

   Perthes disease is five times more common in males with a peak incidence of around 6 years of age; it can affect children from as young as 2 years to those aged 14 years. The majority of children present with a painful hip or limp in the absence of trauma. It is a diagnosis of exclusion and other causes should be excluded first (above).

   This radiograph demonstrates the 'crescent sign' of subchondral lucency in the anterolateral aspect of the right proximal femoral epiphysis, best visualised on the frog-leg lateral projection. Identification of this sign heralds imminent articular collapse and represents stage 2 (of 4) in the radiographic staging of AVN.

Magnetic resonance imaging (MRI) is used to assess the extent of disease, femoral head deformity, and degree of subluxation, in addition to assessing the vascularity on dynamic contrast enhanced sequences. *Both* proximal femoral epiphyses will be affected in up to approximately 15% of cases, usually asymmetrically, with one side affected before the other.

Tip for the viva:
- Cases of AVN are common exam fodder; the causes are myriad and should be learned *ad nauseum*! Remember the 2B viva adage: *common pathologies in uncommon places*.

4. **Oblique # left tibial diaphysis**
An oblique or spiral fracture of the left tibial diaphysis in an ambulant toddler is also known as a 'toddler's fracture', a common accidental injury. A toddler's fracture is not always witnessed and the absence of a history does not necessarily imply abuse. Children may be presented to the Emergency Department (ED), either not moving their leg or refusing to walk/weight bear; often, there is no memorable history of injury. Occasionally, a definitive fracture line may not be visualised if the fracture is not displaced. If present in isolation in the appropriate age group and clinical context, it should not always be regarded as suspicious. However, the same fracture in a *pre-ambulant* infant is highly suspicious for physical abuse and evidence of other physical abuse should be sought.

7. **# base right fifth metatarsal**
It is important that you are familiar with the normal appearance of the base of the fifth metatarsal apophysis which is aligned in the vertical (longitudinal) plane, i.e. parallel to the orientation of the metatarsal. The normal apophysis is usually best appreciated on the oblique projection. The range of normal appearances can include an angulated or fragmented apophysis. The apophysis usually appears at approximately 10 years of age, fusing between 2 and 4 years later. Conversely, fractures of the base of the fifth metatarsal are horizontally (transversely) orientated, as in this radiograph. There may also be associated focal soft tissue swelling.

When you are next at work, search for and review foot radiographs in children aged 10 to 14 years. Note the variance of the normal base of fifth metatarsal apophysis. Look out for examples of fractures with which you can compare.

Tip for the viva:
- Apophysis = ossification centre which is the site of ligamentous attachment or tendinous insertion, e.g. base of fifth metatarsal apophysis which is the site of the peroneus brevis insertion.
- Epiphysis = ossification centre that contributes to the formation of a joint, e.g. proximal radial head epiphysis.

10. **Bilateral pneumothoraces**

We included this radiograph because the deep sulcus sign is demonstrated beautifully, particularly at the left base. Remember that in neonates who are imaged supine (labelled in the top left corner of the image) in their cots or incubators, a pneumothorax will collect anteriorly at the lung base (as opposed to apically in an upright child) with air collecting in the non-dependant pleural space, deepening the costophrenic angle. This is also demonstrated at the right costophrenic angle but to a lesser extent. Further evidence confirming the presence of pneumothoraces in this radiograph are crisp cardiac, mediastinal and diaphragmatic margins, and depressed hemi-diaphragms (left more than right).

Do not fall into the trap of 'satisfaction of search': once you have identified one pneumothorax, check that there is not one on the other side, as in this radiograph. Whilst not present in this example, do not forget to look for pneumomediastinum. Note the prominence of the right superior mediastinum which is consistent with thymus and is normal.

Tip for the viva:
- Look for supine pneumothoraces on radiographs obtained in the resuscitation room or intensive therapy unit (ITU) in both children and adults (they will usually be labelled), typically in the context of becoming increasingly difficult to ventilate/increasing airway pressures. The same radiographic principles discussed above will apply. Also, when present, check all lines and tubes for satisfactory or malposition.

11. **Joint effusion right elbow**

Once a joint effusion has been identified, you should look for the associated fracture. The presence of an intra-articular fracture is inferred by the presence of the joint effusion; however, sometimes a bony injury cannot be identified and therefore is radiographically occult. Commonly, only elevation of the anterior fat pad is seen but if the posterior fat pad is also elevated/visualised then a joint effusion is *definitely* present. Furthermore, alignment should be assessed on *every* elbow radiograph. In this radiograph, both the anterior and posterior fat pads are elevated but no bony injury is identified.

Tip for the viva:
- In children, the commonest intra-articular elbow fracture is supracondylar followed by radial head/neck. These areas should be carefully examined in the presence of an elbow joint effusion.

15. **Right supracondylar #**

Following on from the explanation for Image 11 above, it is important that any anteroposterior (AP) projection of the elbow is thoroughly assessed alongside the contemporaneous lateral projection. In this case, as seen in the magnified image below, the horizontally-orientated supracondylar fracture line can be visualised:

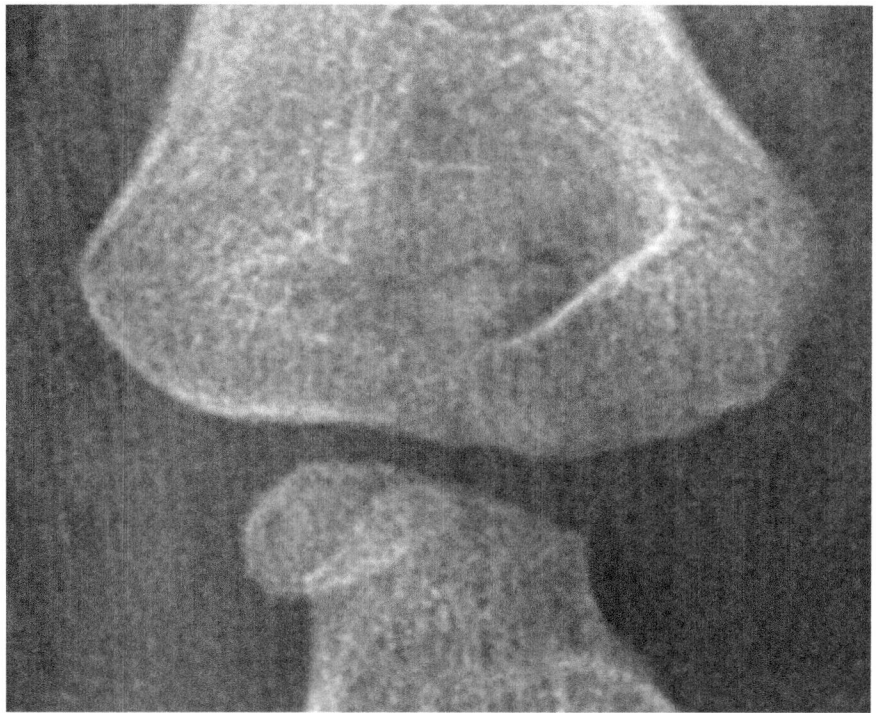

Note also the associated soft tissue swelling indicated by the 'blurring' of the supracondylar fat-muscle planes in the original radiograph.

16. **Normal left foot radiograph**
    Note the normal apophysis at the base of the fifth metatarsal which is aligned in the vertical plane (longitudinally) to the orientation of the metatarsals.

18. **Buckle #s left distal radius and ulna**
    In the examination, there will usually be only one significant diagnosable abnormality per radiograph. However, in those radiographs which demonstrate a well-recognised fracture pattern in which two fractures frequently occur together, you would be expected to identify and write down *both* fractures to get the mark. See the Introduction section.

19. **Bowel obstruction**
    This 10-month infant was presented to the ED with vomiting and was found to have a 'firm abdomen' on examination. The radiograph shows several dilated loops of bowel in the central abdomen with a paucity of bowel gas elsewhere consistent with bowel obstruction. Occasionally, it can be difficult to differentiate between dilated small and large bowel in neonates and young infants on radiography. Often it is more helpful to describe the relative number of dilated loops, their position and whether the imaging appearances are more in keeping with a proximal (high) or distal (low) obstruction. In this case, the calibre of the dilated bowel loops and their

central position indicates that the obstruction is of the small bowel. An intussusception was confirmed on ultrasound.

The aetiology of bowel obstruction in children is dependent on the age. A neonate refers to a newborn baby in their first 28 days of life. An infant (from the Latin *infans*, meaning 'unable to speak' or 'speechless') generally refers to a young child from 1 to 12 months of age. The term toddler is used for those who are walking unsteadily or 'toddling' from the age of 12 to 36 months. Thereafter, the terms young and older child can be used. A 'school-aged child' is usually one from the age of 5 years onwards.

Neonatal bowel obstruction can be categorised into proximal (high) or distal (low):

- Proximal: the 'double bubble sign' describes the appearance when the stomach and first part of the duodenum are distended with gas and no distal gas is visualised indicating duodenal atresia. Where gas is visualised distal to the first part of the duodenum, other causes of proximal obstruction need to be considered, including: duodenal web; duodenal stenosis; jejunal atresia; and annular pancreas. An upper gastrointestinal (GI) contrast examination is the investigation of choice alongside close liaison with paediatric surgical colleagues—it is often helpful if they observe the contrast examination in real time.
- Distal: the causes can be remembered using the mnemonic, **HAMM**:
  - **H**irschsprung's disease—also known as colonic aganglionosis (short segment affecting the rectum and distal sigmoid in the majority of cases, approximately 75%), it almost always affects *term* neonates (especially boys) and is the most common cause of neonatal bowel obstruction (20% of cases).
  - **A**tresia: ileal; anal. Associated with VACTERL syndrome.
  - **M**econium ileus: the meconium is abnormal, thick/inspissated, and becomes impacted in the distal ileum resulting in obstruction. Approximately 20% of infants with cystic fibrosis present with meconium ileus at birth.
  - **M**econium plug syndrome: also known as small left colon syndrome (the left colon is described as a microcolon as it has never been used), this is a functional obstruction secondary to a meconium plug. Lower GI contrast enema examination can be both diagnostic and therapeutic, facilitating the passage of *normal* meconium (cf. meconium ileus where the meconium is abnormal).
- Necrotising enterocolitis (NEC) is a consideration in premature infants. Obstruction can result from strictures as a long-term complication in those infants in whom NEC has been medically managed. Whilst prematurity is a significant risk factor in the development of NEC (approximately 90% of cases affect premature infants and the more premature the infant, the higher the risk and mortality), term babies can also be affected although this is uncommon.

Bowel obstruction in older infants and children is more likely to be secondary to an acquired aetiology. Late presentations of those entities in the neonatal period should also be considered in the appropriate clinical context. **AAIIMM** is a mnemonic which can be used to remember the common causes of bowel obstruction in children:

- **A**ppendicitis
- **A**dhesions: from previous surgery
- **I**ntussusception
- **I**ncarcerated inguinal hernia
- **M**eckel's diverticulum: do not forget the '*Rule of 2's*':
  - 2% of the population.
  - 2 inches (5 cm) long.
  - 2 feet (60 cm) from the ileocaecal valve.
  - 2/3rds contain ectopic mucosa.
  - 2 types of ectopic tissue are commonly present (gastric and pancreatic).
  - 2 years old at presentation.
  - 2% become symptomatic.
  - 2 times more common in boys.
- **M**alrotation/midgut volvulus

Tip for the viva:
- Every clinical radiologist should be familiar with the clinical presentation and imaging findings of malrotation and midgut volvulus. See the references for further reading.

20. **Transverse # left ring finger metacarpal**

21. **Left lower lobe round pneumonia**
   There is a rounded area of left lower lobe opacification consistent with consolidation. In round pneumonia, the consolidation is usually well circumscribed but can have irregular margins, appearing 'roundish'. The presence of an air bronchogram in this case helps to establish the radiological diagnosis of consolidation as opposed to a solid pulmonary mass. The border/dome of the left hemidiaphragm is obliterated localising the pathology to the left lower lobe. The appearance is typical of infective consolidation in children.

   The rounded appearance results from the not-yet-developed collateral airways (pores of Kohn and canals of Lambert) in the paediatric lung. These are more developed in adults facilitating lateral air drift between subsegments in the same lobe which allows infection to disseminate and form lobar consolidation. As such, round pneumonia is more commonly identified in young school-aged children (aged between 5 and 8 years) as these collateral airways are not yet fully established. This limits the spread of infection and results in a 'more compact' consolidation and the subsequent rounded radiographic appearance. As the airways develop in older children, this finding becomes less common as they develop a more 'lobar' pattern of consolidation.

Follow-up chest radiographs are not usually obtained in children in the same way as they are in adults. In cases of round pneumonia, follow-up radiographs may be obtained to ensure that it has resolved or does not develop into lobar consolidation. However, given that the overwhelming majority have usually resolved on follow-up imaging, some centres may only perform a further radiograph in those children who have either not clinically improved or have worsened.

Tip for the viva:
- You may be asked why this pattern of consolidation develops (rounded versus lobar) which is why you should understand the pathology behind this radiographic appearance. Discuss the radiographic follow-up of round pneumonia with your local paediatric radiologists. If questioned, you can state what you do locally.

23. **Buckle # left distal tibia**
    The buckle fracture is seen as an acute 'step' in the medial distal tibial metadiaphyseal cortex, better appreciated in the magnified image below:

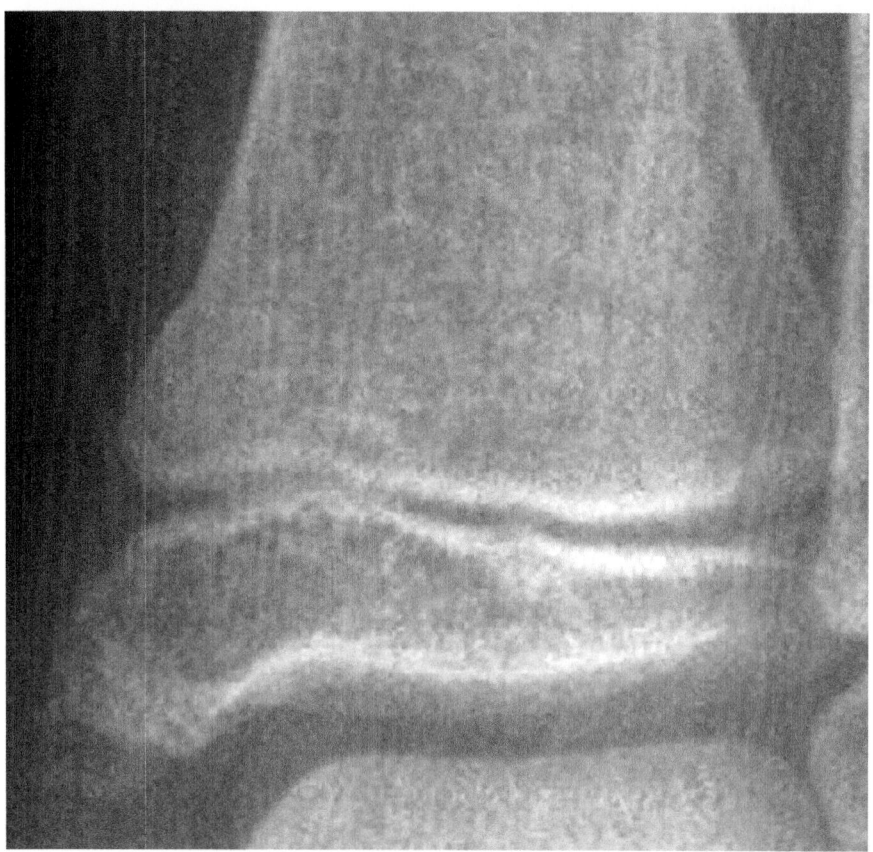

Remember, in the examination you will be able to magnify the images which is recommended when assessing for subtle cortical abnormalities. The fragmentation of the medial aspect of the distal tibial epiphysis/medial malleolus is normal. Epiphyseal ossification can have variable appearances at all ages.

24. **Spiral # left tibial diaphysis and buckle # left proximal fibula**
    Did you also spot the proximal fibular fracture?

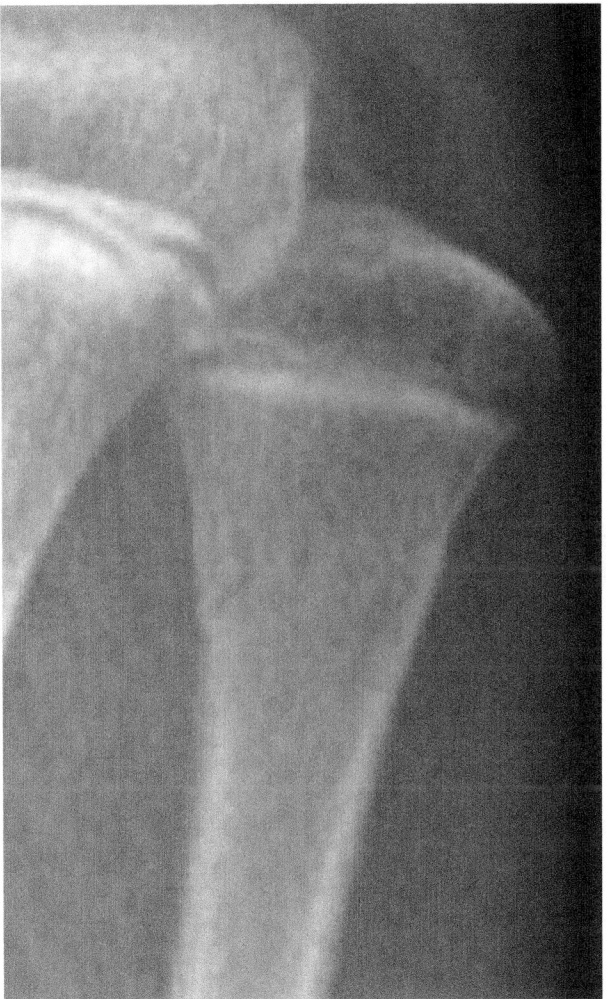

Whilst there is a spiral fracture of the left tibial distal diaphysis, there is also a proximal fibular buckle fracture (proximal medial metadiaphysis). Do not suffer 'satisfaction of search'; once you have seen the relatively obvious tibial fracture you must carefully examine every single bone for a further/associated fracture. Spiral tibial fractures more often occur in isolation than with an associated fibular fracture, but these fractures can occur together because the force is transmitted from the tibia (the weight-bearing bone) along the interosseous membrane to the proximal fibula where the force is dissipated.

This is not the Maisonneuve fracture complex—which is the combination of a proximal fibular fracture (usually proximal third) and a distal tibial fracture (usually medial malleolus/deltoid ligament with widening of the distal tibio-fibular syndesmosis).

25. **Normal facial bone radiograph**

26. **Lipohaemarthrosis**
A lipohaemarthrosis is an important radiographic sign. Its presence indicates an intra-articular fracture which may be radiographically occult. It represents a fat-fluid level in the suprapatellar bursa resulting from the fatty marrow, which is less dense, floating on top of the haemorrhage. When identified, it should prompt the search for a tibial plateau or spine fracture, a distal femoral fracture, osteochondral defect or less commonly, a patella fracture. Importantly however, the absence of a lipohaemarthrosis does *not* exclude an intra-articular fracture.

Tip for the viva:
• A lipohaemarthrosis can be identified on other imaging modalities: look for the fat-fluid level.

28. **Left radial head dislocation**
In the presence of a joint effusion, a bony injury should be sought—see the explanation for Image 11 in this test. Additionally, both the anterior humeral and radiocapitellar alignment should be assessed on every lateral elbow radiographic projection. In this radiograph, the anterior humeral alignment is normal however, the radiocapitellar alignment is not. An imaginary line should be drawn along the radial neck which should bisect the capitellum ossification centre on both the AP and lateral elbow projections. If this is not the case, there is radial head subluxation/dislocation. Children usually present with an unwillingness to use their arm after a fall on an outstretched hand (FOOSH).

Tip for the viva:
• In the presence of a radial head dislocation, a concomitant ulnar shaft fracture should be sought as part of the Monteggia fracture-dislocation pattern, and vice versa. Formal forearm radiographs should be recommended if they have not yet been obtained.

29. **Bilateral nephrocalcinosis**
The renal outlines, alongside those of the other intra-abdominal organs, should not be overlooked on the abdominal radiograph. Nephrocalcinosis is

categorised depending on where the calcium salts are deposited in the renal parenchyma: medullary, being the more common and representing 95% of cases; with cortical comprising the remainder. Both conditions are associated with nephrolithiasis (renal calculi) which may be present anywhere along the urinary tract.

The aetiology of nephrocalcinosis can be best remembered using the mnemonics below:

Medullary—HAM HOP
- **H**yperparathyroidism
- (renal tubular) **A**cidosis
- **M**edullary sponge kidney
- **H**ypercalcaemia/**H**ypercalciuria
- **O**xalosis
- **P**apillary necrosis: think of this in patients with a long-standing history of pain requiring analgesia/non-steroidal anti-inflammatory drug (NSAID) use; in the setting of infection (pyelonephritis, tuberculosis); or those with sickle cell disease.

Cortical—COAG
- **C**ortical necrosis
- **O**xalosis
- **A**lport syndrome: an X-linked recessive disease affecting type IV collagen production. This is found in the eyes, ears, and kidneys and explains why patients present with ocular anomalies, high frequency sensorineural hearing loss, and basement membrane glomerulonephritis.
- (chronic) **G**lomerulonephritis

In this case, the underlying cause was medullary sponge kidney (following recurrent presentations of abdominal pain and urinary tract infection).

Tip for the viva:
- Whilst not present in this case, search for additional radiographic features of the underlying cause of the nephrocalcinosis, e.g. osteopaenia, rugger jersey spine, subchondral resorption of the sacroiliac joints, and Brown's tumours, in the context of hyperparathyroidism. Cases of hyperparathyroidism and renal osteodystrophy (secondary hyperparathyroidism in patients with chronic renal failure) are particularly common in the examination setting.

30. **Salter-Harris 2 # distal phalanx left thumb**
    The Salter-Harris classification is the most widely used system to describe physeal (growth plate) fractures and can be remembered using the mnemonic, **SALTER**:
    - **S**lipped, type 1: the fracture passes through the physis *only* and not through the adjacent bone. There may be an associated shift (slip) about the physis

with an associated widening of its medial or lateral aspect with focal overlying soft tissue swelling at the level of the physis. These fractures do not occur if the growth plate is fused.

- **A**bove, type 2: the fracture passes through and *above* the physis into the metaphysis. These are the most common injury, accounting for approximately 75% of all physeal injuries.
- **L**ower/be**L**ow, type 3: the fracture passes through and *below* the physis into the epiphysis.
- **T**hrough **E**verything/**T**ogether, type 4: the fracture passes through *everything*; the metaphysis, the physis, and the epiphysis.
- **R**ammed/c**R**ush, type 5: the physis is damaged by *direct compression* from the metaphysis and epiphysis. These injuries are uncommon and account for <1% of physeal fractures.

It is important that the physis and adjacent metaphysis and epiphysis are scrutinised for Salter-Harris injury on every skeletal radiograph. The prognosis worsens progressively from type 1 to type 5 Salter-Harris fractures.

Tip for the viva:
- Do not forget that a slipped upper femoral epiphysis (SUFE) is a Salter-Harris 1 injury and that Tillaux and triplanar fractures of the distal tibia are Salter-Harris 3 and 4 fractures, respectively.

Further Reading

Image 1

Bell DJ, Gaillard F et al (2018a) Avascular necrosis causes (mnemonic). https://radiopaedia.org/articles/avascular-necrosis-causes-mnemonic. Accessed April 2018

Bell DJ, Venkatesh M et al (2018b) Caisson disease. https://radiopaedia.org/articles/caisson-disease-1. Accessed April 2018

Bomer J, Holscher H (2018) Hip pathology in children. http://www.radiologyassistant.nl/en/p557dccf34fb1a/hip-pathology-in-children.html. Accessed July 2018

Dillman JR, Hernandez RJ (2009) MRI of Legg-Calve-Perthes disease. AJR Am J Roentgenol 193(5):1394–1407

Di Muzio B, Gaillard F et al (2018) Erlenmeyer flask deformity. https://radiopaedia.org/articles/erlenmeyer-flask-deformity-1. Accessed April 2018

Sharma R, Oozeerally Z et al (2018) Gaucher disease. https://radiopaedia.org/articles/gaucher-disease. Accessed April 2018

Weishaupt D, Exner GU, Hilfiker PR, Hodler J (2000) Dynamic MR imaging of the hip in Legg-Calvé-Perthes disease: comparison with arthrography. AJR Am J Roentgenol 174(6):1635–1637

Image 4

Donnelly LF (2000) Toddler's fracture of the fibula. AJR Am J Roentgenol 175(3):922

Thomas SA, Rosenfield NS, Leventhal JM et al (1991) Long-bone fractures in young children: distinguishing accidental injuries from child abuse. Pediatrics 88:471e6

Image 7

Strayer SM, Reece SG, Petrizzi MJ (1999) Fractures of the proximal fifth metatarsal. Am Fam Physician 59(9):2516–2522

Image 10

Ho ML, Gutierrez FR (2009) Chest radiography in thoracic polytrauma. AJR Am J Roentgenol 192(3):599–561

Yoon H (2016) Interpretation of neonatal chest radiography. J Korean Soc Radiol 74(5):279–290

Image 19

Bell DJ, Hacking C et al (2018c) Rule of 2s in Meckel diverticulum. https://radiopaedia.org/articles/rule-of-2s-in-meckel-diverticulum-1. Accessed May 2018

Gaillard F et al (2018) Double bubble sign (duodenum). https://radiopaedia.org/articles/double-bubble-sign-duodenum. Accessed July 2018

Hacking C, Agrawal R et al (2018) Hirschsprung disease. https://radiopaedia.org/articles/hirschsprung-disease. Accessed May 2018

Minima J (2012a) Neonatal low bowel obstruction differential diagnosis. http://www.theradiologyblog.com/2012/04/bowel-obstruction-in-children.html. Accessed May 2018

Minima J (2012b). Bowel obstruction in children: differential diagnosis #4. http://www.theradiolo-gyblog.com/2012/04/bowel-obstruction-in-children.html. Accessed April 2018

Skandhan AKP, Weerakkody Y et al (2018a) https://radiopaedia.org/articles/meconium-ileus. Accessed May 2018

Skandhan AKP, Weerakkody Y et al (2018b) https://radiopaedia.org/articles/necrotising-enteroco-litis-1. Accessed May 2018

Reid JR (2012) Practical imaging approach to bowel obstruction in neonates: a review and update. Semin Roentgenol 47(1):21–31

Weerakkody Y et al (2018) https://radiopaedia.org/articles/meconium-plug-syndrome. Accessed May 2018

Malrotation and Midgut Volvulus

Applegate KE, Anderson JM, Klatte EC (2006) Intestinal malrotation in children: a problem-solving approach to the upper gastrointestinal series. Radiographics 26(5):1485–1500

Long FR, Kramer SS, Markowitz RI et al (1996) Radiographic patterns of intestinal malrotation in children. Radiographics 16(3):547–556; discussion 556–560

Ortiz-Neira CL (2007) The corkscrew sign: midgut volvulus. Radiology 242(1):315–316

Image 21

Kim YW, Donnelly LF (2007) Round pneumonia: imaging findings in a large series of children. Pediatr Radiol 37(12):1235–1240

McCrossan P, McNaughten B, Shields M, Thompson A (2017) Is follow up chest X-ray required in children with round pneumonia? Arch Dis Child 102(12):1182–1183

Image 24

Beutel BG (2012) Monteggia fractures in pediatric and adult populations. Orthopedics 35(2):138–144

Image 29

Bell D, St-Amant M et al (2018d) Cortical nephrocalcinosis. https://radiopaedia.org/articles/corti-cal-nephrocalcinosis-mnemonic. Accessed March 2018

Dähnert W (2007) Hereditary chronic nephritis. In: Radiology review manual. Lippincott Williams & Wilkins, Philadelphia, p 948

Glick Y, Gaillard F et al (2018) Medullary nephrocalcinosis. https://radiopaedia.org/articles/med-ullary-nephrocalcinosis-mnemonic. Accessed March 2018

Patel CN, Scarsbrook AF (2009) Multimodality imaging in hyperparathyroidism. Postgrad Med J 85(1009):597–605

Test 2

2.1   Images

Image 1

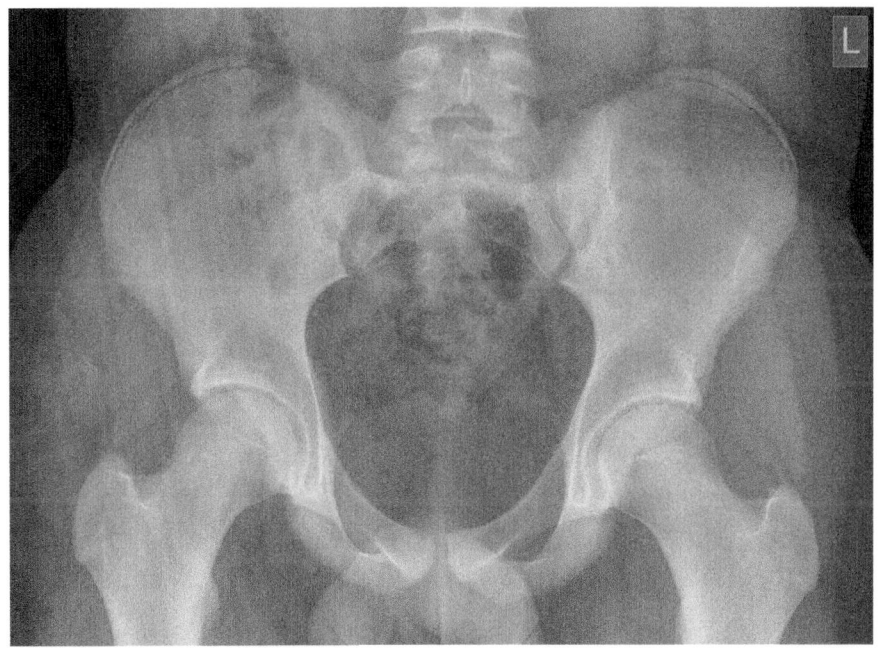

Normal	Abnormal	Diagnosis/Abnormality (only if abnormal)

Image 2

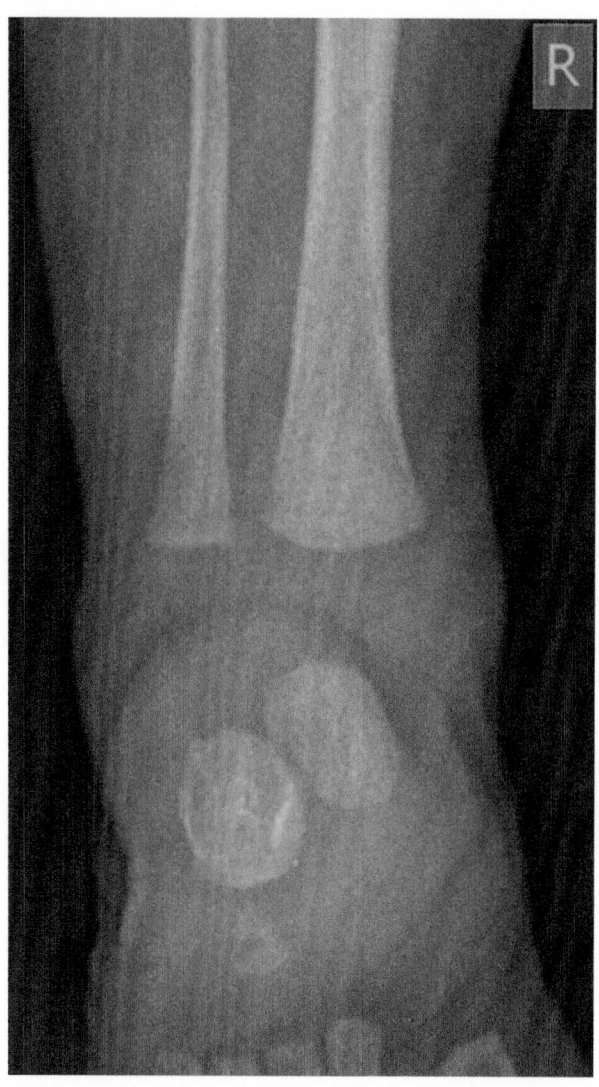

Normal	Abnormal	Diagnosis/Abnormality (only if abnormal)

Image 3

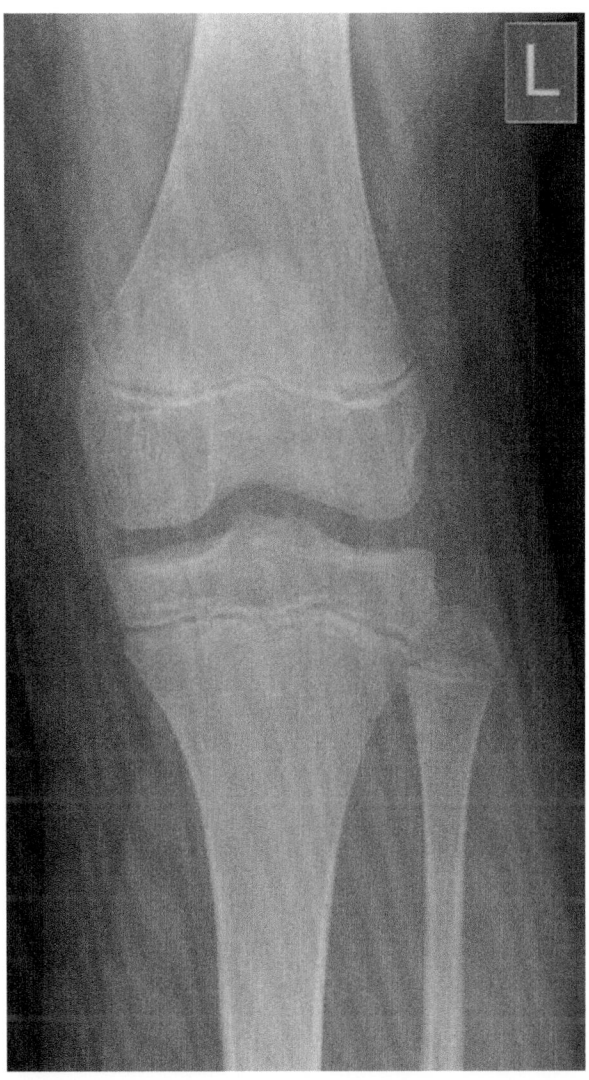

Normal	Abnormal	Diagnosis/Abnormality (only if abnormal)

Image 4

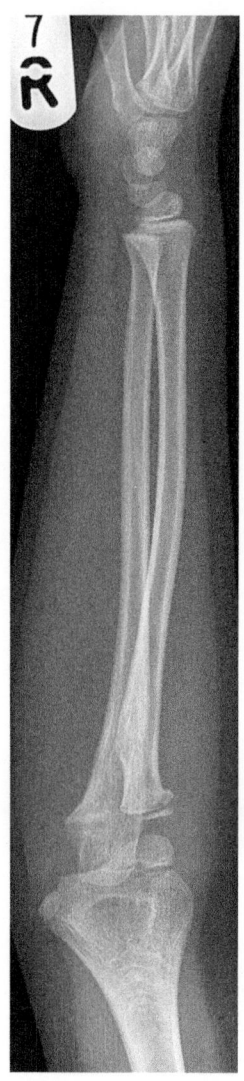

Normal	Abnormal	Diagnosis/Abnormality (only if abnormal)

Image 5

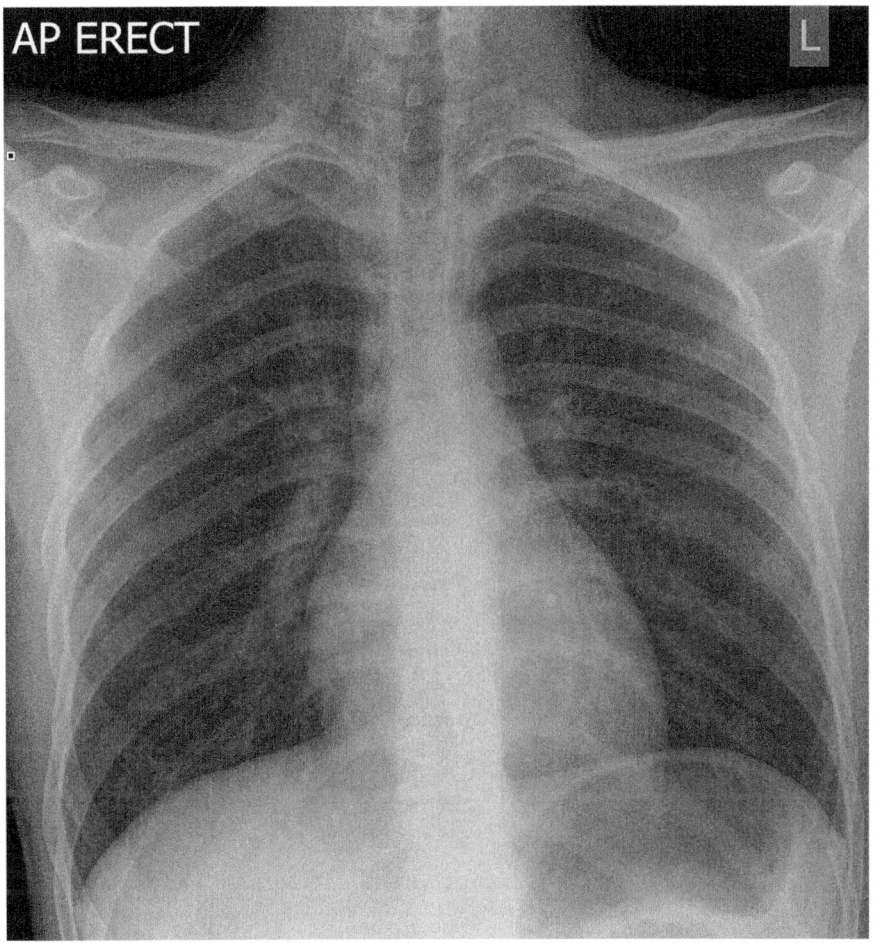

Normal	Abnormal	Diagnosis/Abnormality (only if abnormal)

Image 6

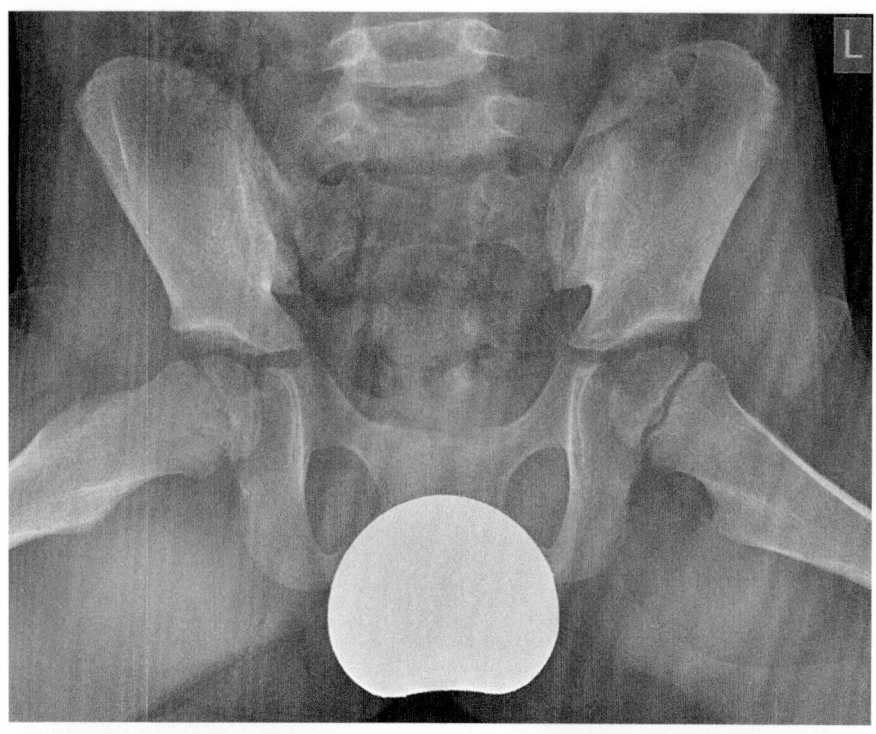

Normal	Abnormal	Diagnosis/Abnormality (only if abnormal)

Image 7

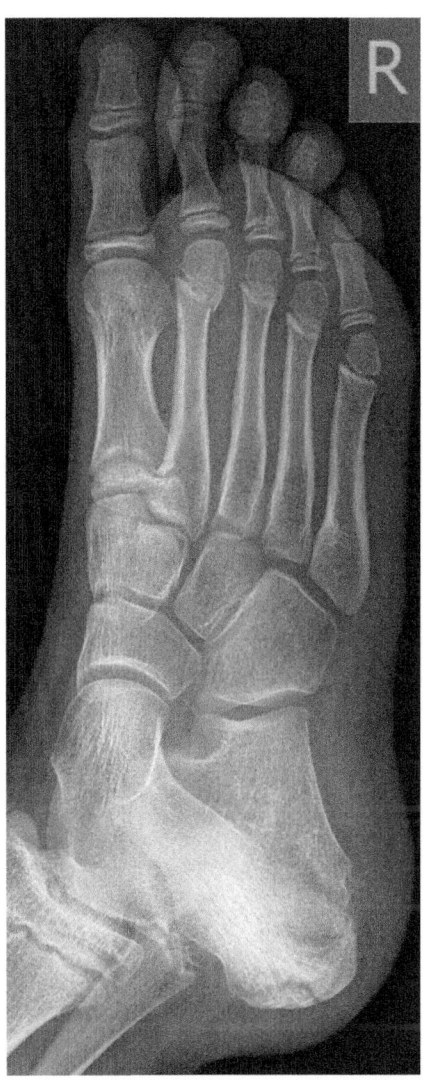

Normal	Abnormal	Diagnosis/Abnormality (only if abnormal)

Image 8

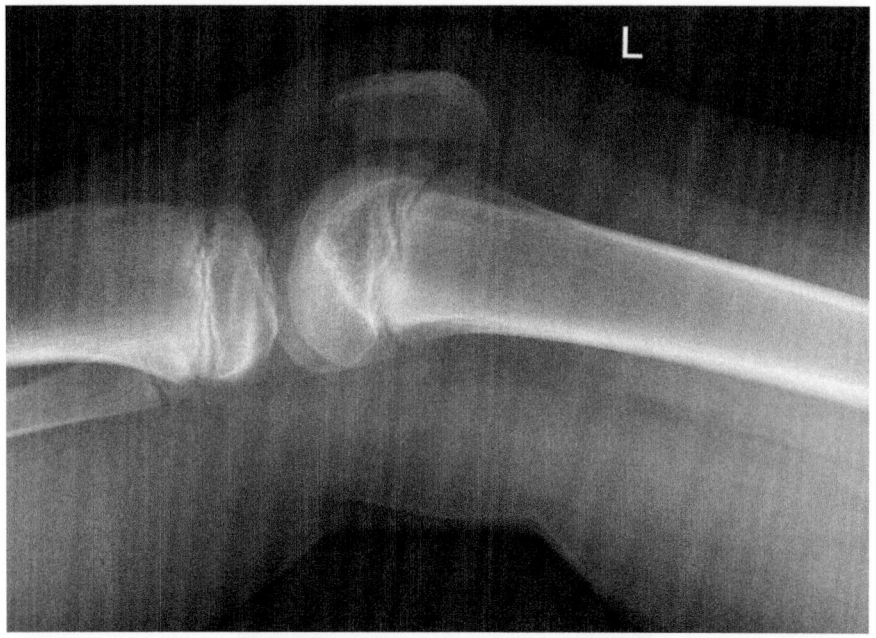

Normal	Abnormal	Diagnosis/Abnormality (only if abnormal)

Image 9

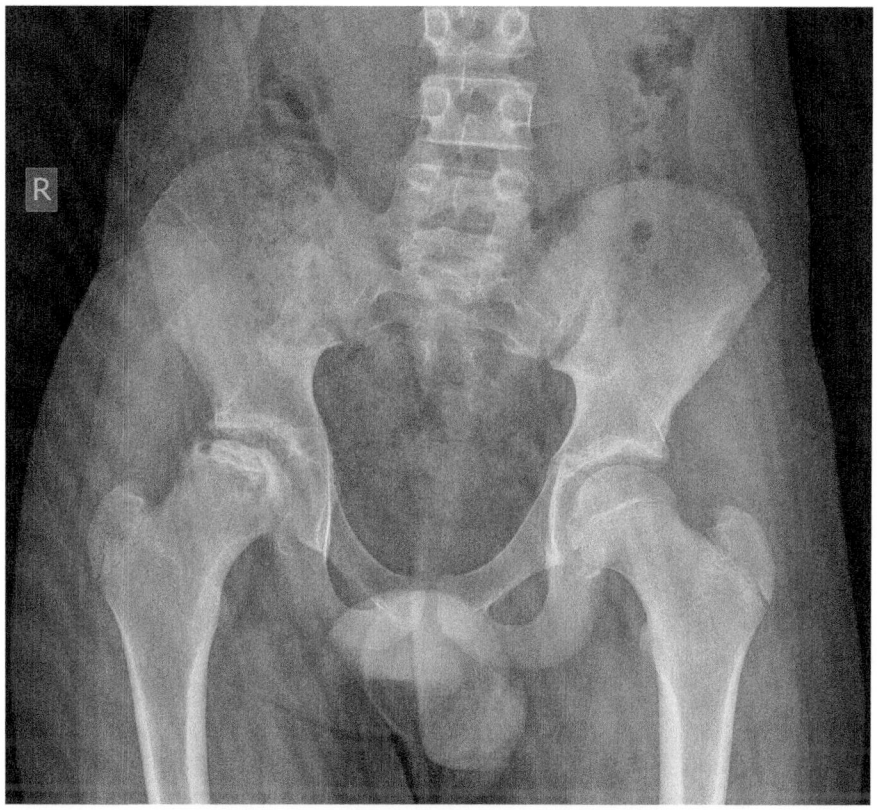

Normal	Abnormal	Diagnosis/Abnormality (only if abnormal)

Image 10

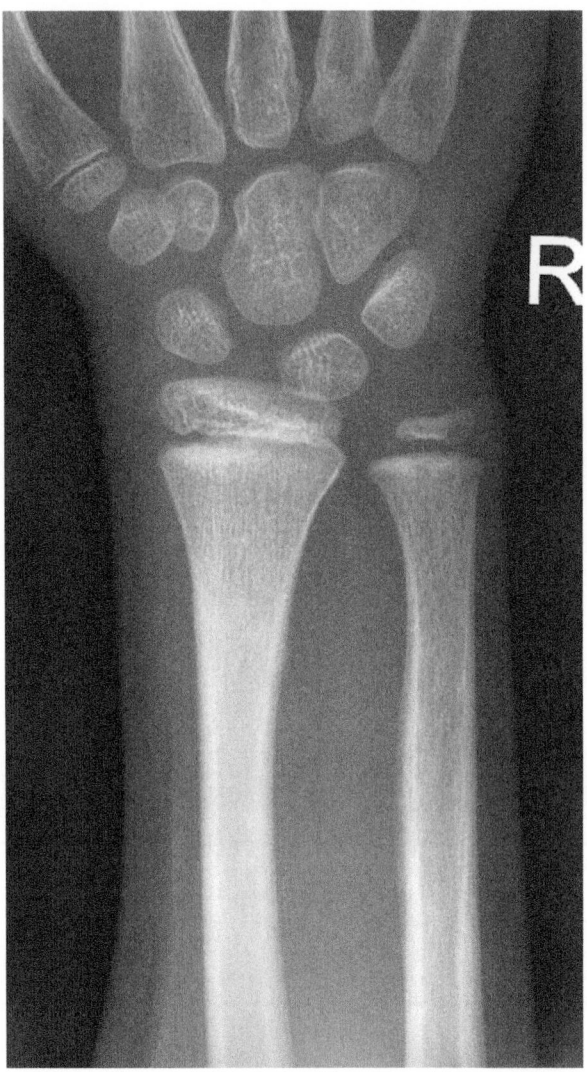

Normal	Abnormal	Diagnosis/Abnormality (only if abnormal)

Image 11

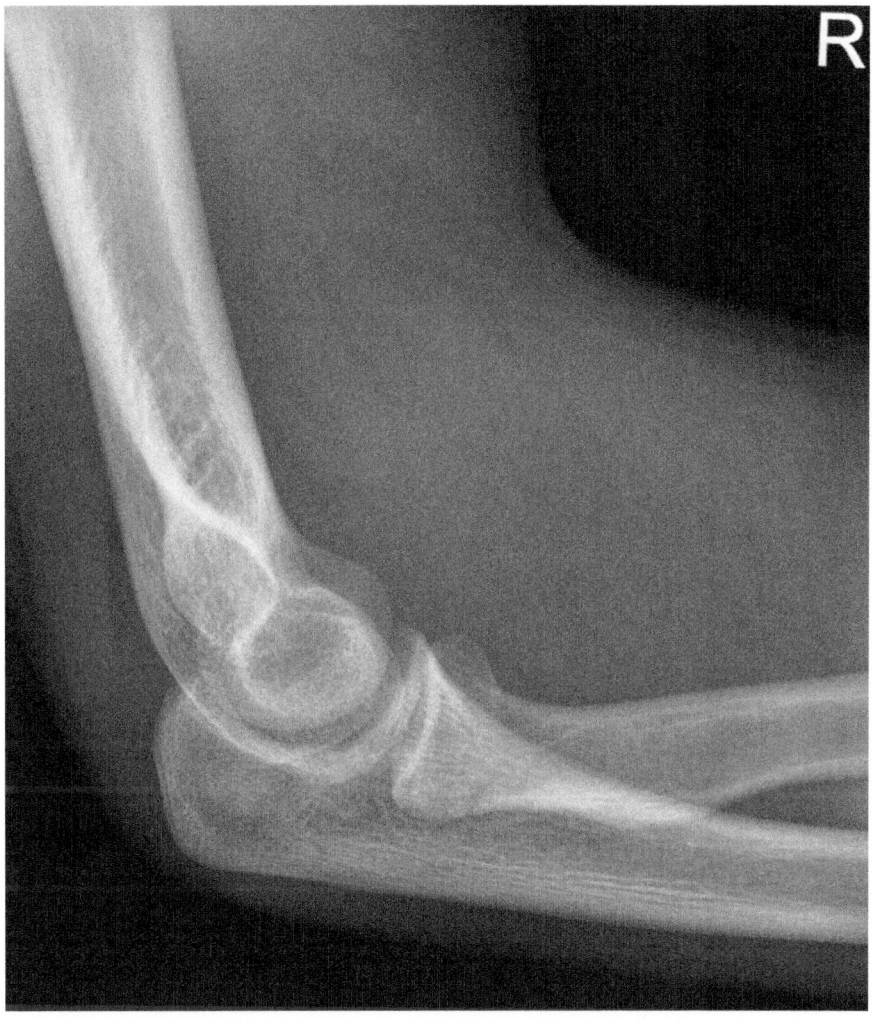

Normal	Abnormal	Diagnosis/Abnormality (only if abnormal)

Image 12

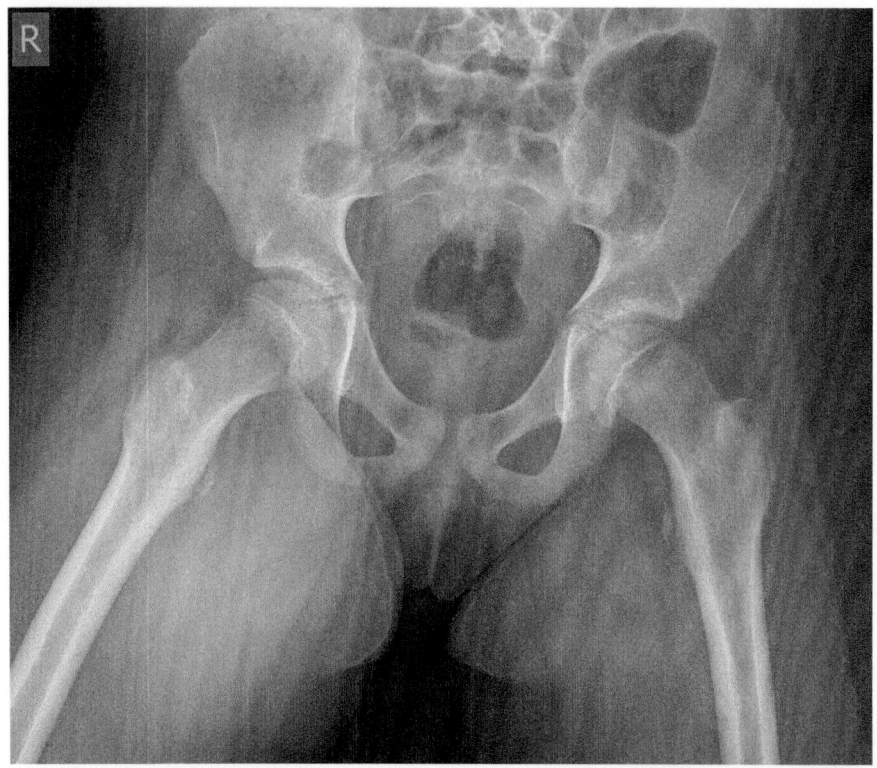

Normal	Abnormal	Diagnosis/Abnormality (only if abnormal)

Image 13

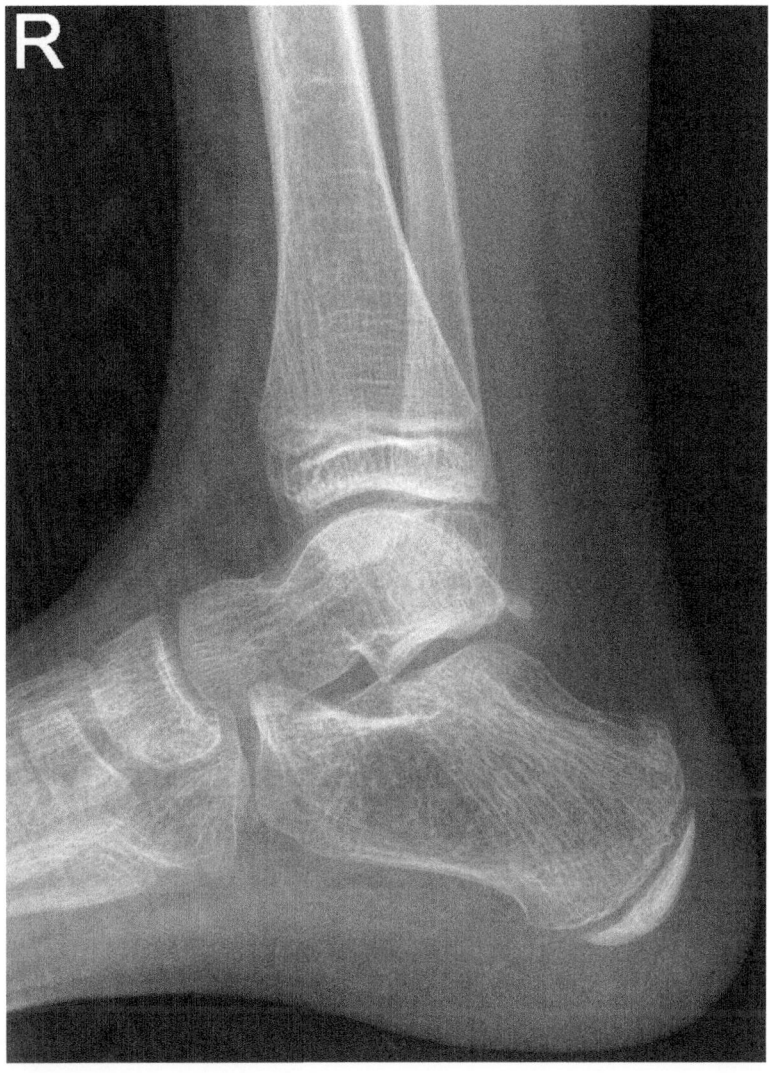

Normal	Abnormal	Diagnosis/Abnormality (only if abnormal)

Image 14

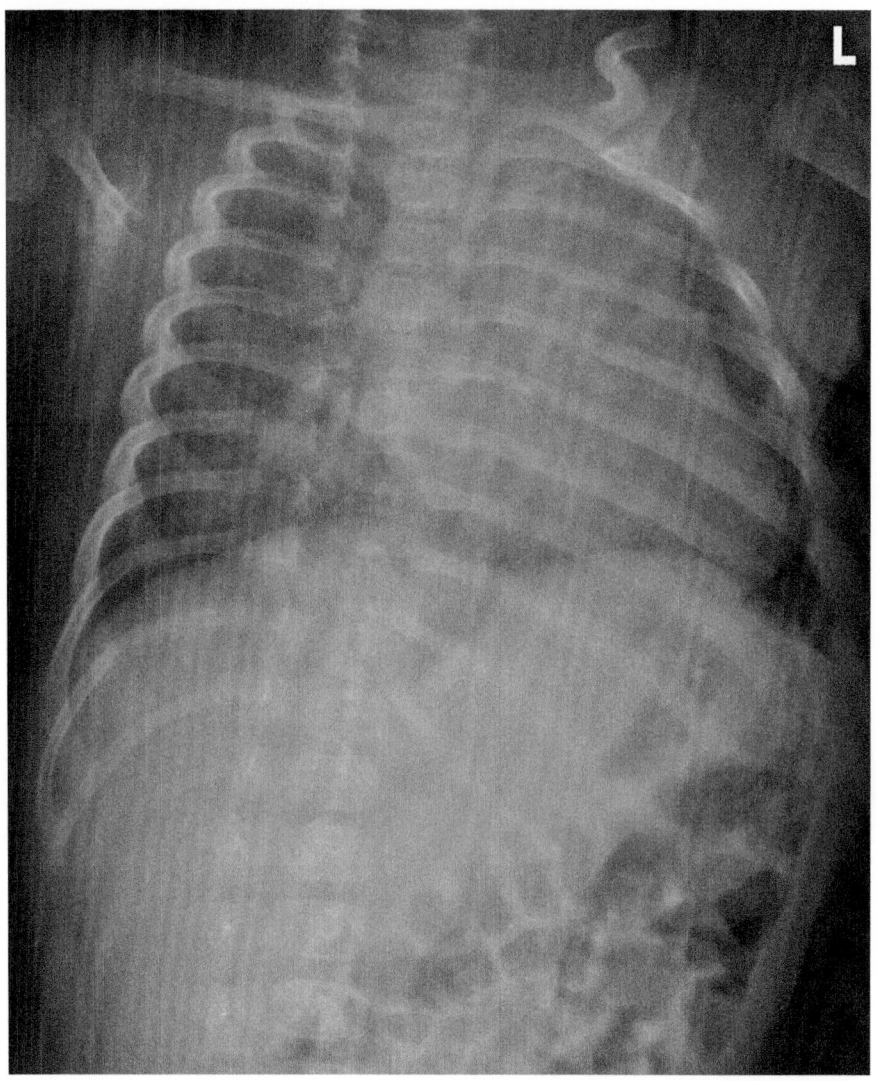

Normal	Abnormal	Diagnosis/Abnormality (only if abnormal)

Image 15

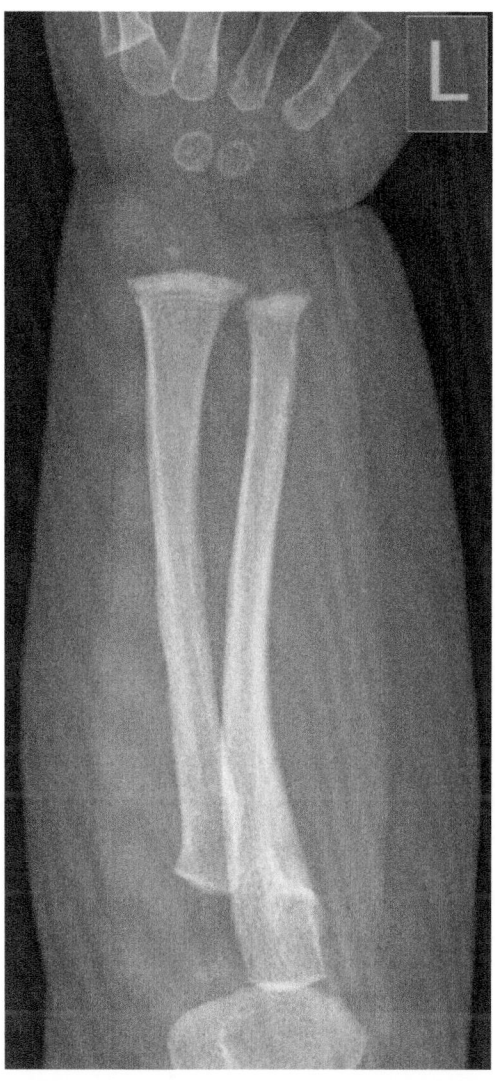

Normal	Abnormal	Diagnosis/Abnormality (only if abnormal)

Image 16

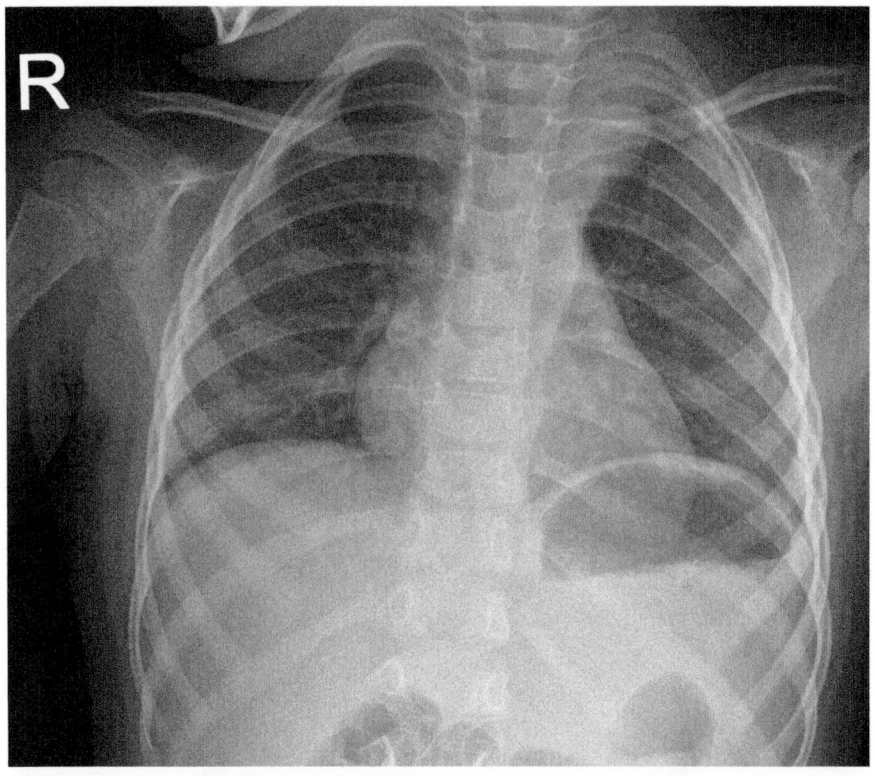

Normal	Abnormal	Diagnosis/Abnormality (only if abnormal)

Image 17

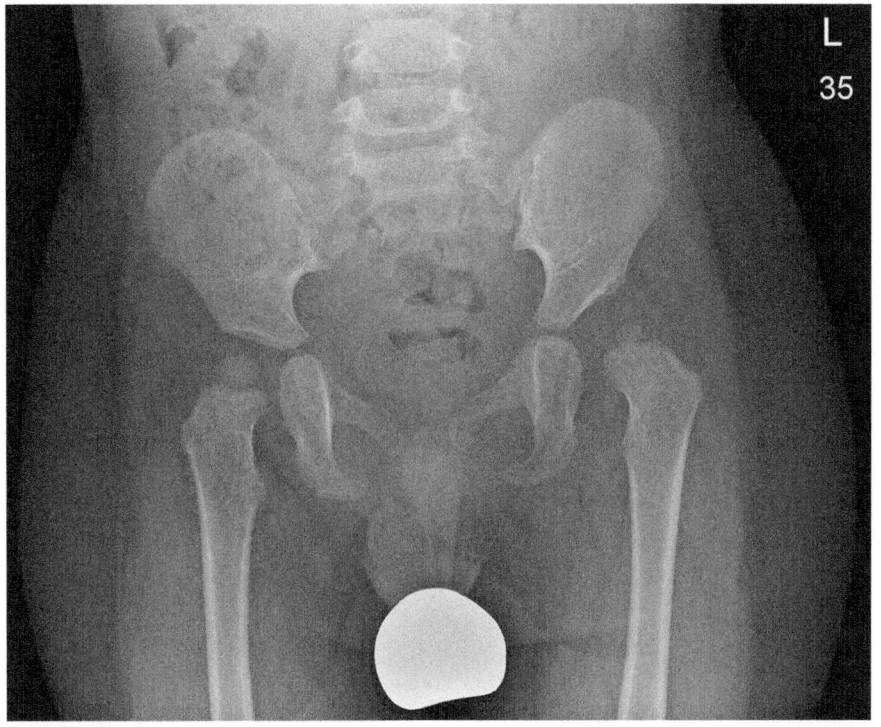

Normal	Abnormal	Diagnosis/Abnormality (only if abnormal)

Image 18

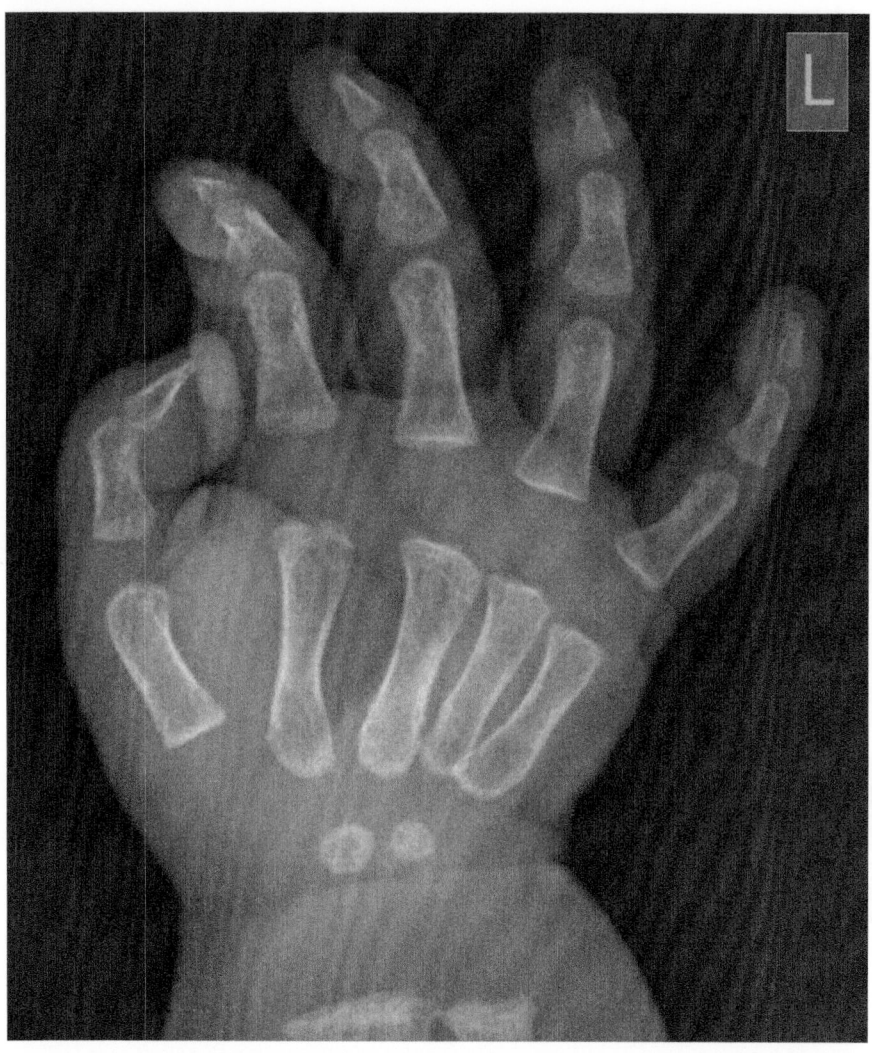

Normal	Abnormal	Diagnosis/Abnormality (only if abnormal)

Image 19

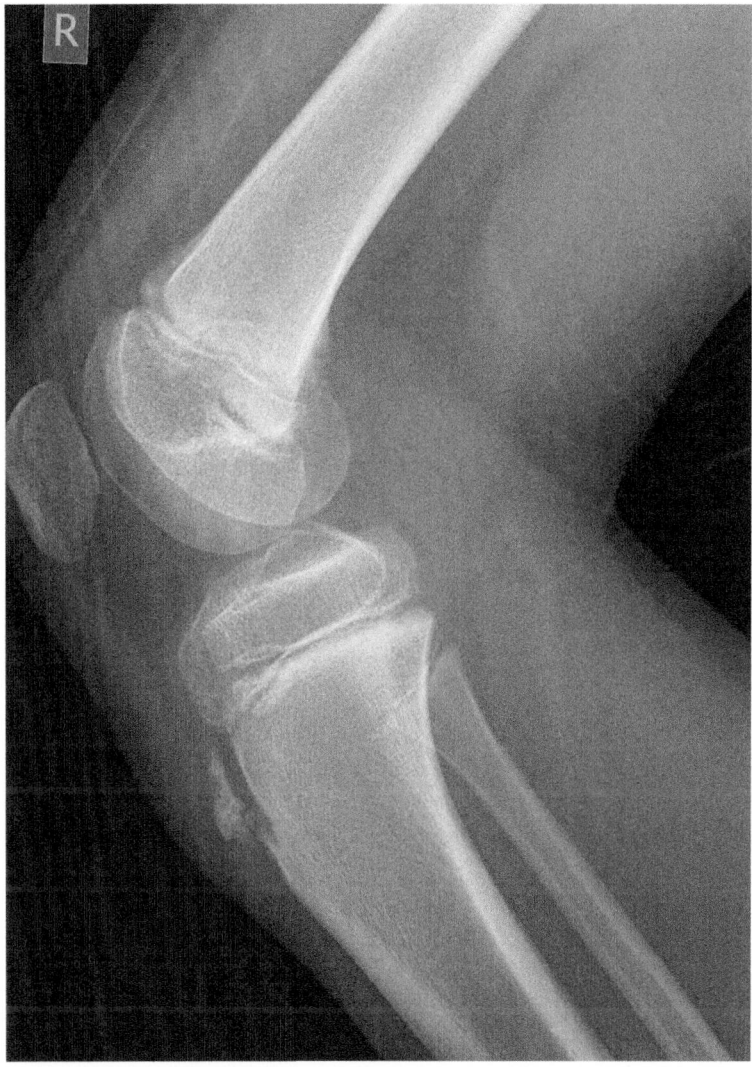

Normal	Abnormal	Diagnosis/Abnormality (only if abnormal)

Image 20

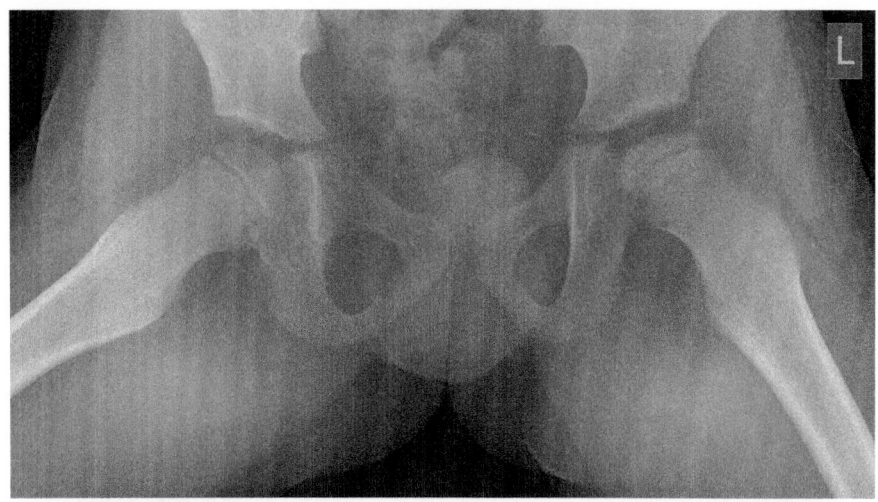

Normal	Abnormal	Diagnosis/Abnormality (only if abnormal)

Image 21

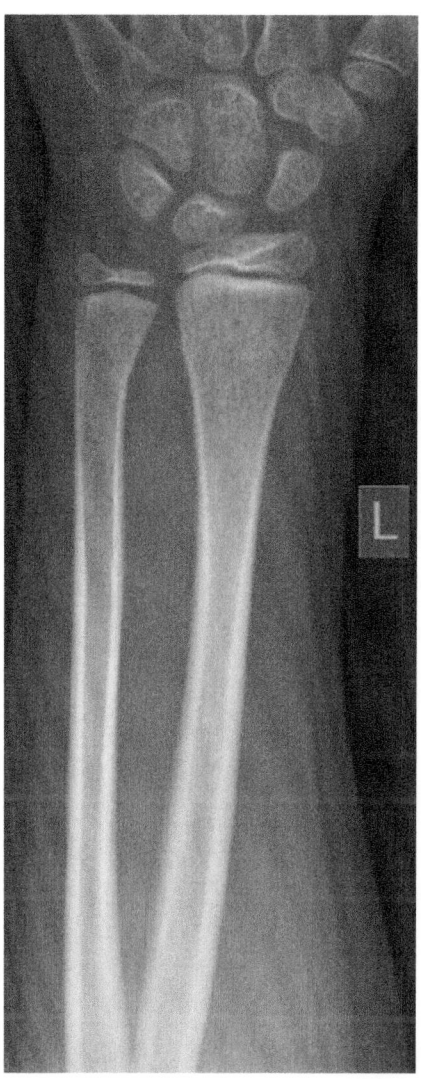

Normal	Abnormal	Diagnosis/Abnormality (only if abnormal)

Image 22

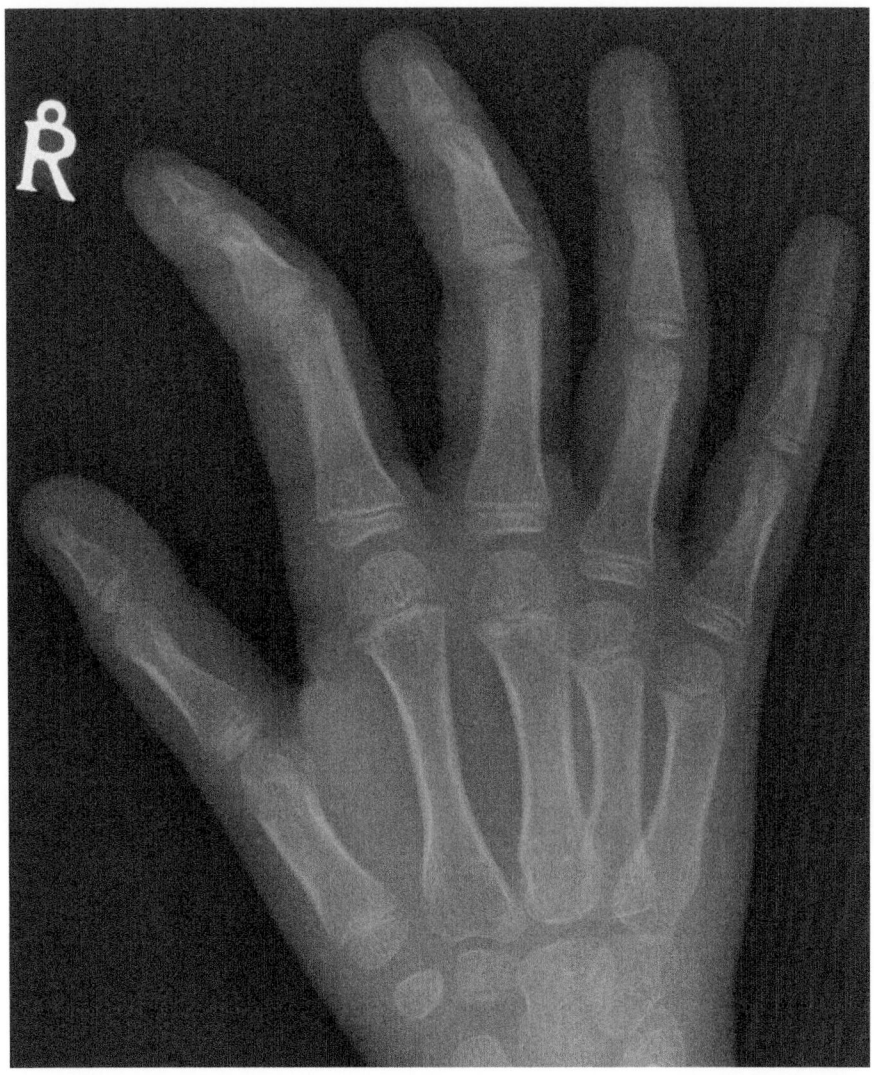

Normal	Abnormal	Diagnosis/Abnormality (only if abnormal)

Image 23

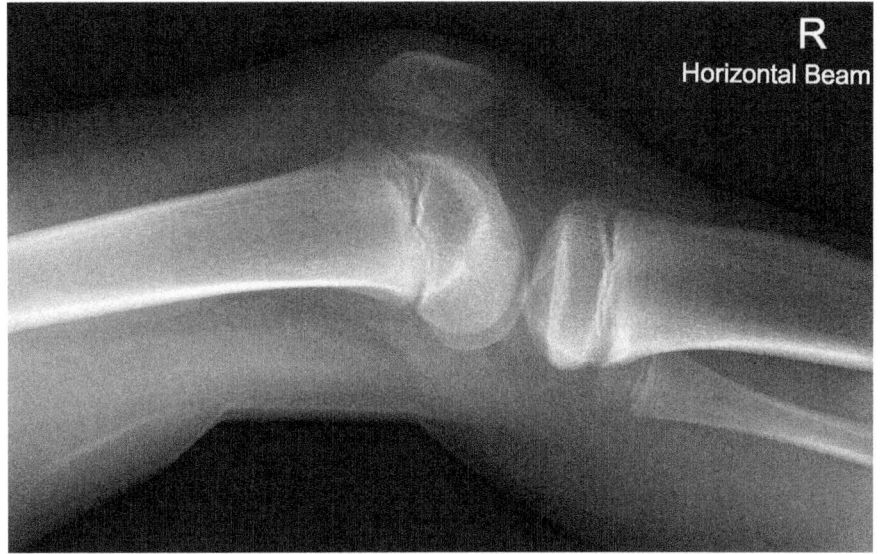

Normal	Abnormal	Diagnosis/Abnormality (only if abnormal)

Image 24

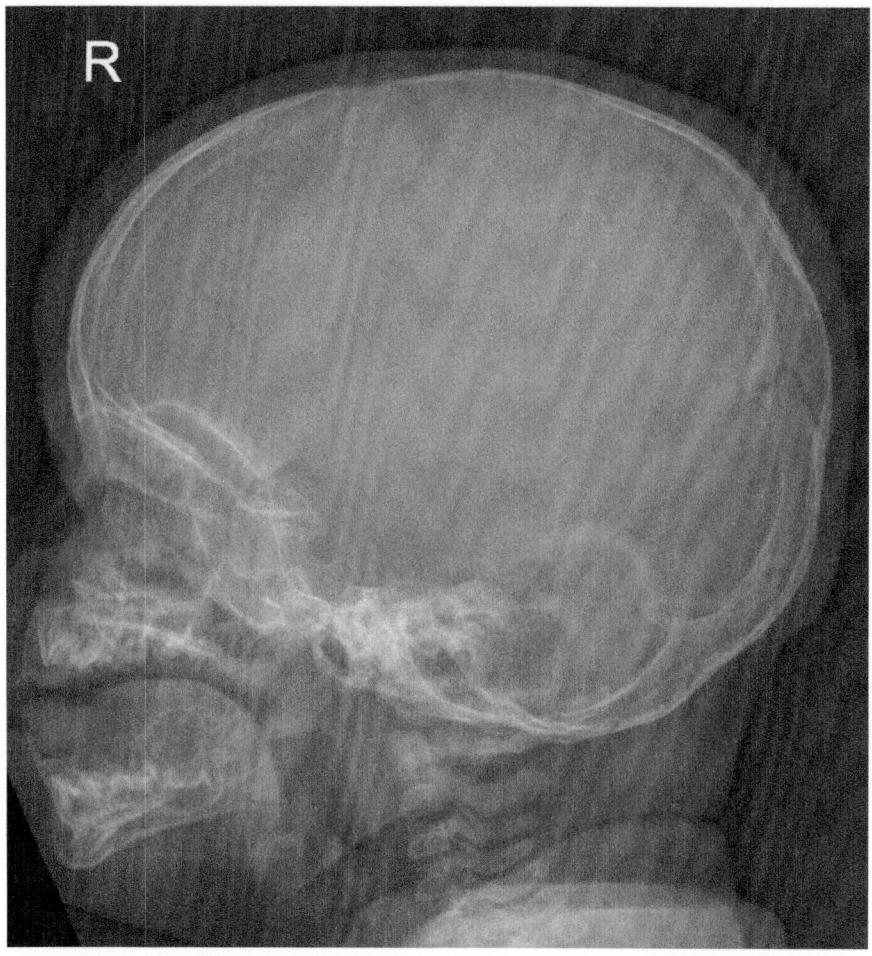

Normal	Abnormal	Diagnosis/Abnormality (only if abnormal)

Image 25

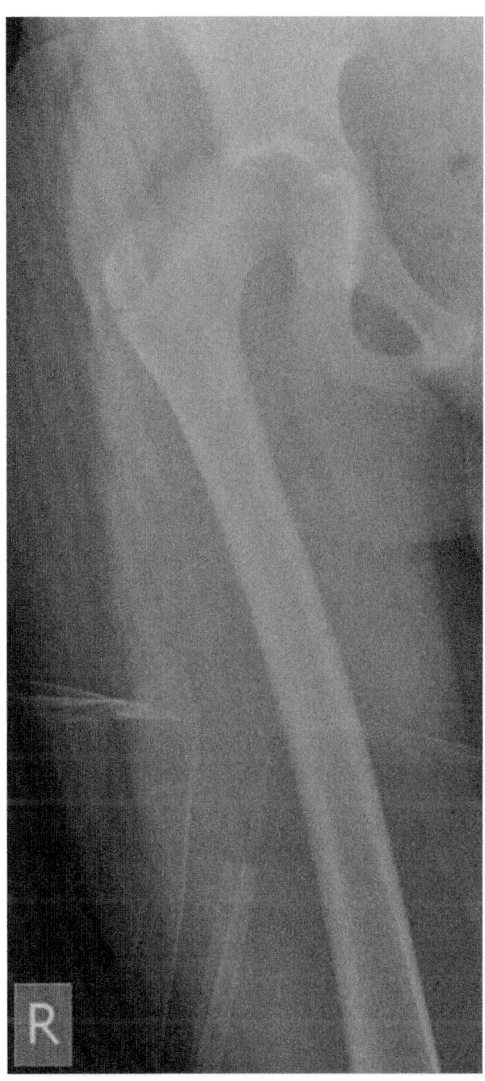

Normal	Abnormal	Diagnosis/Abnormality (only if abnormal)

Image 26

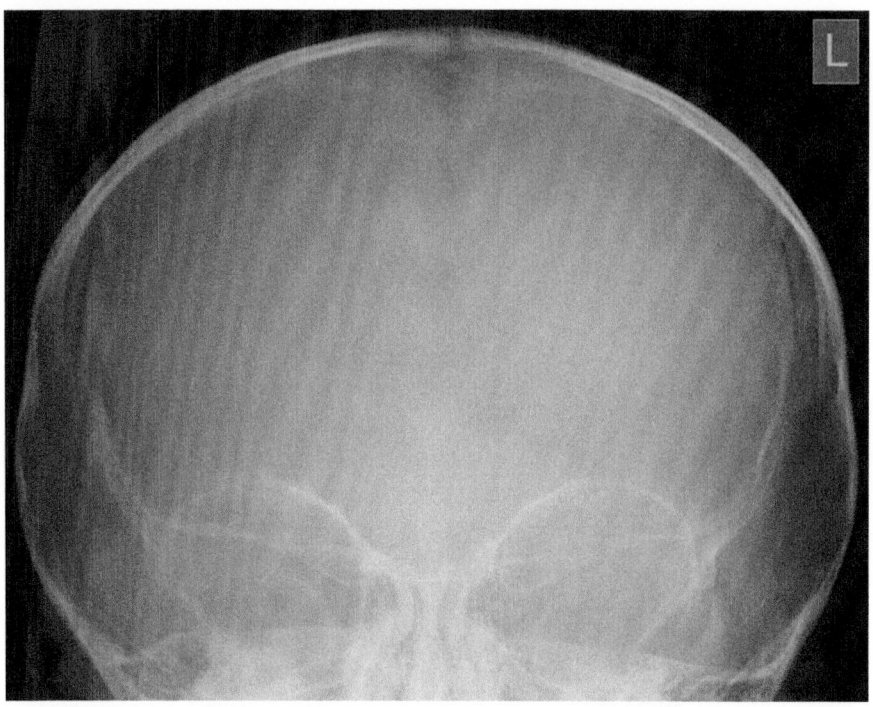

Normal	Abnormal	Diagnosis/Abnormality (only if abnormal)

Image 27

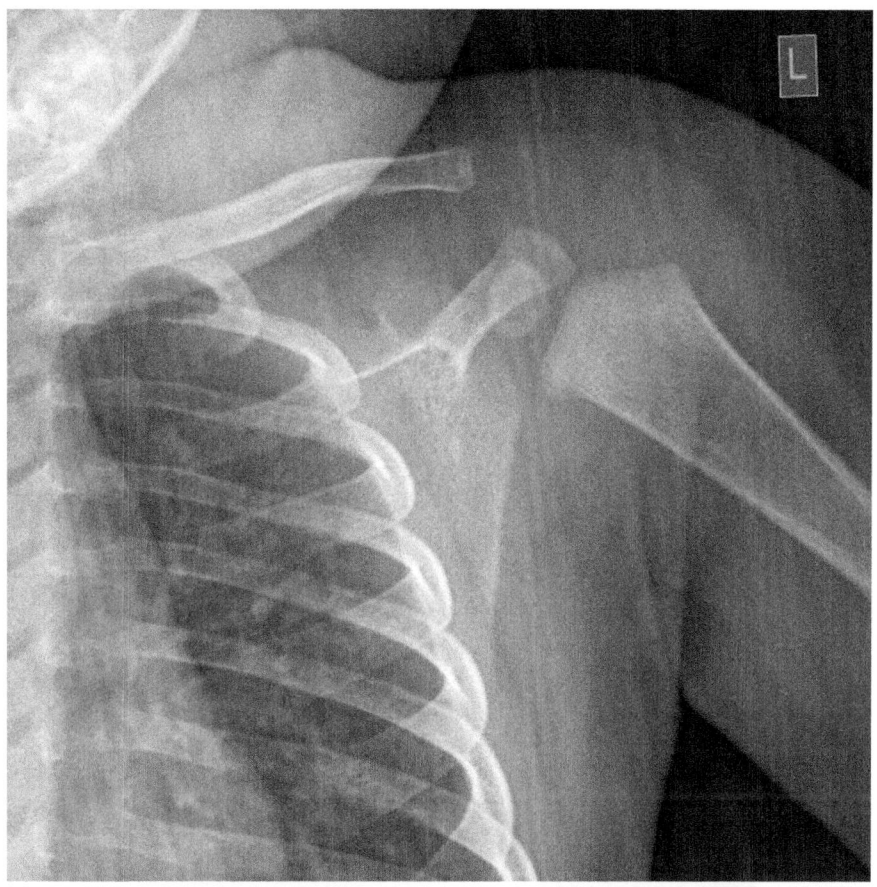

Normal	Abnormal	Diagnosis/Abnormality (only if abnormal)

Image 28

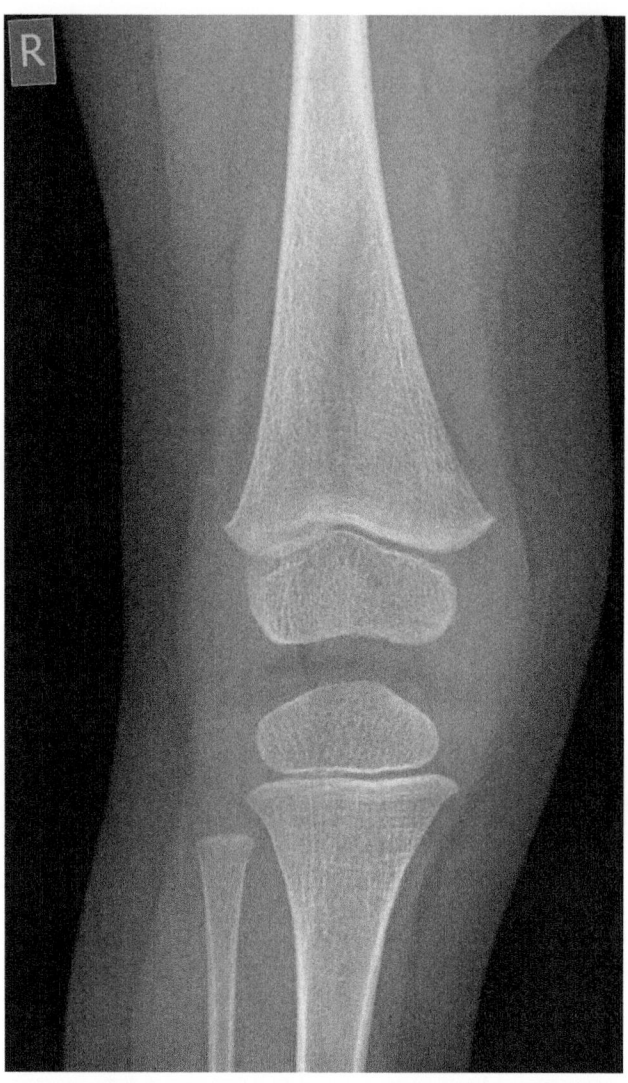

Normal	Abnormal	Diagnosis/Abnormality (only if abnormal)

Image 29

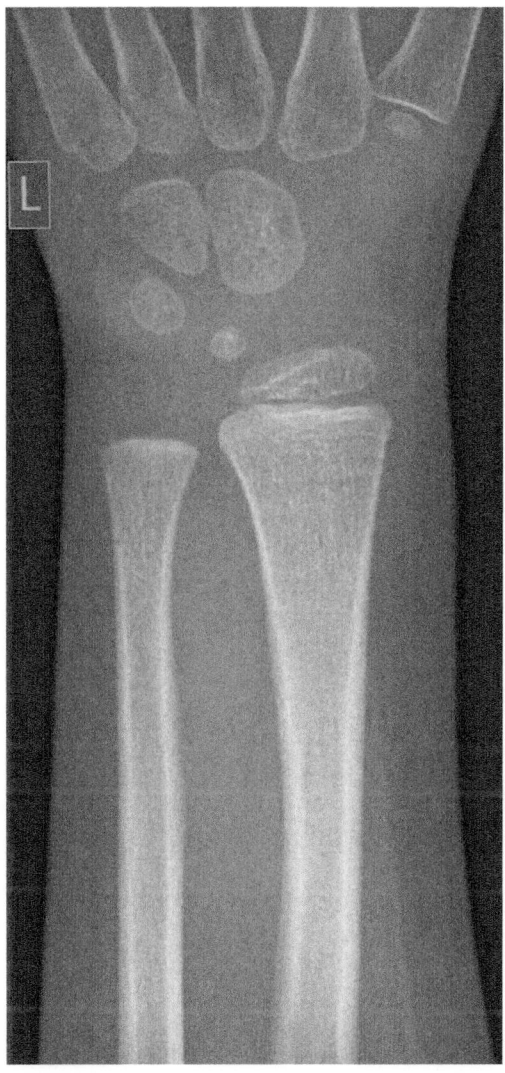

Normal	Abnormal	Diagnosis/Abnormality (only if abnormal)

Image 30

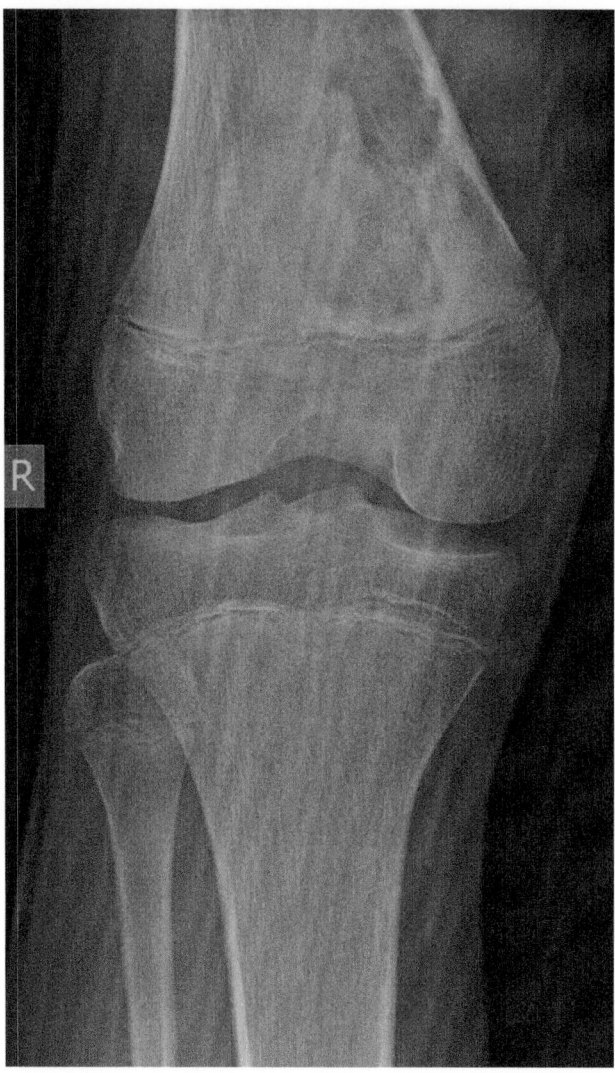

Normal	Abnormal	Diagnosis/Abnormality (only if abnormal)

2.2 Answers

Number	Normal	Abnormal	Diagnosis/abnormality (only required if abnormal column ticked)
1	✓		
2	✓		
3	✓		
4		✓	Salter-Harris 2 # right radial neck
5		✓	Pneumomediastinum
6		✓	Avascular necrosis right proximal femoral epiphysis
7		✓	Salter-Harris 2 # right second metatarsal
8	✓		
9		✓	Avascular necrosis right proximal femoral epiphysis
10		✓	Healing stress # right distal radius
11		✓	# right radial neck
12		✓	Left slipped upper femoral epiphysis
13	✓		
14		✓	Acute # right seventh posterior rib
15	✓		
16		✓	Left posterior mediastinal/paraspinal mass
17		✓	Developmental dysplasia left hip
18	✓		
19		✓	Osgood-Schlatter disease right knee
20		✓	Avascular necrosis left proximal femoral epiphysis
21		✓	Buckle #s left distal radius and ulna
22	✓		
23	✓		
24	✓		
25		✓	Right posterior hip dislocation
26	✓		
27	✓		
28	✓		
29	✓		
30		✓	Aggressive bone lesion right distal femur

2.3   Explanations

1. **Normal pelvic radiograph**

   This radiograph is normal. Note the iliac crest apophyses which have not yet fused and are normal. The iliac crest apophyses ossify lateral to medial, i.e. from the anterior superior iliac spine (ASIS) to the posterior superior iliac spine (PSIS).

   The Risser classification is a system which grades skeletal maturity based upon the degree of fusion of the iliac crest apophyses and can be used as a surrogate marker for the skeletal maturity/ossification of the spinal vertebrae, which generally parallels that of the iliac crest. The higher the Risser grade, the greater the extent of skeletal maturity. As such, this can be used to predict the progression of scoliosis based on the amount of skeletal maturation that remains and can be used when planning corrective surgery. The Risser classification is comprised of the following stages:

   - Stage 0: no ossification centre at the level of iliac crest apophysis
   - Stage 1: apophysis under 25% of the iliac crest
   - Stage 2: apophysis from 25 to 50% of the iliac crest
   - Stage 3: apophysis from 51 to 75% of the iliac crest
   - Stage 4: apophysis from 76 to 100% of the iliac crest
   - Stage 5: complete ossification and fusion of the iliac crest apophysis

3. **Normal left knee radiograph**

   This radiograph is normal. The subtle lucency projected over the proximal tibial metadiaphysis is the tibial tuberosity ossification centre imaged *en face* and is normal.

4. **Salter-Harris 2 # right radial neck**

   The outline of every bone must be traced for cortical irregularity. Whilst there is no appreciable effusion, scrutiny of the right radial neck reveals an acute fracture, seen in the magnified image below:

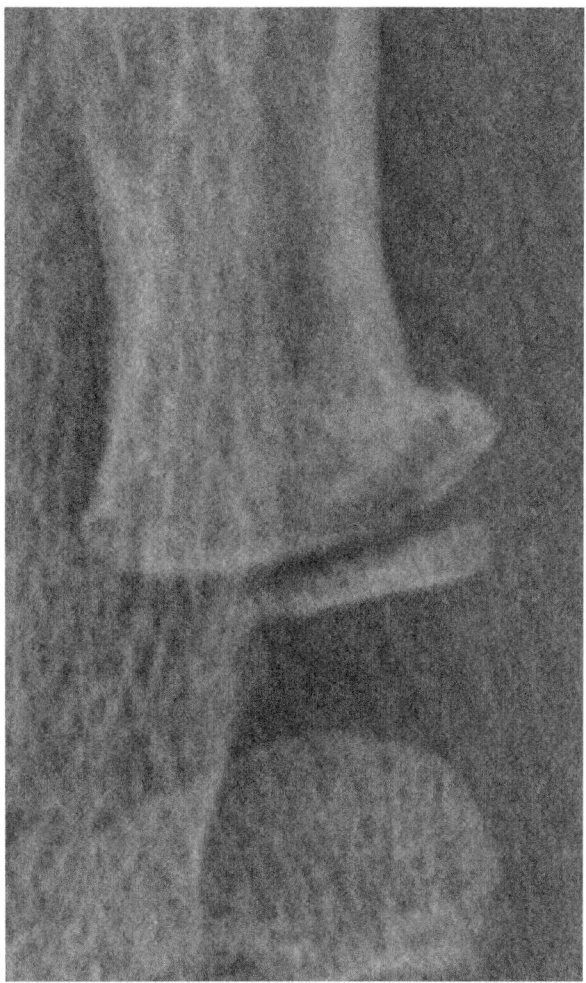

As previously discussed in the explanation for Test 1, Image 11, alignment must be assessed on every elbow radiograph and its accompanying orthogonal projection for subluxation/dislocation.

5. **Pneumomediastinum**

   This is a subtle but important finding. Note the streaky linear paratracheal lucencies projected at the level of the lower cervical spine/thoracic inlet and at the level of the carina/right main bronchus. The left heart border at the level of pulmonary-aortic window is well demarcated. See the magnified image below:

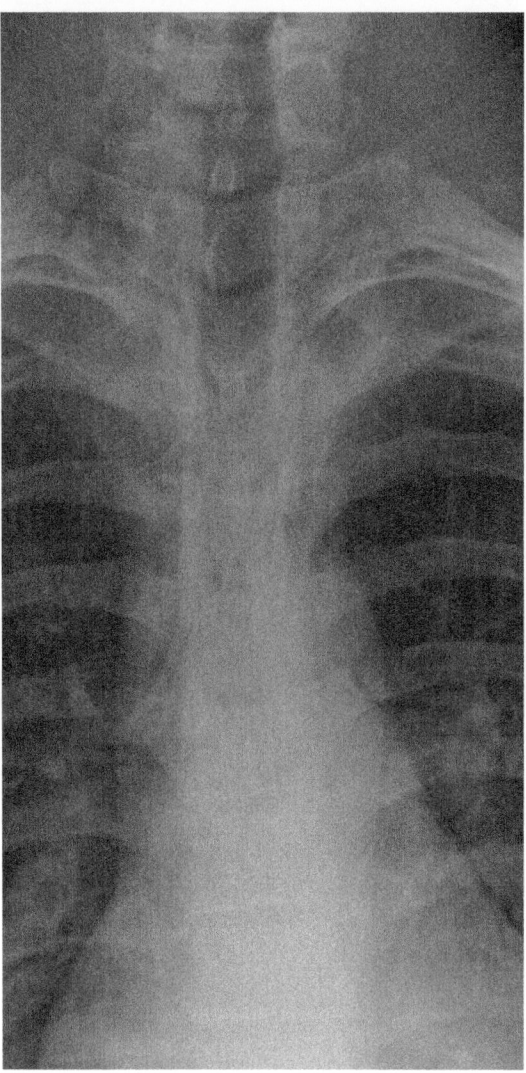

   This child with a known history of asthma (the cause of the pneumomediastinum) presented with chest pain. He was managed conservatively: a follow-up chest radiograph performed several days later demonstrated near-complete resolution.

   The Rapid Reporting examination is made more difficult by the absence of clinical information. However, this is not unlike actual clinical practice on occasion! Therefore, you must ensure that you adopt a structured approach to radiographic interpretation to ensure that important findings are not overlooked.

Tip for the viva:
- Once a pneumomediastinum has been identified, look for an associated pneumothorax (uni- or bilateral), and vice versa; particularly in the context of wheeze, chest pain, or when provided with a history of asthma.

6. **Avascular necrosis right proximal femoral epiphysis**
   Note the subtle increased sclerosis and mild loss of height of the right proximal femoral epiphysis compared to the left. See the explanation for Test 1, Image 1.

7. **Salter-Harris 2 # right second metatarsal**
   This minimally displaced fracture reinforces the point that the physis *and* the adjacent metaphysis and epiphysis must be scrutinised on every radiograph. The Salter-Harris classification is discussed in the explanation for Test 1, Image 30. In the examination, as in clinical practice, you would magnify the image to better evaluate the acute fracture which is seen below:

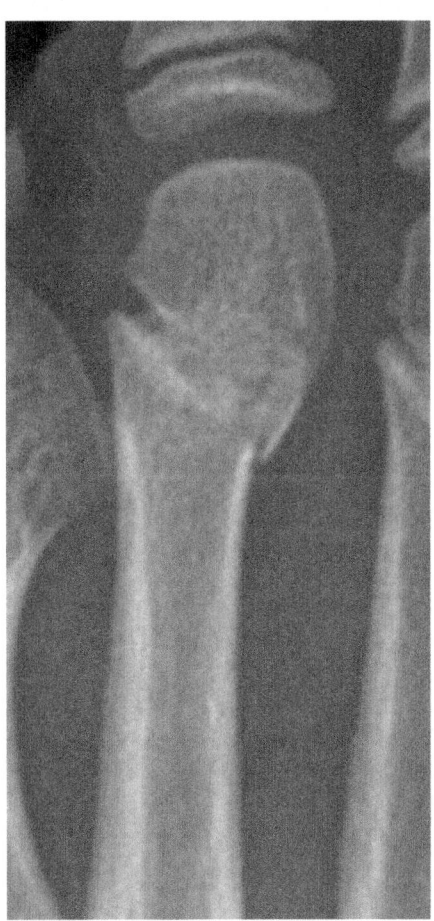

Tip for the viva:
- When presented with an extremity/musculoskeletal radiograph, you must ask for the contemporaneous orthogonal projection to complete your evaluation.

8. **Normal accessory ossification centre inferior pole left patella**

   This radiograph is normal. The patella can have variable ossification at all ages: on occasion, it can appear fragmented and can have multiple centres of ossification which may result in a bi- or multi-partite patella. An accessory ossification centre at the inferior pole of the patella is a well-recognised normal variant which in the examination you should denote as 'normal' (see the Introduction section at the start of this book). Furthermore, secondary signs of injury are absent with no overlying soft tissue swelling and no effusion or lipohaemarthrosis.

   Tip for the viva:
   - If presented with a similar appearance *plus* the presence of associated soft tissue swelling and/or other acute findings, consider these diagnoses:
     - **Patella sleeve fracture**: also known as an osteochondral avulsion fracture. Accompanied by an appropriate history, this is an acute avulsion injury at the inferior pole of the patella where the proximal portion of the patella tendon inserts, and which results from forceful contraction of the quadriceps tendon in a flexed knee. These fractures may be difficult to discern on radiography given the occasional variable appearance of patella ossification. Moreover, this fracture is extra-articular, so a joint effusion may not be present. Evaluation with MRI is essential to assess the extent of the osteochondral defect, the extensor mechanism of the knee, and the presence of anterior soft tissue swelling.
     - **Sinding-Larsen-Johansson syndrome**: also known as 'jumper's knee'. This is often thought of as the 'Osgood-Schlatter equivalent' at the inferior patella pole and represents a chronic traction injury. Children usually present with focal soft tissue swelling and point tenderness. If radiography is performed, appearances may be normal. However, positive findings may include soft tissue swelling, thickening of the proximal portion of the patella tendon, stranding of the infrapatellar fat pad (of Hoffa), and irregular/dystrophic calcification at the inferior patella pole.

9. **Avascular necrosis right proximal femoral epiphysis**

   See the explanation for Test 1, Image 1.

   This 12-year-old boy was referred for radiography by his General Practitioner (GP) for long-standing atraumatic right hip pain. This was his first radiograph: he was otherwise fit and well, and he walked into the radiology department (albeit with a painful limp).

The changes in this radiograph correspond to stage 4 in the radiographic staging of AVN and include:

- Subarticular collapse of the right proximal femoral epiphysis which is flattened and sclerotic.
- Widening of the right hip joint space with acetabular remodelling and sclerosis.
- The right proximal femoral metaphysis is starting to flatten/widen (coxa magna) with lateral uncovering of the epiphysis.

Children are usually quite robust and may tolerate significant symptom burden before presenting. Perthes disease may present at any time and if not investigated promptly, children can present late with significant changes, as in this case. One must always assess the contralateral hip as Perthes disease may affect *both* hips in approximately 15% of cases. In this image, the left proximal femoral epiphysis is of normal size, morphology and radiographic density, and lies within the joint.

Tip for the viva:
- *Both* proximal femoral epiphyses must be carefully inspected on *every* paediatric pelvic radiograph for early radiographic changes of AVN.
- In the appropriate clinical context, the late sequelae of a septic hip joint could have similar radiographic appearances.
- Bilateral symmetrical "Perthes" should raise the suspicion of a skeletal dysplasia.

10. **Healing stress # right distal radius**
    The findings in this radiograph include increased sclerosis, cortical thickening, and associated subtle benign/non-aggressive periosteal reaction of the distal radial shaft. If you had been presented with these findings with respect to the second metatarsal on an oblique foot radiograph in an adult, you would not hesitate in calling it a healing stress fracture.

    This 7-year-old female gymnast presented with recurrent right wrist pain. Even though the radiographic features are entirely consistent with healing stress fracture, an MRI was performed which demonstrated the fracture line.

Tip for the viva:
- Remember the 2B viva adage: *common pathologies in uncommon places.*

11. **# right radial neck**
    Note the joint effusion and acute cortical step in the volar aspect of the radial neck, the latter is better visualised in the magnified image below:

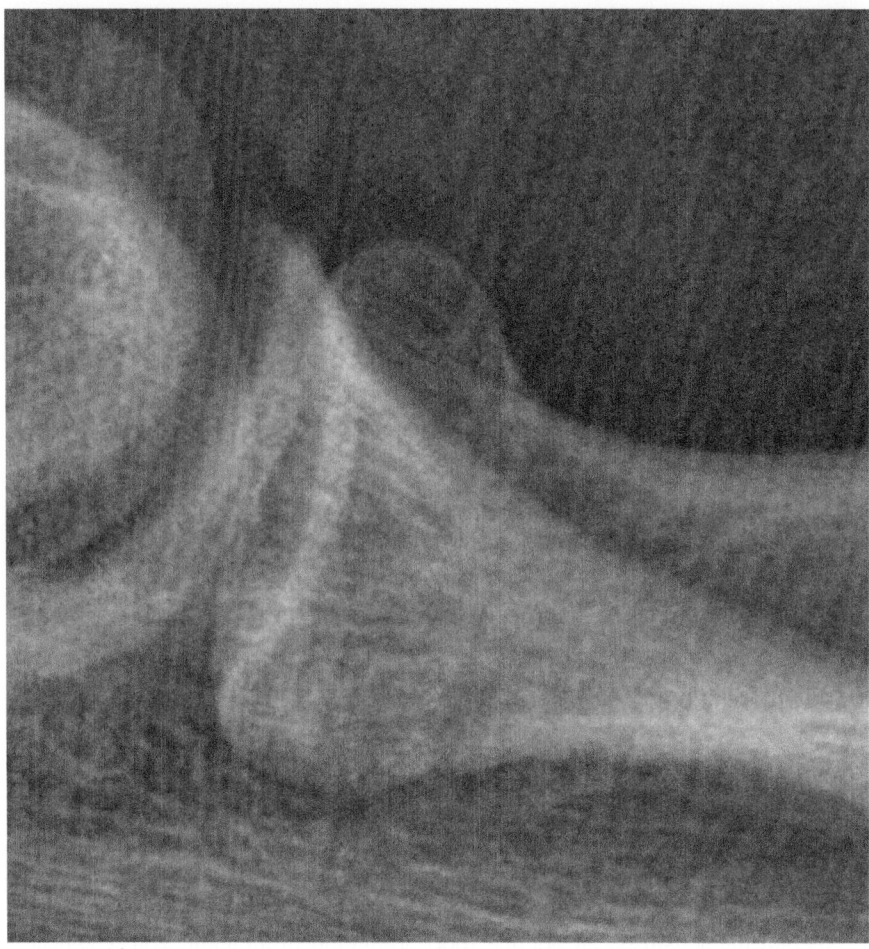

12. **Left slipped upper femoral epiphysis**

Slipped upper femoral epiphysis (SUFE), also known as slipped capital femoral epiphysis (SCFE), is one of the more common hip pathologies in adolescence. As a Salter-Harris 1 injury, it is thought to result from repeated biomechanical stress/trauma but may also occur acutely.

It is more common in boys than girls, although boys typically present later (10–17 years) than girls (8–15 years), in addition to being more common in Afro-Caribbean children than Caucasians. Obesity is a significant risk factor and there may be predisposing endocrine conditions (e.g. hypothyroidism, hyperparathyroidism).

As the slip is *posteromedial* (often more posterior than medial), the most sensitive radiographic projection is the frog-leg lateral and is often the only projection performed; the AP projection rarely adds any further diagnostic information.

Early changes include widening, blurring, and increased lucency of the physis. As the changes progress, the metaphysis may be displaced laterally such that it may no longer overlap the posterior lip of the acetabulum—this is known as the metaphyseal extrusion sign. As the changes become more chronic, the physis becomes sclerotic with metaphyseal widening/flattening resulting in coxa magna (enlargement and deformation of the femoral head and neck) on the affected side(s). The chronic changes are sequelae of AVN.

Tip for the viva:
- In this case, the SUFE is evident on the left but careful evaluation of the right hip is required because *both* hips can be affected in up to 20% of cases. Discuss the imaging protocol used (frog-leg lateral and/or AP projections) with your local paediatric radiologists.

13. **Normal right ankle radiograph**
    This radiograph is normal. There is increased ill-defined lucency in the calcaneus representing atrophic trabeculae. This is a normal variant and is termed pseudotumour of the calcaneus. Recognition of this normal appearance is important so as to not overcall it as genuine pathology given that it may mimic a tumour. If the lucency is more well defined with a sclerotic margin, an intraosseous lipoma or bone cyst should be considered. The axial projection of the calcaneum can be extremely helpful in excluding a tumour.

    There is an ossicle posterior to the talus—if this does not fuse with the lateral tubercle of the posterior talar process, it persists as an *os trigonum*.

14. **Acute # right seventh posterior rib**
    Posterior rib fractures, along with complex skull and metaphyseal fractures, are highly specific for physical abuse in infants and young children below the age of 2 years. Suspected physical abuse is also termed suspected inflicted injury and was previously known as non-accidental injury (NAI). In this case (and indeed, on every paediatric radiograph), every rib and bony structure must be assessed for evidence of acute or healing fracture(s). The acute fracture is magnified below:

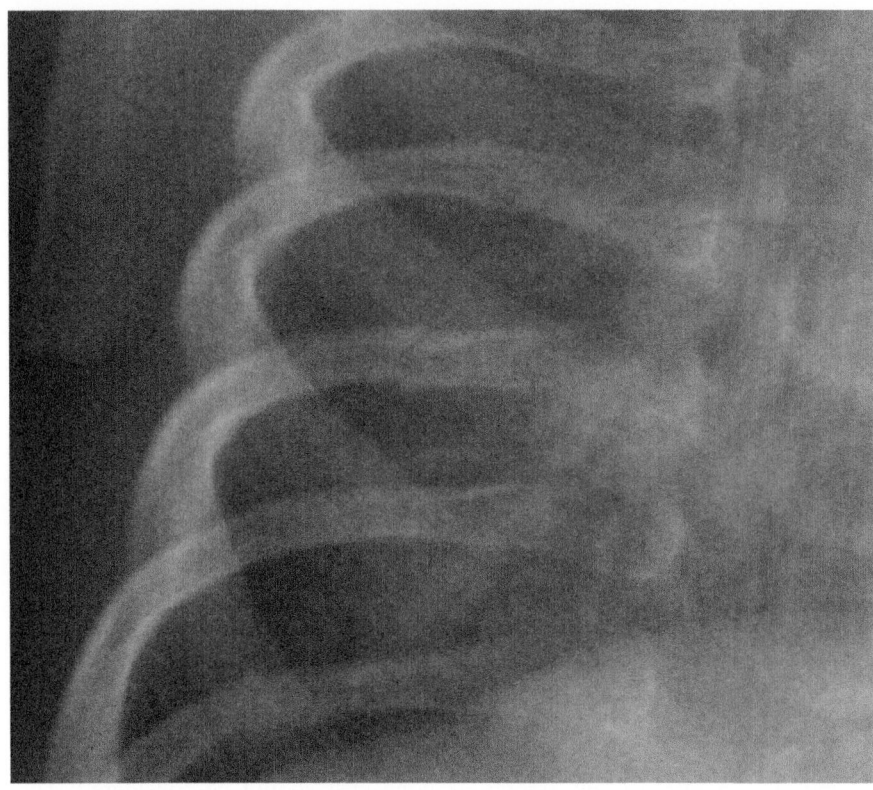

Oblique chest radiograph projections (left and right) increase the specificity for identifying rib fractures, as they allow visualisation of the ribs in two further planes. They form part of the skeletal survey—the standard series of radiographs performed in the investigation of suspected physical child abuse.

Candidates *must* be familiar with the recently updated national guidance on the radiological investigation of suspected physical abuse in children, published in late 2017 and which is freely available on the Royal College of Radiologists website:

https://www.rcr.ac.uk/publication/radiological-investigation-suspected-physical-abuse-children

The authors have published key pictorial reviews in this area which provide a comprehensive overview of this topic and which we encourage you to read—please see the references.

Tip for the viva:
• Given that oblique chest radiographs in infants and young children are specifically obtained to better visualise the ribs, look very carefully for acute/displaced or healing rib fractures when presented with an oblique chest radiograph. Do not mistake the sternal segments for healing rib fractures on an oblique chest radiograph.

16. **Left posterior mediastinal/paraspinal mass**

The left apical mass traverses the thoracic plane (of Ludwig) which is the imaginary line used to separate the superior and inferior mediastinum at the level of the T4 vertebral body/manubriosternal joint. Given that the mass extends above the superior aspect of the left clavicle (the imaginary border of the anterior mediastinum and known as the positive *cervicothoracic sign*), it must lie either in the neck and/or the posterior mediastinum. Furthermore, the left hilar vessels (the hilum overlay sign) *and* the left heart border are visualised (i.e. not obliterated) because the mass is *posterior* to the pericardium. Thus, this mass lies in the posterior mediastinum in addition to traversing the superior/inferior mediastinum. Whilst not evident on this radiograph, widening of the paravertebral stripes further localise the pathology to the posterior mediastinum.

In the examination, you will have approximately 1 min to decide whether the radiograph is normal or abnormal; although 'left posterior mediastinal mass' is more accurate, 'left paraspinal mass' would be sufficient.

Lateral radiographs to confirm/further localise a mediastinal mass are not routinely obtained in children (and diminishingly so in adults); both to reduce radiation burden but also because a suspected mediastinal mass will require investigation with CT. However, this does not preclude the examiner from presenting you with one in the viva examination! If one has been obtained and is presented to you, the examiner will expect you to be able to interpret it before moving on to the inevitable CT.

In children, the most common mediastinal masses (all compartments) are:

- Neurogenic tumours: comprising the majority of cases, these arise from sympathetic ganglia (neuroblastoma) or nerve roots (schwannoma or neurofibroma).
- Malignant germ cell tumours: mature teratomas (a type of germ cell tumour containing several different types of tissue) account for the majority of tumours in the anterior mediastinum. Correlation with serum tumour markers is required (both AFP and β hCG are elevated in germ cell tumours).
- Foregut duplication cysts: these may be bronchogenic (usually mediastinal in location but can be intrapulmonary, are often asymptomatic, and do not communicate with the tracheobronchial tree); oesophageal (may be symptomatic causing dysphagia due to oesophageal compression. These can be lined by gastric mucosa and are prone to infection, perforation, and haemorrhage); or neurogenic (rare, <1%; these result from incomplete resorption of the neuroenteric canal).
- Extramedullary haematopoiesis: this is the deposition of normal blood cells outside the bone marrow from a failure of erythropoiesis. Consider this in patients with thalassemia, sickle cell disease, or myelofibrosis in the context of smooth, well-defined, lobulated paraspinal masses which may be unilateral or bilateral.

In this case, CT confirmed the presence of a posterior mediastinal mass, iodine-123 metaiodobenzylguanidine (MIBG) scintigraphy demonstrated corresponding high uptake and CT guided biopsy confirmed the suspected radiological diagnosis of thoracic neuroblastoma.

The majority of neuroblastomas (approximately two-thirds) arise from the adrenal glands and the retroperitoneum; posterior mediastinal thoracic neuroblastoma comprises approximately 20% of cases. Intrathoracic neuroblastoma is much less common.

Tip for the viva:
- If presented with a suspected mediastinal mass on chest radiography, you must first localise it *to* and then *within* the mediastinum. You may be presented with some clinical information which is often necessary to contextualise the radiographic findings to enable you to order/limit the differential diagnosis.
- If no history is initially given by the examiner, in the context of a mediastinal mass remember to look for "H-shaped" vertebrae on the chest radiograph, AVN of the humeral head(s), and/or cardiomegaly as clues to a diagnosis of sickle cell disease.

17. **Developmental dysplasia left hip**
    The key radiographic features in this image are:
    - A small left ossific nucleus
    - A shallow and dysplastic left acetabulum
    - Lateral subluxation of the left hip joint
    - Broadening/widening of the left proximal femoral metaphysis

    The appearances are consistent with developmental dysplasia of the left hip.

    Developmental dysplasia of the hip (DDH) describes an abnormally developed hip joint with a subsequent abnormal relationship between the proximal femoral epiphysis and the acetabulum. It is thought to result from abnormal *in utero* positioning. Oligohydramnios and breech positioning during pregnancy are associated risk factors, alongside a previous family history. There is a female predominance being approximately eight times more common than in males.

    DDH is suggested clinically by asymmetric thigh creases and, positive Barlow manoeuvre (hip adduction followed by posterior/downward force to dislocate the femoral head posteriorly) and Ortolani test (flexing then gently abducting the hips to relocate the [possibly dislocated] femoral head anteriorly back into the acetabulum with a positive 'clunk').

    Ultrasound is the modality of choice in those infants under the age of 6 months given that the proximal femoral epiphyses are not yet ossified. After this age, radiographic evaluation is usually required to assess the hip joints, including:
    - Symmetry, size, shape, and radiographic density of the proximal femoral ossific nuclei—a delay in ossification, i.e. smaller and more lucent proximal femoral epiphysis is a feature of DDH.

- Acetabular morphology—a shallow or dysplastic acetabulum is more likely to subluxate/dislocate.
- A subluxed (as in this case) or frankly dislocated joint

It is important to remember that DDH is a dynamic disease, and it is not always present or clinically apparent at birth. It is important to evaluate the pelvis and both hip joints on every radiograph, particularly if it has been performed for an unrelated clinical indication.

Tip for the viva:
- In this case, radiographic changes are evident on the right hip but careful evaluation of *both* hips is required given that both can be affected in *up to one-third of cases.*

19. **Osgood-Schlatter disease right knee**
    This is a chronic traction apophysitis of the distal portion of the patellar tendon at its insertion onto the tibial tuberosity ossification centre. It is more commonly seen in young active adolescent boys who kick and jump, typically affecting those aged 10–15 years. It can be bilateral in up to 50% of cases. Affected children typically present with focal soft tissue swelling and point tenderness over the tibial tuberosity which is exacerbated by exercise.
    As this is a clinical diagnosis, it does not require investigation with radiography. However, if radiography is performed, focal soft tissue swelling over the tibial tuberosity is usually present and fragmentation of the tibial tuberosity is typically seen. However, it is important to note that fragmentation can be a normal finding in the asymptomatic knee and represents the normal secondary ossification centre. Thus, the radiological diagnosis of Osgood-Schlatter disease should not be made on the basis of fragmentation alone and explains why the diagnosis is largely clinical. The condition typically resolves once the tibial tuberosity physis has fused.

20. **Avascular necrosis left proximal femoral epiphysis**
    See the explanation for Test 1, Image 1.

21. **Buckle #s left distal radius and ulna**
    See explanation for Test 1, Image 18 and the Introduction section.

24. **Normal skull radiograph**
    See the references for an annotated presentation of the radiological anatomy of the normal paediatric skull and of the craniosynostoses.

25. **Right posterior hip dislocation**
    Significant force is required to displace the femoral head from the normal hip joint. As such, traumatic hip dislocations are uncommon in the paediatric population and are only usually seen in the context of high energy impact trauma,

e.g. road traffic accident (RTA). This child fell off a trampoline and landed awkwardly; the contemporaneous lateral projection confirmed the dislocation.

Tip for the viva:
- In the context of an acute traumatic subluxation/dislocation (any joint), look for an associated fracture and do not forget to evaluate any contemporaneous orthogonal projection(s).

29. **Normal left wrist radiograph.**
    This radiograph is normal. Compare with Image 10 from this test.

30. **Aggressive bone lesion right distal femur**
    This radiograph is abnormal. There is a lucent lesion in the right medial distal femoral metadiaphysis with a wide zone of transition (particularly inferiorly and laterally adjacent to the physis) consistent with an aggressive lesion. The contemporaneous lateral projection demonstrated posterior cortical destruction, periosteal reaction, and associated soft tissue swelling. This 14-year-old boy presented with a history of atraumatic medial knee pain. Following this radiograph, he was referred for an urgent paediatric orthopaedic opinion and was eventually diagnosed with primary osteosarcoma.

    Imaging evaluation for suspected/confirmed osteosarcoma includes: MRI of the whole lower limb to assess for skip lesions (a feature of osteosarcoma); technetium-99 bone scintigraphy to assess for distant sites of bony disease; and CT thorax to evaluate for pulmonary metastases.

Tip for the viva:
- Patients should be referred to a specialist paediatric orthopaedic centre experienced in managing suspected cases of osteosarcoma: any biopsy tract will need to be carefully planned to reduce the risk of malignant seeding and which may be included in any subsequent resection. Preoperative chemotherapy may help to downstage the tumour prior to resection.

Further Reading

Image 1

Aziz PAA, Luijkx T et al (2018) Risser criteria. https://radiopaedia.org/articles/risser-classification. Accessed July 2018

Hacquebord JH, Leopold SS (2012) In brief: the Risser classification: a classic tool for the clinician treating adolescent idiopathic scoliosis. Clin Orthop Relat Res 470(8):2335–2338

Image 4

Dupuis CS, Westra SJ, Makris J et al (2009) Injuries and conditions of the extensor mechanism of the pediatric knee. Radiographics 29(3):877–886

Jones J, Gaillard F et al (2018) Patella sleeve fractures. https://radiopaedia.org/articles/patellar-sleeve-fractures. Accessed April 2018

Luiijkx T, Gaillard F et al (2018) Sinding-Larsen-Johansson disease. https://radiopaedia.org/articles/sinding-larsen-johansson-disease. Accessed April 2018

Image 5

el-Khoury GY, Boles CA (1997) Slipped capital femoral epiphysis. Radiographics 17(4):809–823

Thurston M, Gaillard F et al (2018) Slipped upper femoral epiphysis. https://radiopaedia.org/articles/slipped-upper-femoral-epiphysis. Accessed April 2018

Image 13

Jones J et al (2018) Os trigonum. https://radiopaedia.org/articles/os-trigonum. Accessed July 2018

Thurston M, Niknejad MT et al (2018) Pseudotumour of the calcaneus. https://radiopaedia.org/articles/pseudotumour-of-the-calcaneus. Accessed July 2018

Image 14

Bulloch B, Schubert CJ, Brophy PD et al (2000) Cause and clinical characteristics of rib fractures in infants. Pediatrics 105:E48

Cadzow SP, Armstrong KL (2000) Rib fractures in infants: red alert! The clinical features, investigations and child protection outcomes. J Pediatr Child Health 36:322e6

Imaging of Suspected Physical Abuse in Infants and Young Children

Lonergan GJ, Baker AM, Morey MK et al (2003) From the archives of the AFIP. Child abuse: radiologic-pathologic correlation. Radiographics 23:811e45

Offiah A, van Rijn RR, Perez-Rosello JM, Kleinman PK (2009) Skeletal imaging of child abuse (non-accidental injury). Pediatr Radiol 39(5):461–470

Paddock M, Sprigg A, Offiah AC (2017a) Imaging and reporting considerations for suspected physical abuse (non-accidental injury) in infants and young children. Part 1: initial considerations and appendicular skeleton. Clin Radiol 72(3):179–188

Paddock M, Sprigg A, Offiah AC (2017b) Imaging and reporting considerations for suspected physical abuse (non-accidental injury) in infants and young children. Part 2: axial skeleton and differential diagnoses. Clin Radiol 72(3):189–201

Paddock M, Sprigg A, Halliday K, Offiah AC (2018) Re: a comprehensive toolkit for imaging children who may have been abused: new guidance from the Royal College of Radiologists and the Society and College of Radiographers. Clin Radiol 73(7):672–673

Royal College of Radiologists & Society of College of Radiographers (2017) The radiological investigation of suspected physical child abuse. https://www.rcr.ac.uk/publication/radiological-investigation-suspected-physical-abuse-children. Accessed September 2017

Image 16

Bhalla S, Hazewinkel M, Smithuis R (2018) Mediastinum – masses. http://www.radiologyassistant.nl/en/p4620a193b679d/mediastinum-masses.html. Accessed April 2018

Di Mazio B et al (2018) Extramedullary haematopoiesis. https://radiopaedia.org/articles/extramedullary-haematopoiesis. Accessed April 2018

Hacking C, Gaillard F et al (2018) Anterior mediastinal germ cell tumours. https://radiopaedia.org/articles/anterior-mediastinal-germ-cell-tumours. Accessed April 2018

Hacking C, Knipe H et al (2018) Thoracic plane. https://radiopaedia.org/articles/thoracic-plane. Accessed April 2018

Jones J et al (2018) Bronchogenic cyst. https://radiopaedia.org/articles/bronchogenic-cyst. Accessed April 2018

Ranganath SH, Lee EY, Restrepo R, Eisenberg RL (2012) Mediastinal mass in children. AJR Am J Roentgenol 198(3):W197–W216

Skandhan AKP, St-Amant M et al (2018) Neurenteric cyst. https://radiopaedia.org/articles/neurenteric-cyst. Accessed April 2018

Thurston M, Bekhit E et al (2018) Neuroblastoma. https://radiopaedia.org/articles/neuroblastoma. Accessed April 2018

Image 17

Knipe H, Gaillard F et al (2018) Acetabular angle. https://radiopaedia.org/articles/acetabular-angle. Accessed July 2018

Niknejad MT, Gaillard F et al (2018) Developmental dysplasia of the hip. https://radiopaedia.org/articles/developmental-dysplasia-of-the-hip. Accessed July 2018

Robben S, Smithuis R (2018) Developmental dysplasia of the hip – ultrasound. http://www.radiologyassistant.nl/en/p54ba2c50995c5/developmental-dysplasia-of-the-hip-ultrasound.html. Accessed July 2018

Storer SK, Skaggs DL (2006) Developmental dysplasia of the hip. Am Fam Physician 74(8):1310–1316

Tamai J, McCarthy JJ (2018) Developmental dysplasia of the hip. http://learningradiology.com/notes/bonenotes/conghipdysplasiapage.htm. Accessed July 2018

Image 19

Gottsegen CJ, Eyer BA, White EA et al (2008) Avulsion fractures of the knee: imaging findings and clinical significance. Radiographics 28(6):1755–1770

Stevens MA, El-Khoury GY, Kathol MH et al (1999) Imaging features of avulsion injuries. Radiographics 19(3):655–672

Image 24

Eley KA, Johnson D, Sheerin F (2018) Cranial sutures & craniosynostosis. https://www.bir.org.uk/media/76496/cranial_sutures___craniosynostosis_-_ka_eley__f_sheerin__d_johnson__final_.pdf. Accessed July 2018

Image 30

Shah JN, Cohen HL, Choudhri AF et al (2017) Pediatric benign bone tumors: what does the radiologist need to know? Pediatr Imaging 37(3):1001–1002

van der Woude HJ, Smithuis R (2018) Bone tumor – systematic approach and differential diagnosis. http://www.radiologyassistant.nl/en/p494e15cbf0d8d/bone-tumor-systematic-approach-and-differential-diagnosis.html. Accessed July 2018

Yarmish G, Klein MJ, Landa J et al (2010) Imaging characteristics of primary osteosarcoma: nonconventional subtypes. Radiographics 30(6):1653–1672

Test 3

3.1   Images

Image 1

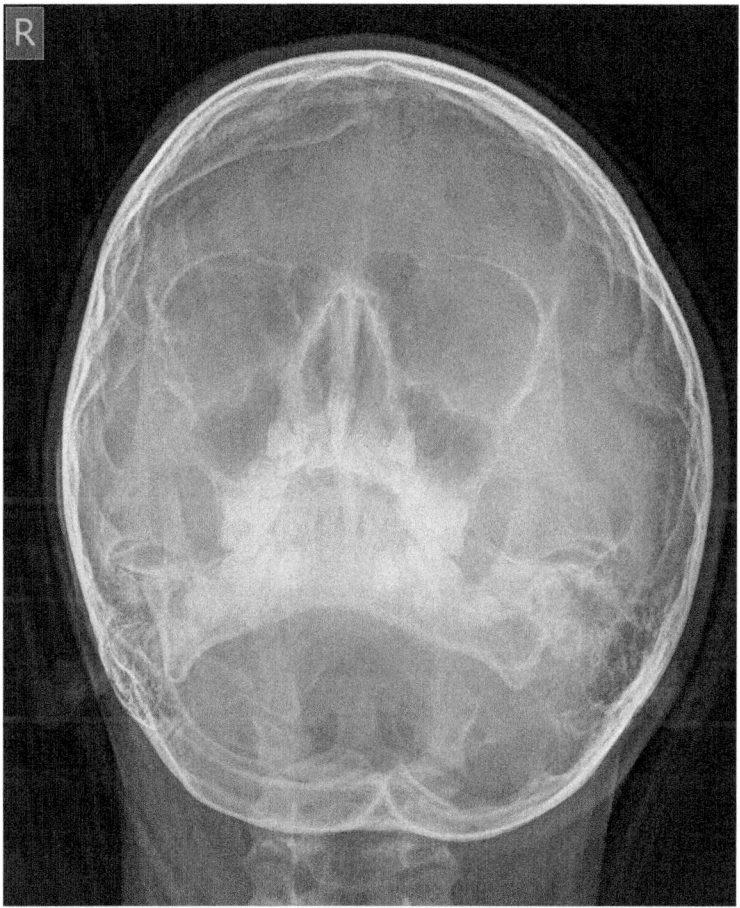

Normal	Abnormal	Diagnosis/Abnormality (only if abnormal)

© Springer Nature Switzerland AG 2019
M. Paddock, A. C. Offiah, *Paediatric Radiology Rapid Reporting for FRCR Part 2B*,
https://doi.org/10.1007/978-3-030-01965-5_3

Image 2

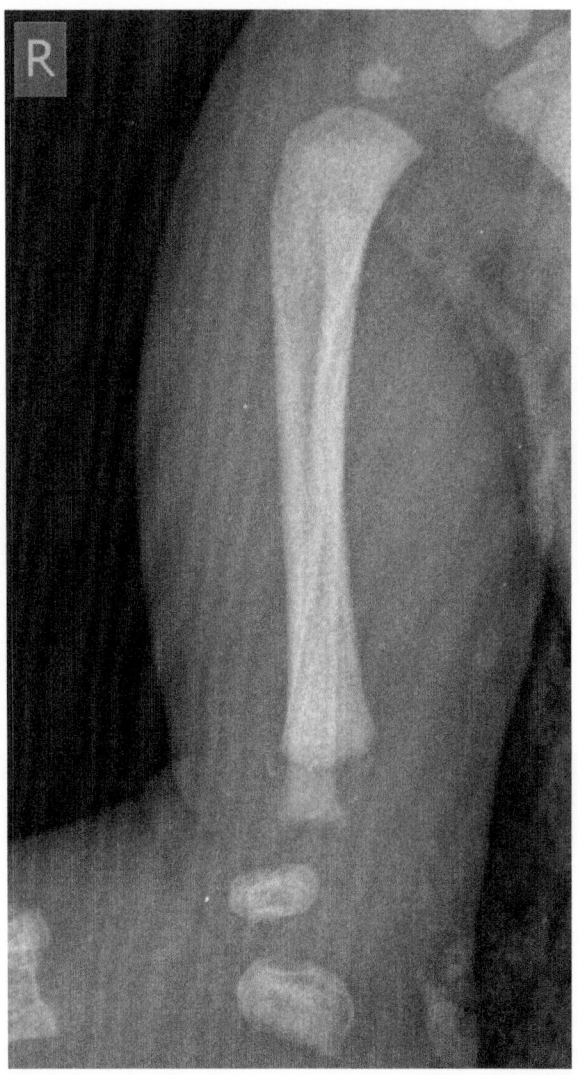

Normal	Abnormal	Diagnosis/Abnormality (only if abnormal)

Image 3

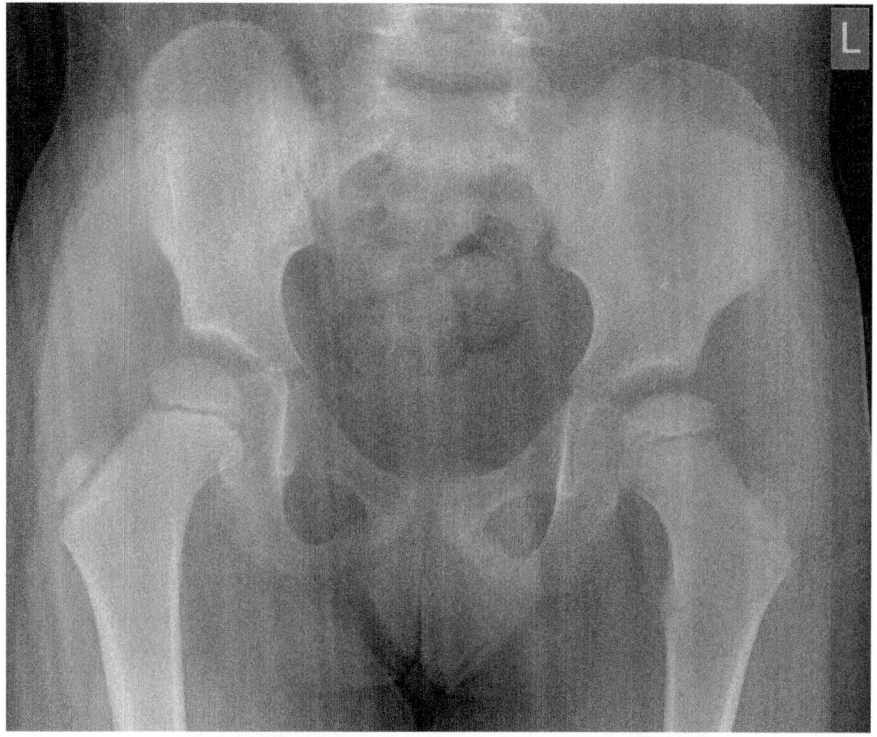

Normal	Abnormal	Diagnosis/Abnormality (only if abnormal)

Image 4

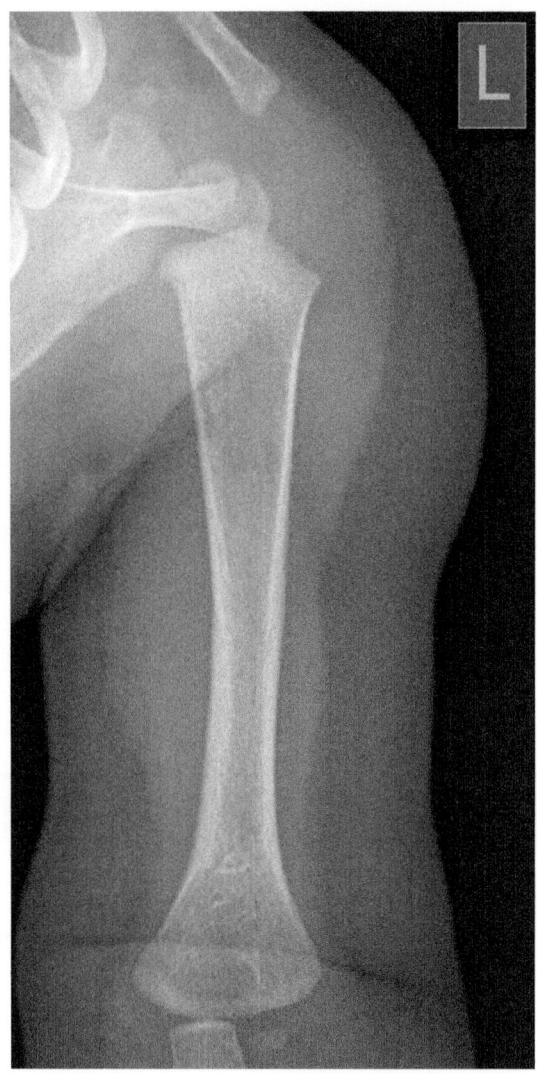

Normal	Abnormal	Diagnosis/Abnormality (only if abnormal)

Image 5

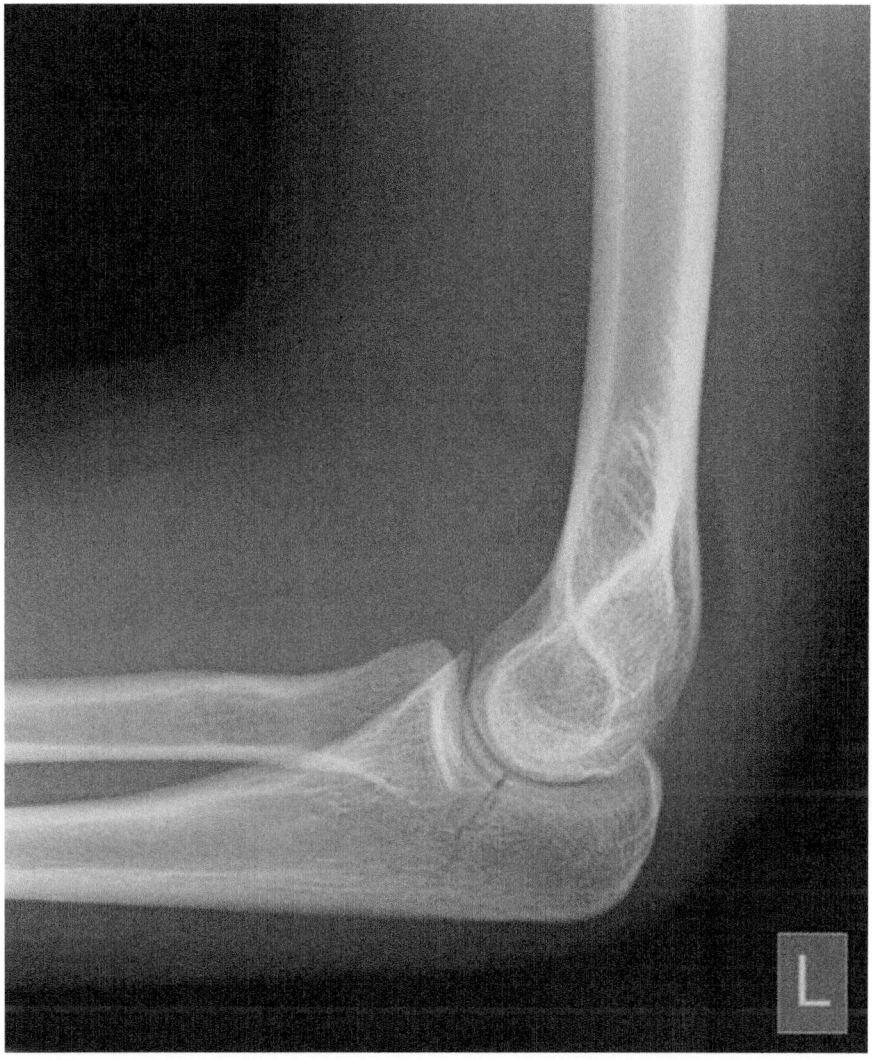

Normal	Abnormal	Diagnosis/Abnormality (only if abnormal)

Image 6

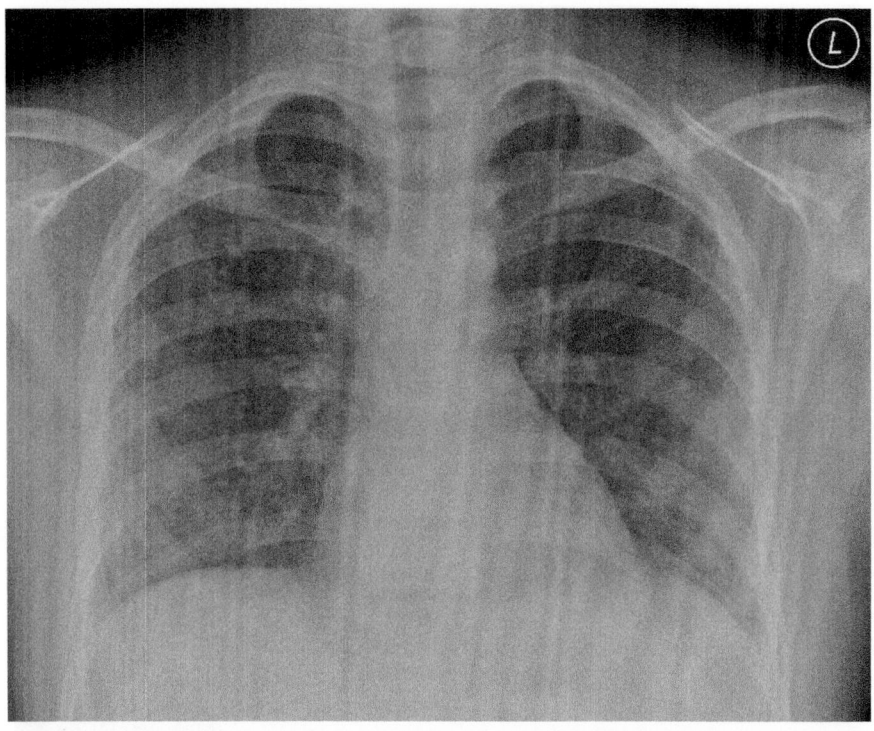

Normal	Abnormal	Diagnosis/Abnormality (only if abnormal)

Image 7

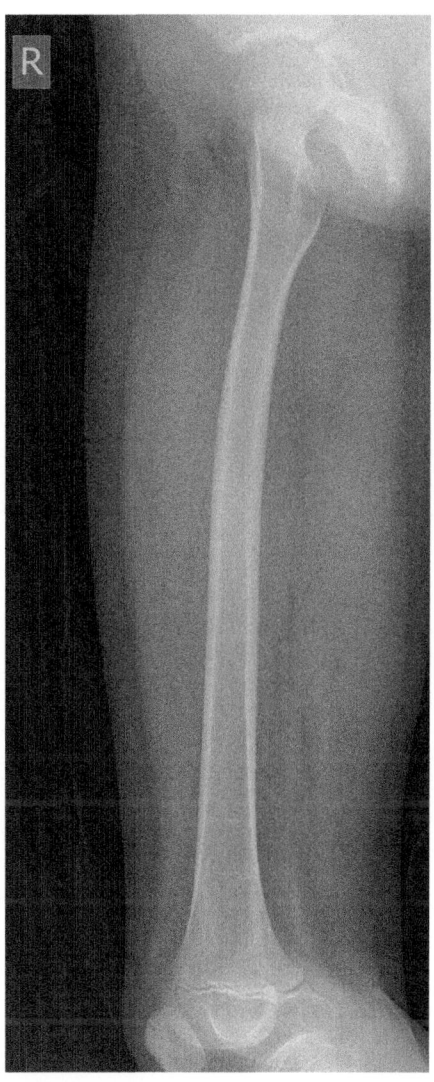

Normal	Abnormal	Diagnosis/Abnormality (only if abnormal)

Image 8

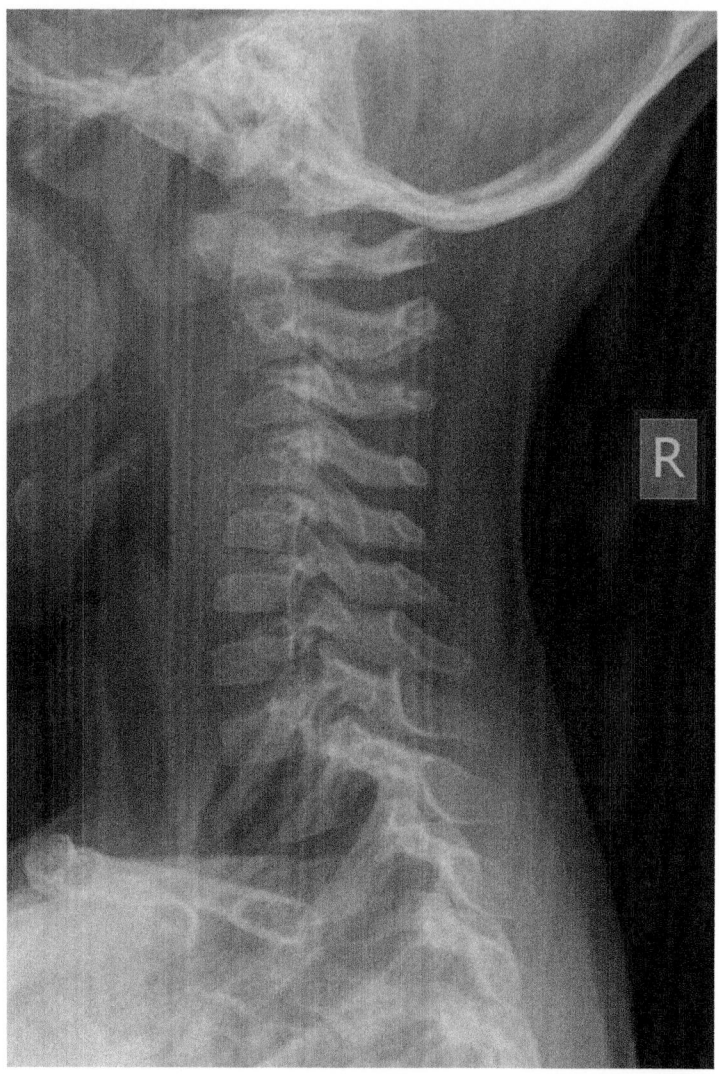

Normal	Abnormal	Diagnosis/Abnormality (only if abnormal)

Image 9

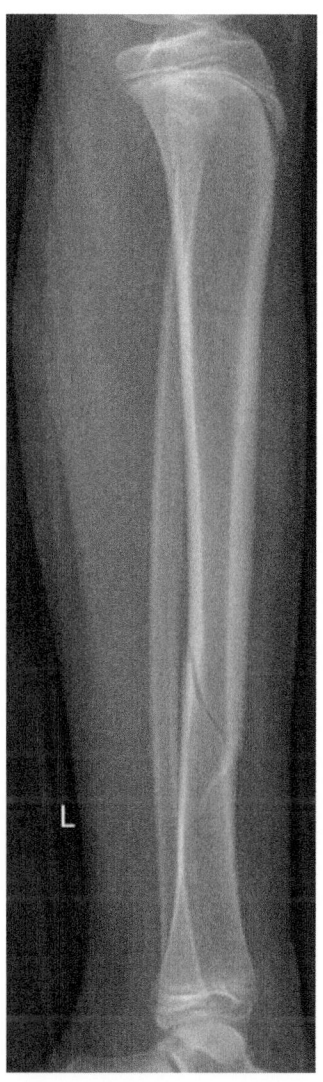

Normal	Abnormal	Diagnosis/Abnormality (only if abnormal)

Image 10

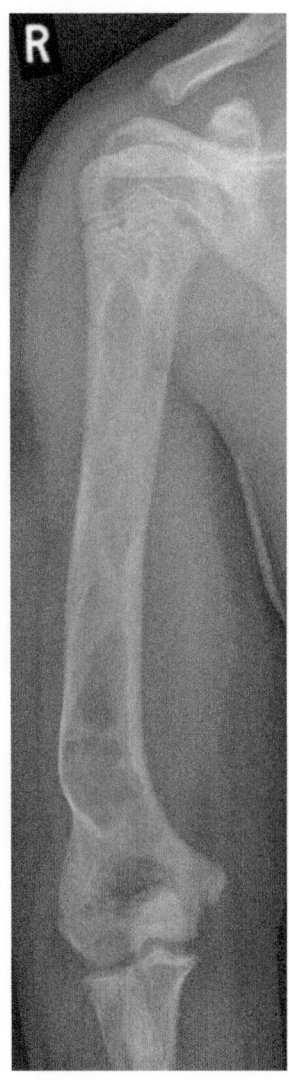

Normal	Abnormal	Diagnosis/Abnormality (only if abnormal)

Image 11

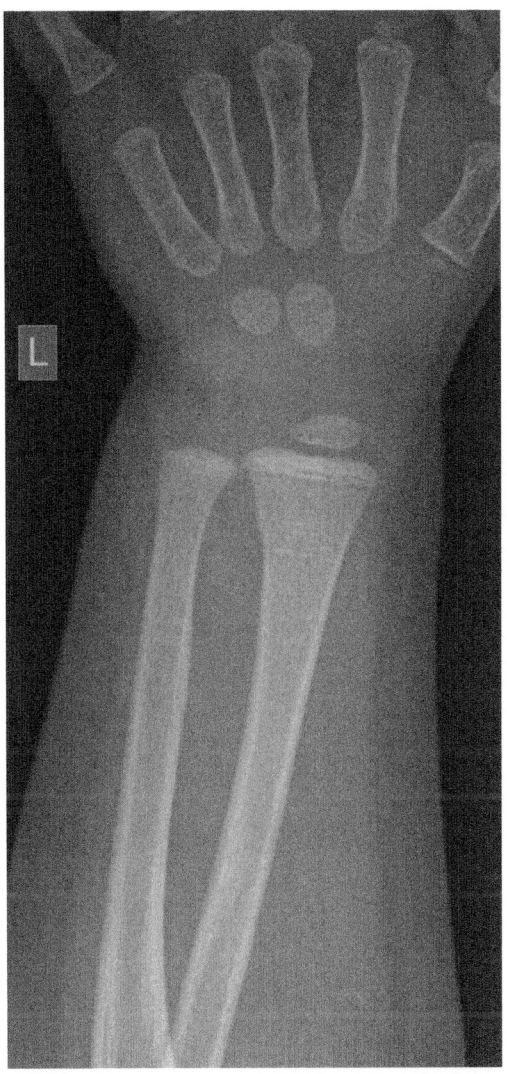

Normal	Abnormal	Diagnosis/Abnormality (only if abnormal)

Image 12

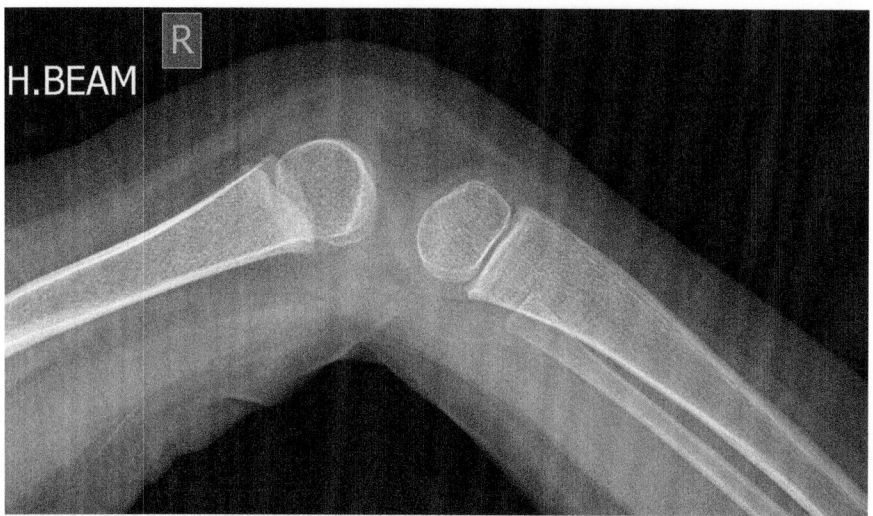

Normal	Abnormal	Diagnosis/Abnormality (only if abnormal)

Image 13

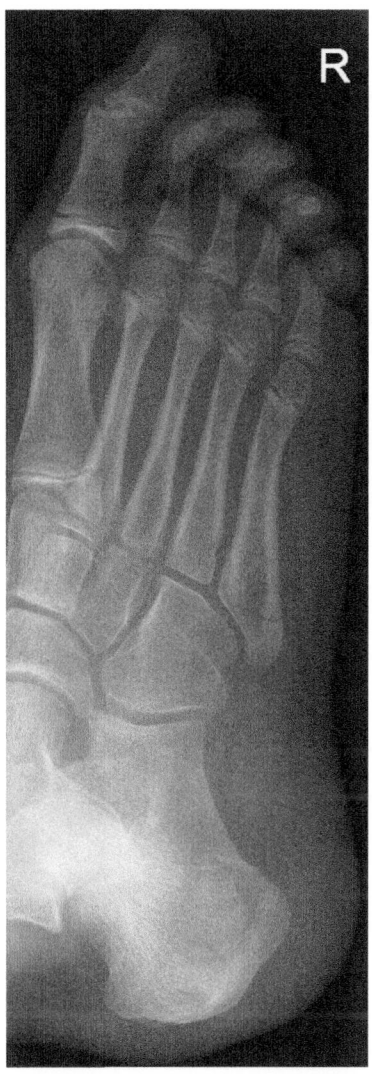

Normal	Abnormal	Diagnosis/Abnormality (only if abnormal)

Image 14

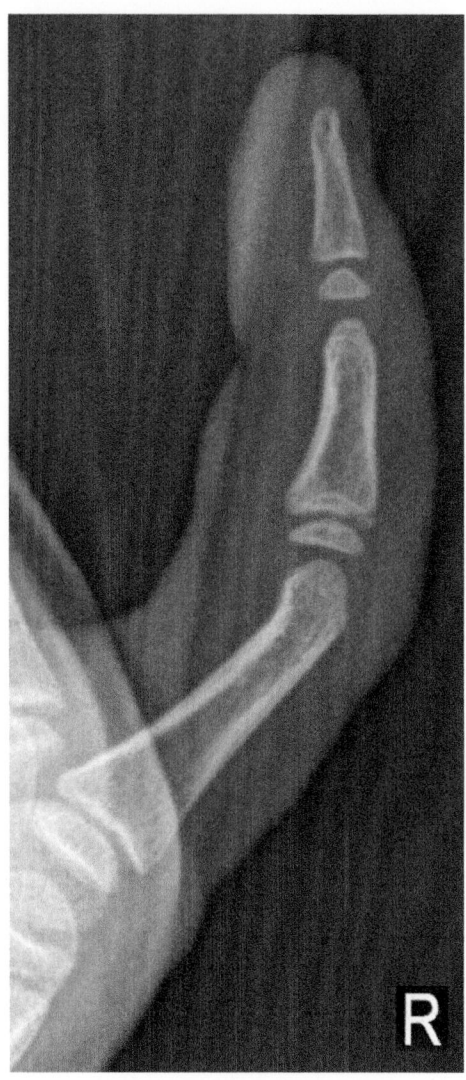

Normal	Abnormal	Diagnosis/Abnormality (only if abnormal)

Image 15

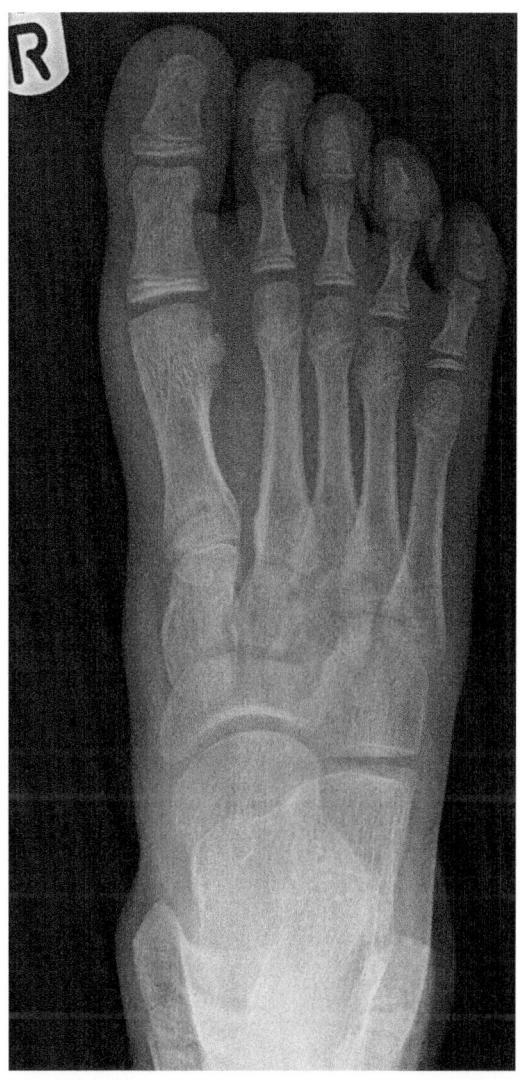

Normal	Abnormal	Diagnosis/Abnormality (only if abnormal)

Image 16

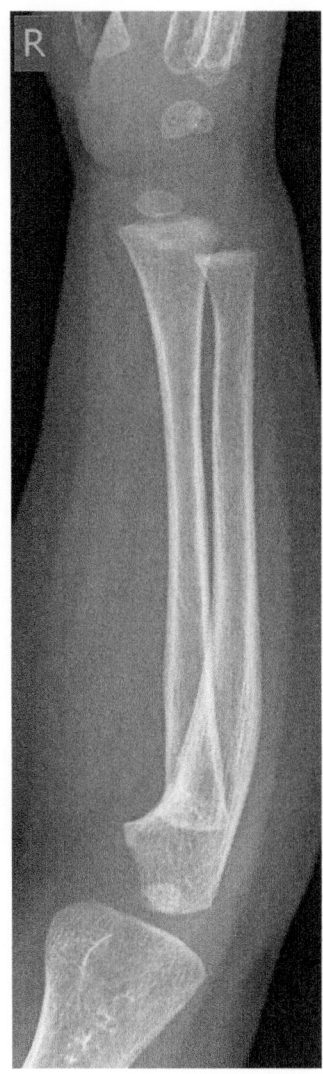

Normal	Abnormal	Diagnosis/Abnormality (only if abnormal)

Image 17

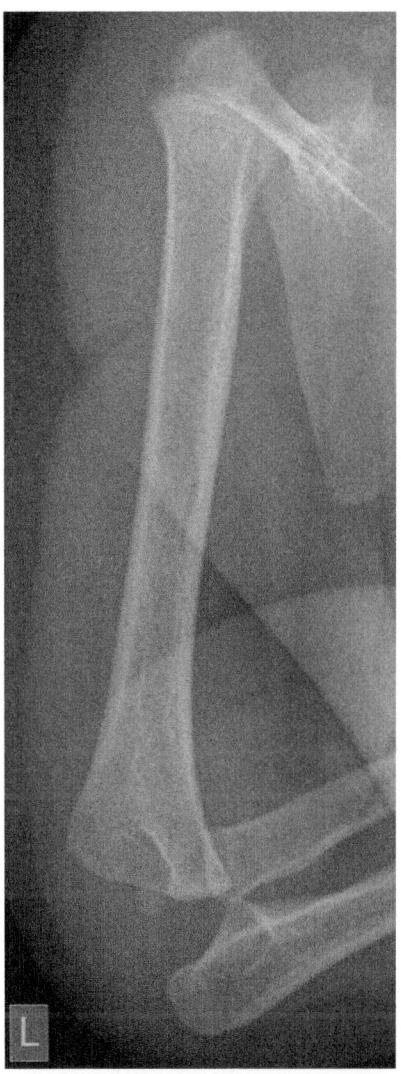

Normal	Abnormal	Diagnosis/Abnormality (only if abnormal)

Image 18

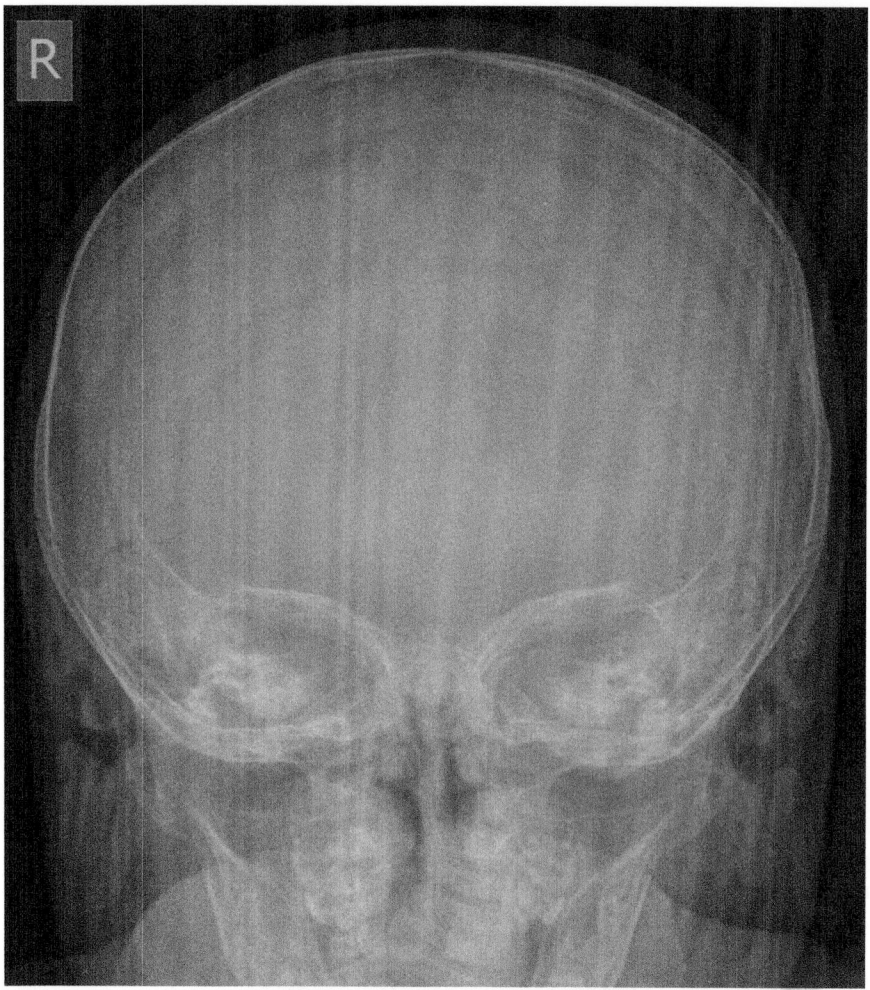

Normal	Abnormal	Diagnosis/Abnormality (only if abnormal)

Image 19

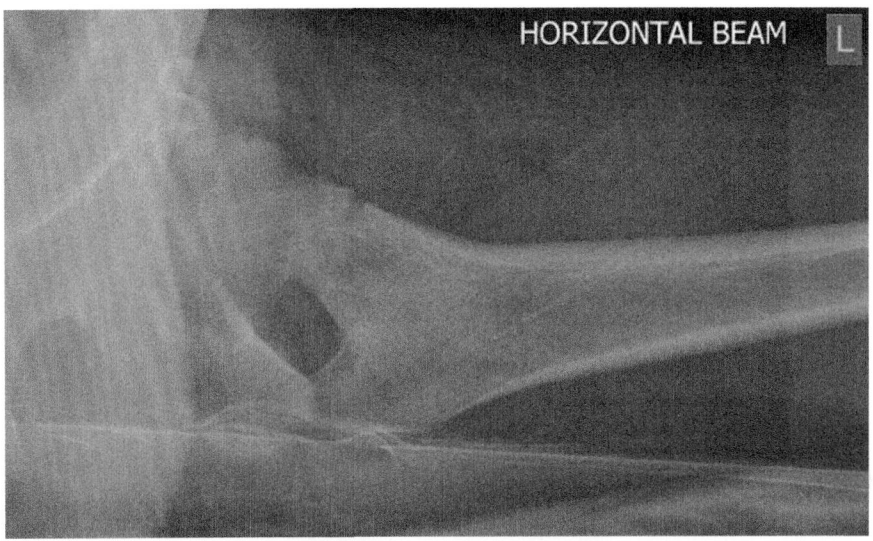

Normal	Abnormal	Diagnosis/Abnormality (only if abnormal)

Image 20

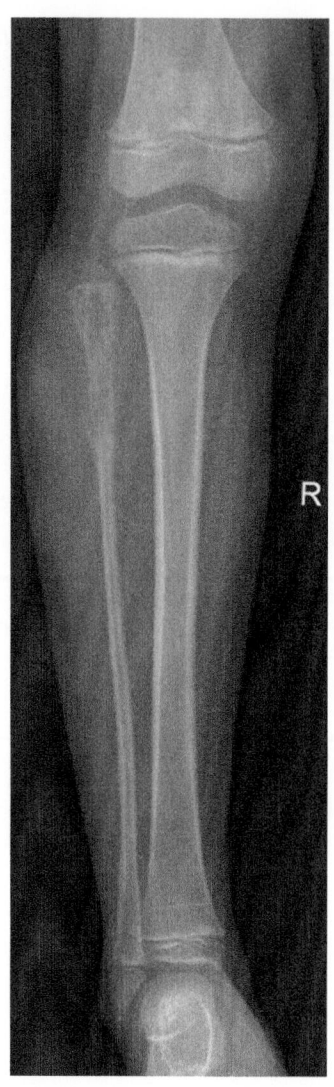

Normal	Abnormal	Diagnosis/Abnormality (only if abnormal)

Image 21

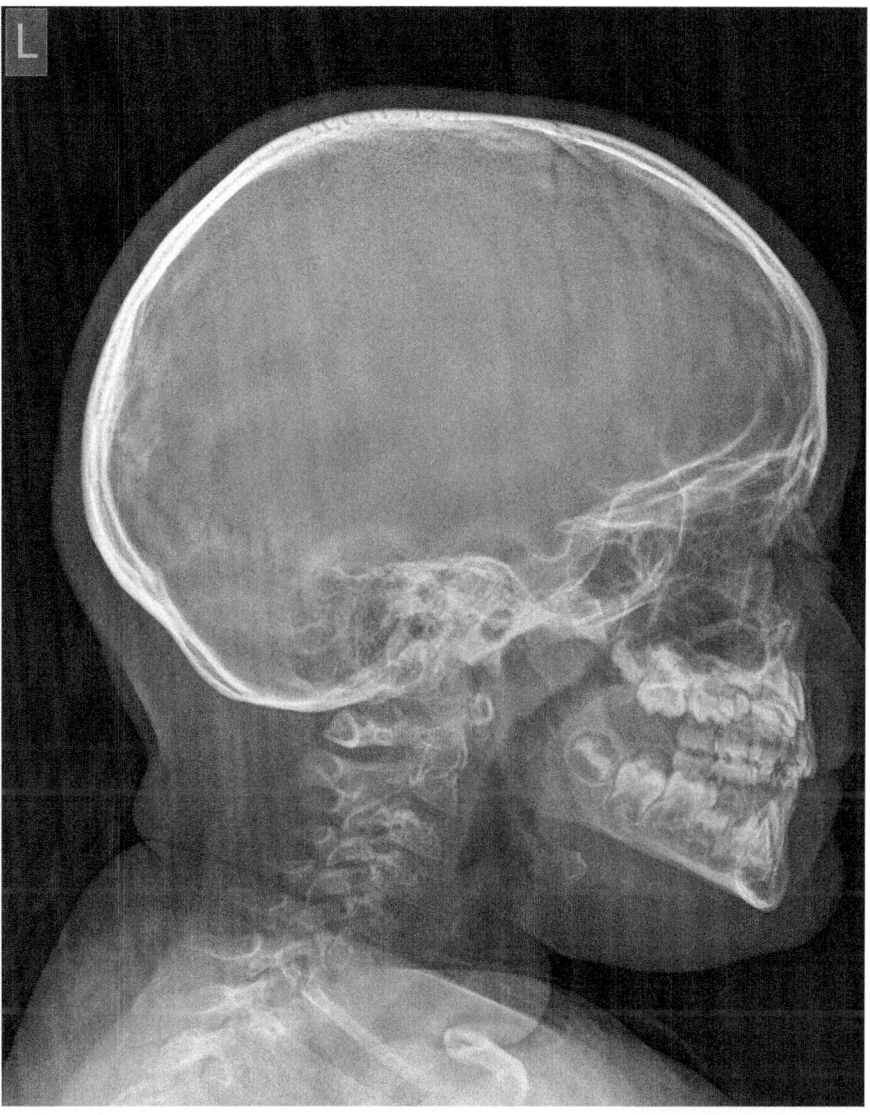

Normal	Abnormal	Diagnosis/Abnormality (only if abnormal)

Image 22

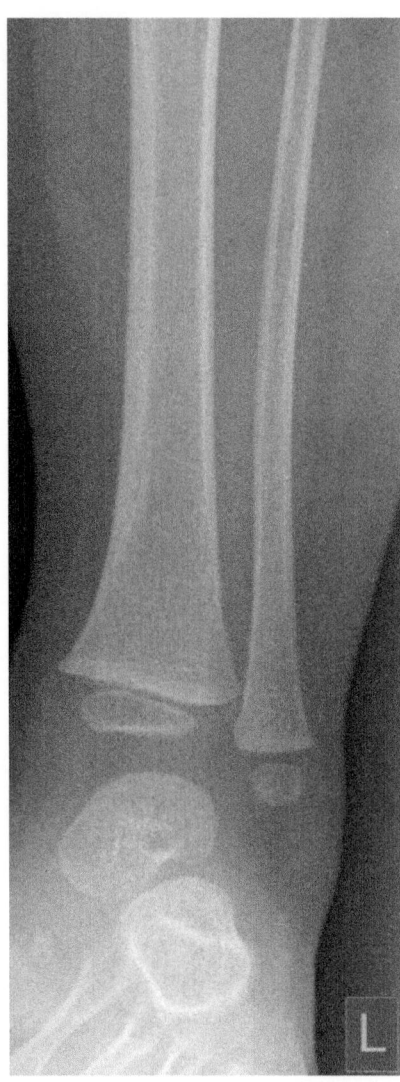

Normal	Abnormal	Diagnosis/Abnormality (only if abnormal)

Image 23

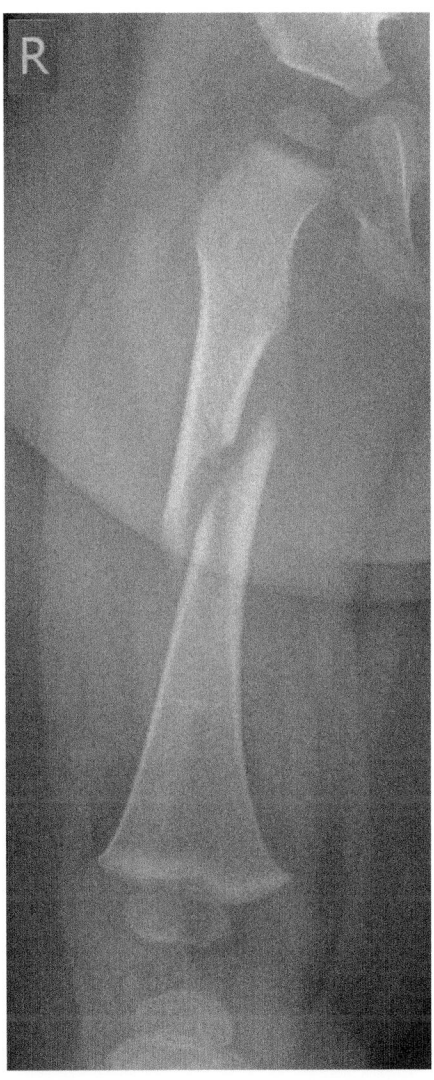

Normal	Abnormal	Diagnosis/Abnormality (only if abnormal)

Image 24

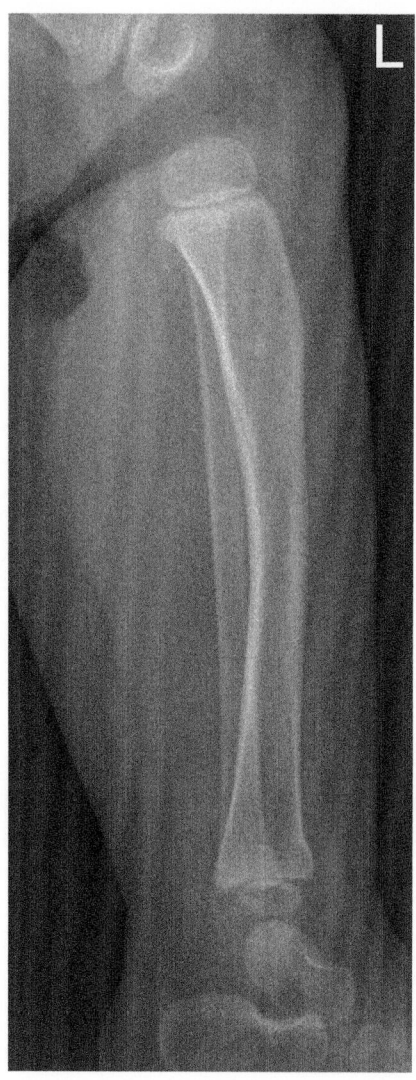

Normal	Abnormal	Diagnosis/Abnormality (only if abnormal)

Image 25

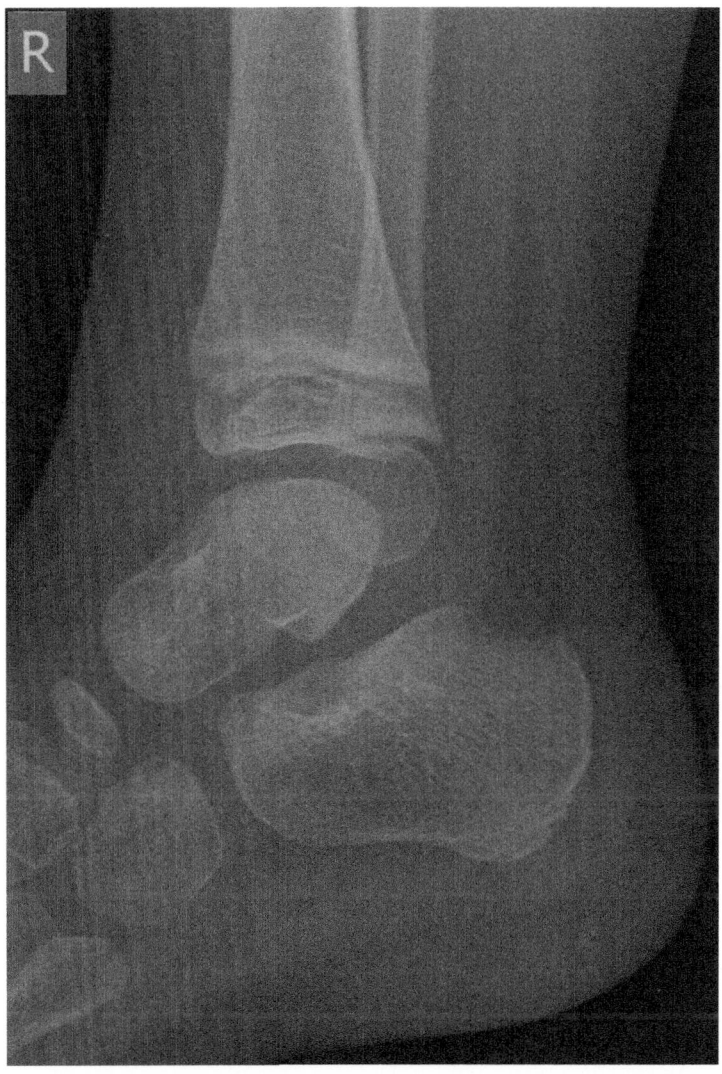

Normal	Abnormal	Diagnosis/Abnormality (only if abnormal)

Image 26

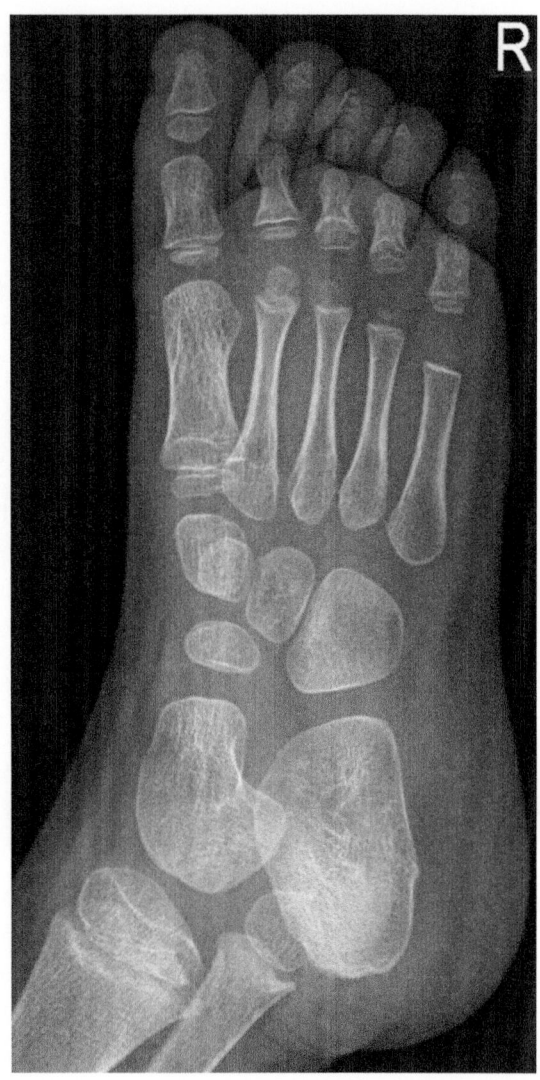

Normal	Abnormal	Diagnosis/Abnormality (only if abnormal)

Image 27

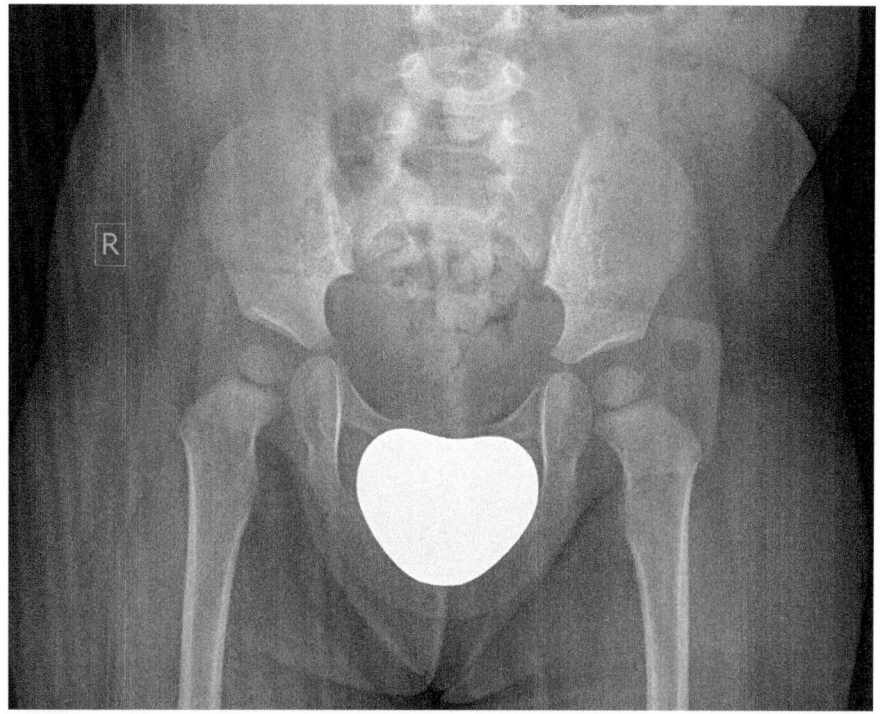

Normal	Abnormal	Diagnosis/Abnormality (only if abnormal)

Image 28

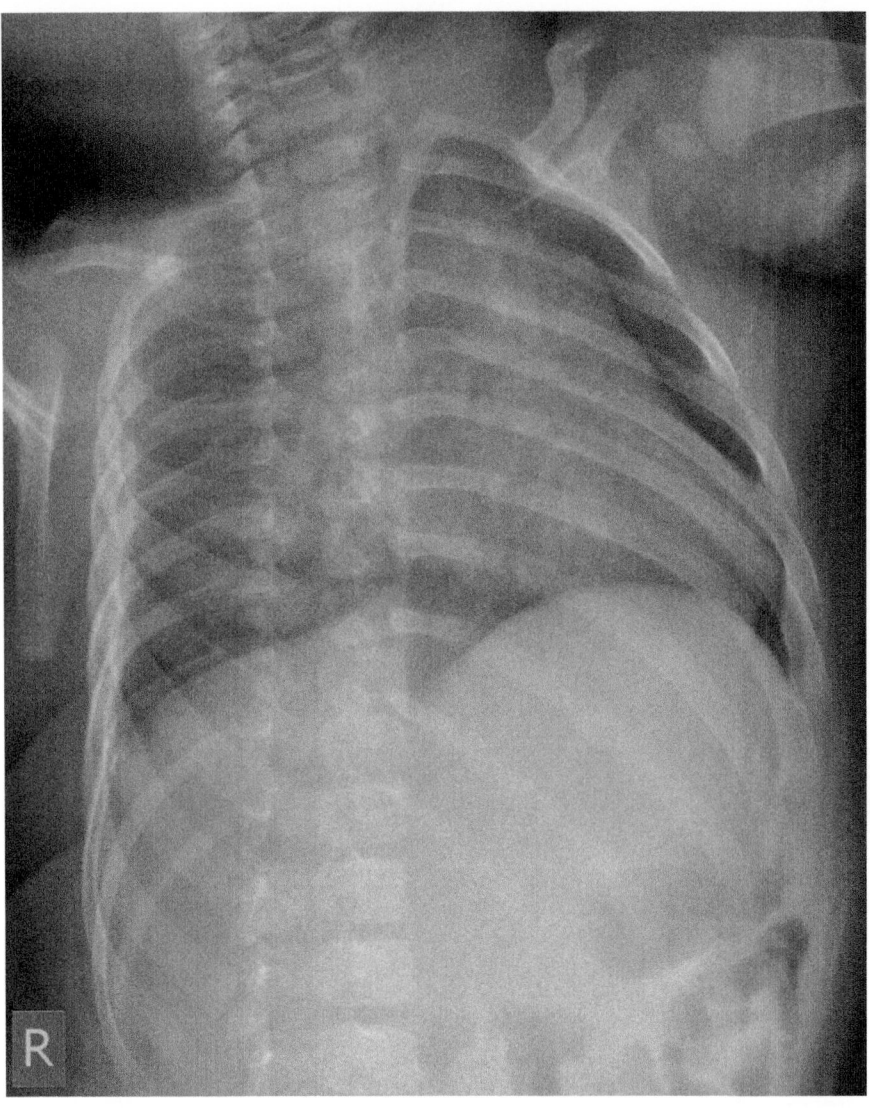

Normal	Abnormal	Diagnosis/Abnormality (only if abnormal)

Image 29

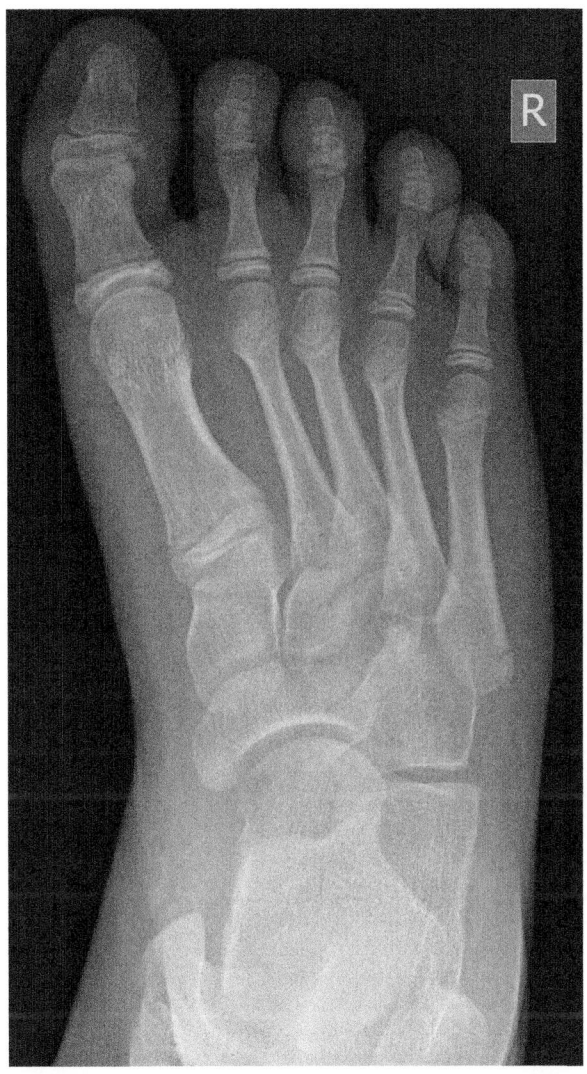

Normal	Abnormal	Diagnosis/Abnormality (only if abnormal)

Image 30

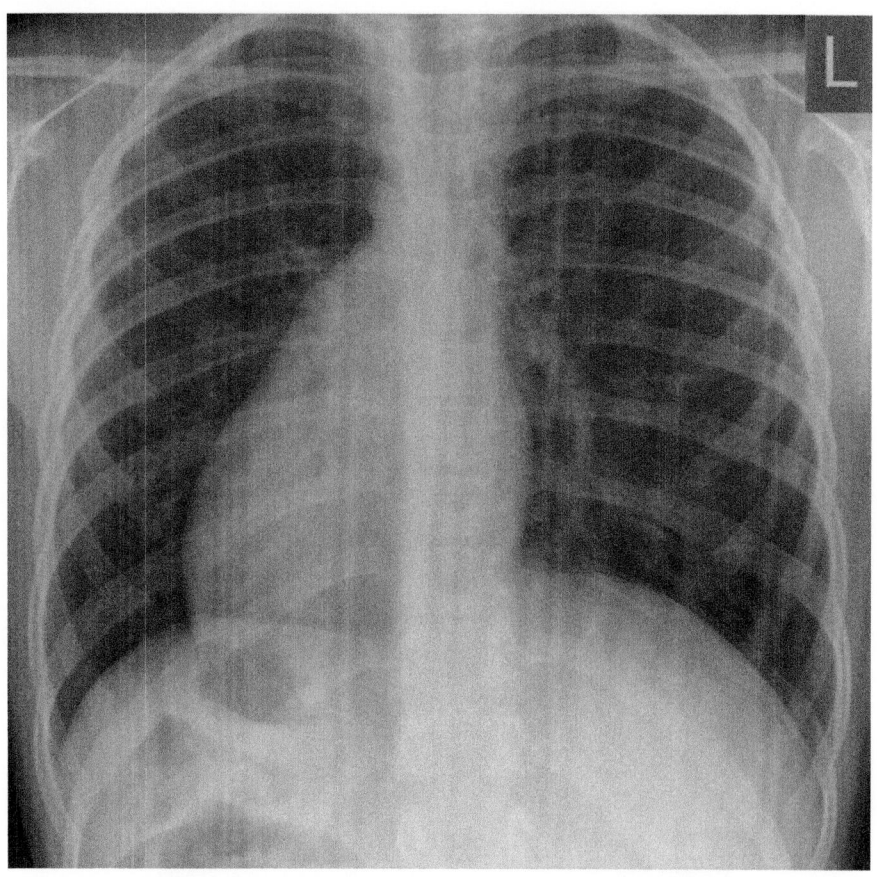

Normal	Abnormal	Diagnosis/Abnormality (only if abnormal)

3.2   Answers

Image	Normal	Abnormal	Diagnosis/abnormality (only if abnormal)
1	✓		
2		✓	Metaphyseal #s right distal tibial and fibula
3		✓	Avascular necrosis left proximal femoral epiphysis
4	✓		
5		✓	# left olecranon
6		✓	Multiple pulmonary nodules both lungs
7	✓		
8		✓	Increased prevertebral soft tissue
9		✓	Butterfly # left tibial diaphysis and buckle # left proximal fibula
10		✓	Fibrous dysplasia right humerus and proximal radius
11		✓	Buckle # left distal radius
12	✓		
13		✓	# base right fifth metatarsal
14		✓	Salter-Harris 2 # dorsal aspect right little finger middle phalanx
15		✓	Salter-Harris 2 # base right fifth toe proximal phalanx
16	✓		
17	✓		
18	✓		
19		✓	# left neck of femur
20		✓	Aggressive bone lesion right proximal fibula
21	✓		
22	✓		
23		✓	Spiral # right femoral diaphysis
24		✓	Volar buckle #s left distal tibia and fibula
25	✓		
26	✓		
27	✓		
28	✓		
29		✓	# base right fifth metatarsal
30		✓	Situs inversus

3.3   Explanations

2. **Metaphyseal #s right distal tibia and fibula**
   Along with posterior rib and complex skull fractures, metaphyseal fractures
   (also known as classic metaphyseal lesions—CMLs) are high specificity fractures for physical abuse in infants and young children. CMLs are rare in the
   context of 'normal handling' of an infant. In an otherwise normal child (i.e. no
   underlying bone dysplasia or metabolic disease) with an inappropriate history
   from the caregiver/parent, CMLs are considered to be pathognomonic for
   inflicted injury. They may be said to have a 'corner fracture' or 'bucket handle'
   configuration, describing the fracture appearance on tangential and angled radiographic projections, respectively.
   Children under the age of 1 year, and in particular less than 4 months, have the
   highest incidence of metaphyseal and abusive fractures. CMLs are less common
   in older, more ambulant children. In the presence of CMLs, there is a strong
   association with further abusive fractures identified on the skeletal survey which
   is why identification of these fractures is paramount. The distal femur, proximal
   and distal tibia, and proximal humeri are the commonest locations for metaphyseal fractures.
   It is important to remember that physical child abuse is insidious,
   transcends racial and socio-economic groups, can present at any time, and
   may do so in an unrelated context. As clinical radiologists, we *must* be vigilant of those radiographic findings that are highly specific for physical abuse
   in order that child protection measures can be initiated promptly. Discuss
   local pathways with your paediatric radiologists and safeguarding/child
   protection team.

3. **Avascular necrosis left proximal femoral epiphysis**
   See the explanation for Test 1, Image 1.

4. **# left olecranon**

5. **Multiple pulmonary nodules both lungs**
   These are multiple pulmonary metastases from a primary rhabdomyosarcoma in
   a 15-year-old male. In children, pulmonary metastases may arise from the fol-
   lowing non-exhaustive list of solid tumours (in order of frequency):
   • Osteosarcoma
   • Ewing's sarcoma
   • Wilms' tumour
   • Hepatoblastoma
   • Neuroblastoma
   • Rhabdomyosarcoma
   • Well-differentiated thyroid cancer
   • Non-rhabdomyosarcoma soft tissue sarcoma (NRSTS)
   • Adrenocortical carcinoma

In a child known to have one of these primary malignancies, the thorax should be evaluated for metastases. See the multiple nodules in the upper zone of the right lung magnified in the image below:

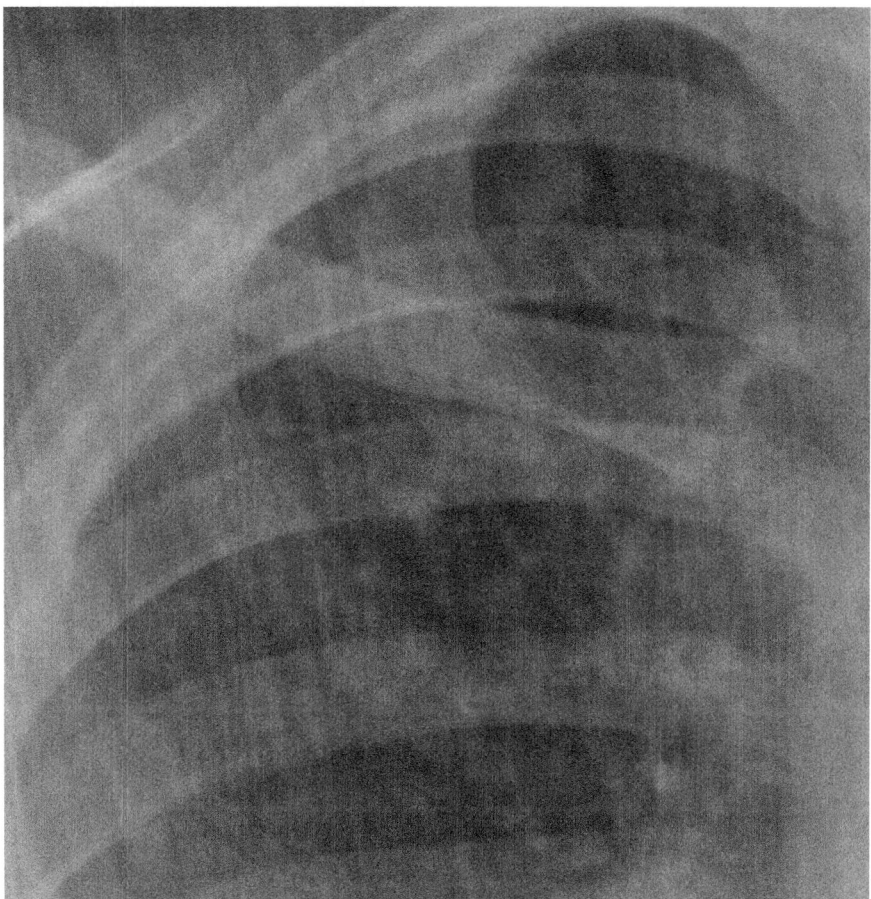

8. **Increased prevertebral soft tissue**

This radiograph is abnormal. There is increased prevertebral soft tissue anterior to the C2–C5 vertebral bodies resulting in loss of the normal cervical lordosis, and an almost kyphotic appearance at the C2/C3 and C3/C4 levels. Note also, the pseudosubluxation of C2 on C3 which refers to the anterior displacement of the C2 vertebral body with respect to the C3 vertebral body. This is a common *normal* finding in children less than 7 years of age due to ligamentous immaturity resulting in laxity.

The horizontal line through the vertebral body of C2 represents the synchondrosis between the ossification of the dens and the anterior body of C2—this is *not* a fracture. Remember that the C2 vertebral body is formed by the fusion of *four* separate ossification centres which is usually complete by the age of 12 years.

Alignment of the upper cervical spine should be assessed on every lateral cervical spine radiograph using Swischuk's line—this is a line connecting the anterior aspects of the posterior arches of C1 and C3. Assessment can be difficult in children where a true lateral projection may not always be obtained due to movement/patient distress, and obliquity can hinder/limit this assessment.

The anterior aspect of the posterior arch of C2 should be assessed with respect to Swischuk's line, and it should lie within 1–2 mm of this line:

- If there is deviation of more than 2 mm, a *true* subluxation is indicated.
- If the deviation is less than 2 mm, this is consistent with a pseudosubluxation; however, this is *not* sufficient to exclude a hangman's fracture—*bilateral pars interarticularis fractures of C2 from a hyperextension and distraction injury resulting in anterior spondylolisthesis.*

Thus, in the appropriate clinical context (i.e. traumatic injury), a CT of the cervical spine may be indicated—consult the National Institute for Health and Care Excellence (NICE) imaging algorithm for the 'Selection of children for imaging of the cervical spine' (Algorithm 4) in the references and maintain close liaison with ED colleagues in an acute setting.

Compare with Image 21 in this test and note the normal radiographic appearance of the paediatric cervical spine. Use Swischuk's line to assess the alignment on the magnified image in the corresponding explanation.

It is important to look for any gas in the increased prevertebral soft tissue which may indicate the presence of gas-forming organisms in a retropharyngeal abscess—as was confirmed on CT in this 3-year-old child and is present on the radiograph following scrutiny. Up to three-quarters of cases in children occur before the age of 5 years. Occasionally, retropharyngeal abscesses may result from foreign body ingestion, an important point to remember when discussing cases with clinical colleagues, as children (being children) may ingest all manner of objects without their parents or caregivers knowledge!

CT better evaluates the extent and nature of any abscess, confirms the retropharyngeal location, and assesses for evidence of mediastinal extension/mediastinitis, in addition to differentiating from retropharyngeal cellulitis. Compression or narrowing of the airway is also better assessed on CT which is an important anaesthetic consideration prior to any planned surgical intervention, if indicated.

Tip for the viva:
Consider the following points:

- Infection: the abscess may lie in the prevertebral space, *not* the retropharyngeal space, which may then extend into the epidural space and result in discitis/osteomyelitis.
- Grisel syndrome: atlanto-axial subluxation from inflammatory ligamentous laxity secondary to a retropharyngeal abscess causing torticollis. Whilst this is a rare cause of torticollis in infants and young children, knowledge of this

condition is imperative given that affected patients are often not able to verbalise their symptoms.

- Lemierre syndrome: internal jugular vein thrombophlebitis and/or thrombosis in the setting of oropharyngeal infection, i.e. retropharyngeal abscess.

9. **Butterfly # left tibial diaphysis and buckle # left proximal fibula**
Butterfly fracture fragments are commonly seen in comminuted long bone fractures. These result from the intersection of two oblique fracture lines between the proximal and distal fragments creating large, triangular fragments resembling a butterfly.

Did you also spot the proximal fibular fracture? You must carefully trace the outline of every bone; doing so reveals the posterior cortical proximal fibular fracture, seen in the magnified image below:

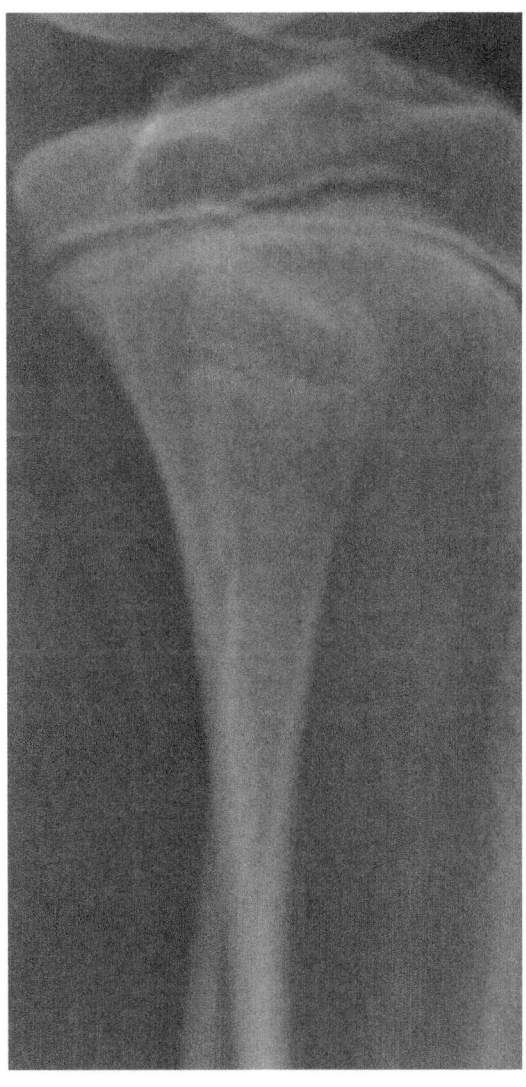

10. **Fibrous dysplasia right humerus and proximal radius**

The radiographic findings include well-circumscribed lucent lesions with an internal ground-glass matrix surrounded by reactive sclerosis/cortical thickening, known as the 'rind sign'. Note also the endosteal scalloping (thinning of the inner cortex by the lesions). Both sides of the joint are affected, as is typical for fibrous dysplasia, and more than one bone is affected—note the involvement of the proximal radius, making the involvement polyostotic. This child has McCune-Albright syndrome, the triad of:

- Polyostotic fibrous dysplasia
- Endocrinopathy (precocious puberty)
- The characteristic *café au lait* cutaneous pigmentation in the shape of the coast of Maine

Tip for the viva:
- If a lucent bone lesion has been identified in the context of pain, it is important to look carefully for a pathological fracture as these may be subtle.

11. **Buckle # left distal radius**

13. **# base right fifth metatarsal**

See explanation for Test 1, Image 7.

14. **Salter-Harris 2 # dorsal aspect right little finger middle phalanx**

15. **Salter-Harris 2 # base right fifth toe proximal phalanx**

This is better visualised on the magnified image below:

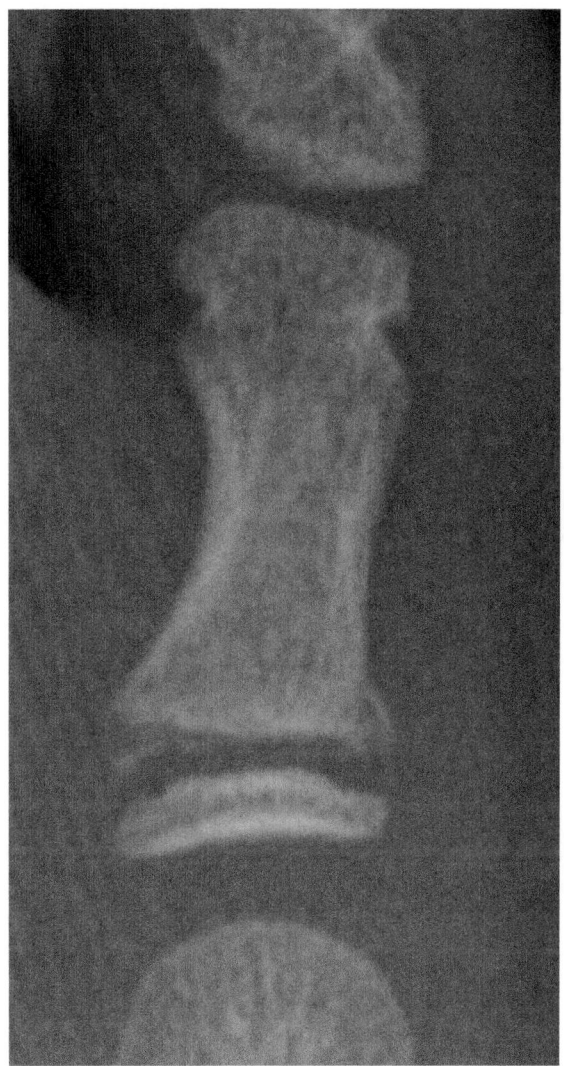

19. **# left neck of femur**

Neck of femur fractures in children are rare and account for less than 1% of all paediatric fractures. These fractures typically result from a high energy impact such as a fall from a height or a RTA. This 13-year-old girl presented to ED with severe left hip pain and decreased range of movement after a fall on ice.

20. **Aggressive bone lesion right proximal fibula**

There is a moth-eaten, destructive, permeative appearance of the right proximal fibular metadiaphysis with a soft tissue component but *without* an osteoid matrix (cf. the tumour matrix calcification seen with osteosarcomas which may be ill-defined and 'cloud-like'). Radiographic findings are consistent with Ewing's sarcoma, diagnosed in this 5-year-old boy presenting with leg pain. Note the associated Codman's triangle periosteal reaction, indicative of an aggressive bone lesion—the periosteum does not have time to ossify given the aggressiveness of the lesion so only the edge of the raised periosteum will ossify. Multilamellated or 'onion skin' type periosteal reaction is typically encountered also although not present in this case.

Following osteosarcoma, Ewing's sarcoma is the second most common primary malignant osseous tumour of childhood and arises from the medullary cavity. There is a slight male predilection with lesions involving the:

- Long bones: the majority of cases, approximately 60%, typically affect the metadiaphysis followed by mid-diaphyseal lesions of the femur, tibia, and humerus.
- Flat bones: the pelvis; scapula; and ribs (with regard to the latter two locations, consider Ewing's sarcoma of the chest wall—formally known as Askin tumour, it is a peripheral primitive neuroectodermal tumour [pPNET] and belongs to the Ewing's sarcoma family of tumours).

Prognosis is significantly impacted by the presence of distant metastases at the time of diagnosis and which can be bony (pelvis, extremities) and/or pulmonary. Imaging evaluation is similar to that for osteosarcoma and typically involves: MRI of the affected limb/area, technetium-99 bone scintigraphy and CT thorax. Positron emission tomography-computed tomography (PET-CT) may also be employed depending on patient age and clinical circumstances to assess extent of tumour and presence of metastases. Systemic chemotherapy is the mainstay of treatment with surgery and consideration of adjuvant radiotherapy depending on the location and size of the primary tumour.

21. **Normal paediatric skull radiograph.**

Compare with Image 8 from this test. Note the subtle anterior displacement of the C2 vertebral body with respect to C3 consistent with pseudosubluxation, a normal finding as described above. Use Swischuk's line to assess the alignment of the upper cervical spine in the magnified image below:

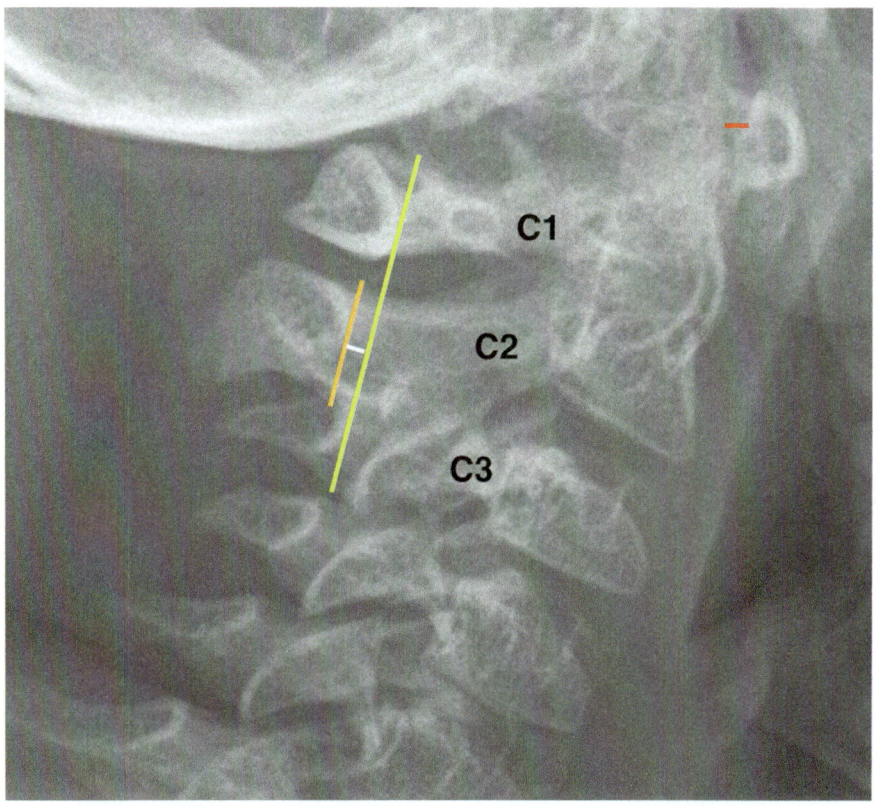

Yellow line—this is Swischuk's line, the line connecting the anterior aspects of the posterior arches of C1 and C3.

Orange line—the anterior aspect of the posterior arch of C2.

White line—the distance between the yellow and orange lines which should normally be 1–2 mm, as on this radiograph. If there is deviation of more than 2 mm, a true subluxation is indicated.

Red line—this corresponds to the atlanto-dental interval and is the horizontal distance between the posterior cortex of the anterior arch of C1 (the atlas) and the anterior cortex of the dens (peg) of C2 (the axis). This value should be less than 5 mm in children: this is greater than the 3 mm limit in adults due to ligamentous laxity in children.

These lines and distances should be assessed on every paediatric lateral cervical spine radiograph, particularly in the context of trauma.

23. **Spiral # right femoral diaphysis**

When considering femoral fractures in infants and young children, one *must* consider the age and developmental status of the child. Broadly, infants can be divided into whether they are ambulant or pre-ambulant, and specifically whether they are able to pull themselves up, cruise, stand or toddle, unaided or with support.

Any fracture in a pre-ambulant infant without an appropriate history is suspicious. In particular, the spiral fracture is the commonest abusive femoral fracture implying a significant torsional force which is uncommon unless inflicted. This 10-month-old female was presented to the Emergency Department after being unsettled since rolling off the bed and landing on the floor; examination revealed right thigh swelling with crepitus. Following this radiograph, she was investigated with an initial and follow-up skeletal survey, and CT of the head as per the RCR national guidance on the radiological investigation of suspected physical abuse in children.

24. **Volar buckle #s left distal tibia and fibula**

The fractures are visualised in the magnified image below:

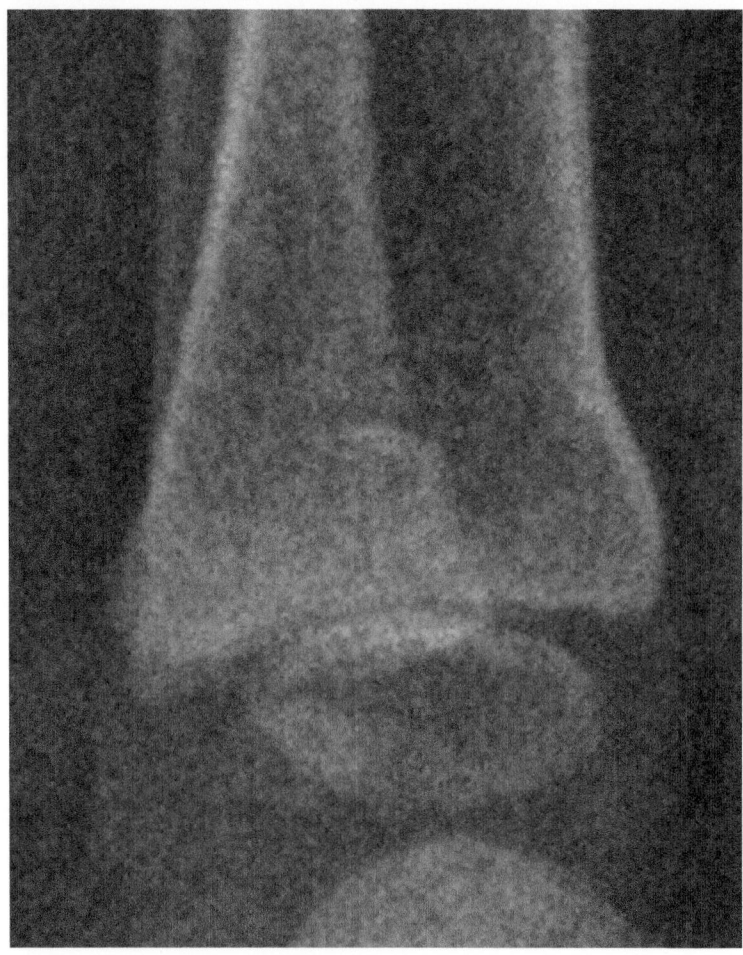

28. **Normal sternal ossification centres**

This radiograph is normal. It is important that the sternal ossification centres (also known as sternal segments or sternebrae) are not mistaken for healing rib fractures on oblique chest projections. Occasionally, these segments can line up perfectly along the ribs simulating callus from healing rib fractures but in fact represent *normal* sternal ossification. See the magnified image below—we have included an asterisk on each of the sternal ossification centres:

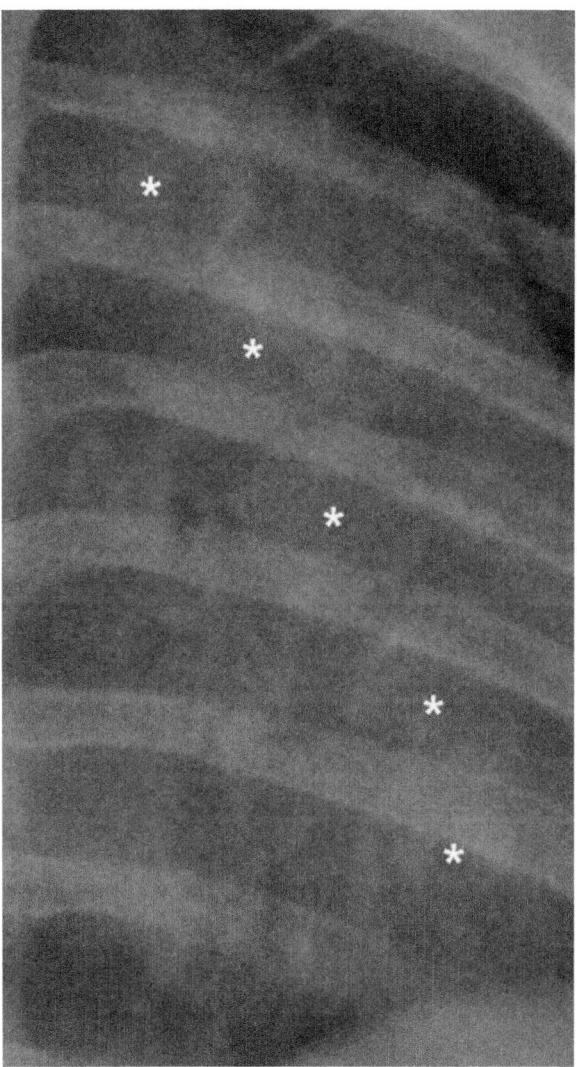

Overcalling these segments as healing fractures can have a significant impact on management, not only for the child but for the family, which is why we have included this radiograph to emphasise the recognition of this normal finding.

Tip for the viva:
- Remember to look at the anteroposterior and contralateral oblique chest projections to confirm/exclude healing rib fractures.

29. **# base right fifth metatarsal**

30. **Situs inversus**

This is situs inversus and *not* dextrocardia because of the positions of the cardiac apex, the aortic knuckle, *and* the stomach bubble which lies under the right hemidiaphragm. Dextrocardia may exist in isolation, i.e. not in the context of situs inversus, in which case the stomach bubble will lie under the left hemidiaphragm.

Up to 20% of patients with situs inversus may have Kartagener syndrome, a primary ciliary dyskinesia, which comprises of the following triad:
- Situs inversus
- Chronic sinusitis/nasal polyposis
- Bronchiectasis

Males with Kartagener syndrome may experience subfertility and females have an increased rate of ectopic pregnancy because of the underlying ciliopathy which affects the fallopian tubes.

Further Reading

Image 2

Dwek JR (2011) The radiographic approach to child abuse. Clin Orthop Relat Res 469(3):776–789
Lonergan GJ, Baker AM, Morey MK et al (2003) From the archives of the AFIP. Child abuse: radiologic-pathologic correlation. Radiographics 23(4):811–845

Image 6

Davidoff AM, Heaton TE (2016) Surgical treatment of metastases in pediatric solid tumors. Semin Pediatr Surg 25(5):311–317

Image 8

Craig FW, Schunk JE (2003) Retropharyngeal abscess in children: clinical presentation, utility of imaging, and current management. Pediatrics 111(6):1394–1398
Gaillard F et al (2018) Lemierre syndrome. https://radiopaedia.org/articles/lemierre-syndrome. Accessed April 2018
Knipe H, Babu AS et al (2018) Grisel syndrome. https://radiopaedia.org/articles/grisel-syndrome-2. Accessed April 2018
Knipe H, Hacking C et al (2018) Pseudosubluxation of the cervical spine. https://radiopaedia.org/articles/pseudosubluxation-of-the-cervical-spine. Accessed April 2018
National Institute for Health and Care Excellence (2014) 'Head injury', NICE clinical guideline 176. National Clinical Guideline Centre, London. https://www.nice.org.uk/guidance/cg176. Algorithm 4: selection of children from imaging of the cervical spine. https://www.nice.org.uk/guidance/cg176/resources/imaging-algorithm-pdf-498950893. Accessed April 2018
O'Brien TW Sr, Shen P, Lee P (2015) The dens: normal development, developmental variants and anomalies, and traumatic injuries. J Clin Imaging Sci 30(5):38
St-Amant M, Gaillard F et al (2018) Hangman fracture. https://radiopaedia.org/articles/hangman-fracture. Accessed April 2018
Swischuk LE (1977) Anterior displacement of C2 in children: physiologic or pathologic. Radiology 122(3):759–763

Image 10

Fitzpatrick KA, Taljanovic MS, Speer DP et al (2004) Imaging findings of fibrous dysplasia with histopathologic and intraoperative correlation. AJR Am J Roentgenol 182(6):1389–1398
Knipe H, Gaillard F et al (2018) McCune-Albright syndrome. https://radiopaedia.org/articles/mccune-albright-syndrome. Accessed April 2018
Yongjing G, Huawei L, Zilai P et al (2001) McCune-Albright syndrome: radiological and MR findings. JBR-BTR 84(6):250–252

Image 19

Al Khatib N, Younis MH, Hegazy A et al (2018) Early versus late treatment of paediatric femoral neck fractures: a systematic review and meta-analysis. Int Orthop 2018. https://doi.org/10.1007/s00264-018-3998-4 [Epub ahead of print]

Image 20

Di Muzio D, Weerakkody Y (2018) Askin tumour. https://radiopaedia.org/articles/askin-tumour-1. Accessed July 2018

Sharma R, Gaillard F et al (2018) Ewing sarcoma. https://radiopaedia.org/articles/ewing-sarcoma. Accessed April 2018

Tatco V, Amini B et al (2018) Codman triangle periosteal reaction. https://radiopaedia.org/articles/codman-triangle-periosteal-reaction. Accessed April 2018

Image 21

Knipe H, Hacking C et al (2018) Pseudosubluxation of the cervical spine. https://radiopaedia.org/articles/pseudosubluxation-of-the-cervical-spine. Accessed April 2018

Swischuk LE (1977) Anterior displacement of C2 in children: physiologic or pathologic. Radiology 122(3):759–763

Image 23

Hui C, Joughin E, Goldstein S et al (2008) Femoral fractures in children younger than three years: the role of nonaccidental injury. J Pediatr Orthop 28:297e302

Kemp AM, Dunstan F, Harrison S et al (2008) Patterns of skeletal fractures in child abuse: systematic review. BMJ 337:a1518

Paddock M, Sprigg A, Offiah AC (2017) Re: Imaging and reporting considerations for suspected physical abuse (non-accidental injury) in infants and young children. Part 1: initial considerations and appendicular skeleton. A reply. Clin Radiol 72(5):422

Image 28

McAloon J, O'Neill C (2011) Ossification centres, not rib fractures. Arch Dis Child 96(3):284

Image 30

Berdon WE, Willi U (2004) Situs inversus, bronchiectasis, and sinusitis and its relation to immotile cilia: history of the diseases and their discoverers-Manes Kartagener and Bjorn Afzelius. Pediatr Radiol 34(1):38–42

Knipe H, Wahba M et al (2018) Kartagener syndrome. https://radiopaedia.org/articles/kartagener-syndrome-1. Accessed April 2018

Test 4

4.1   Images

Image 1

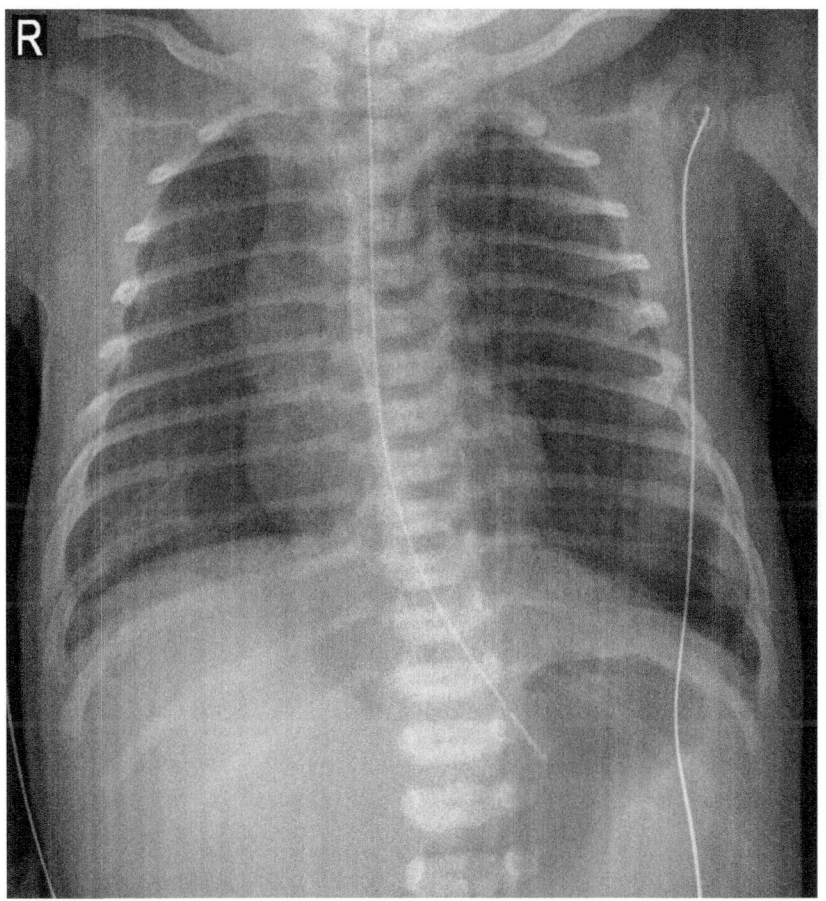

Normal	Abnormal	Diagnosis/Abnormality (only if abnormal)

M. Paddock, A. C. Offiah, *Paediatric Radiology Rapid Reporting for FRCR Part 2B*,
https://doi.org/10.1007/978-3-030-01965-5_4

Image 2

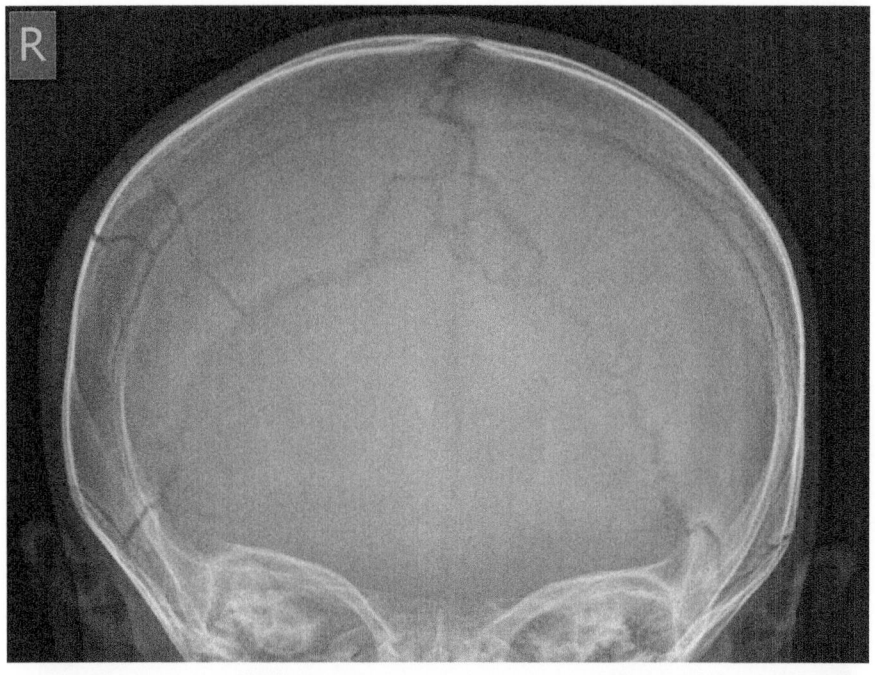

Normal	Abnormal	Diagnosis/Abnormality (only if abnormal)

Image 3

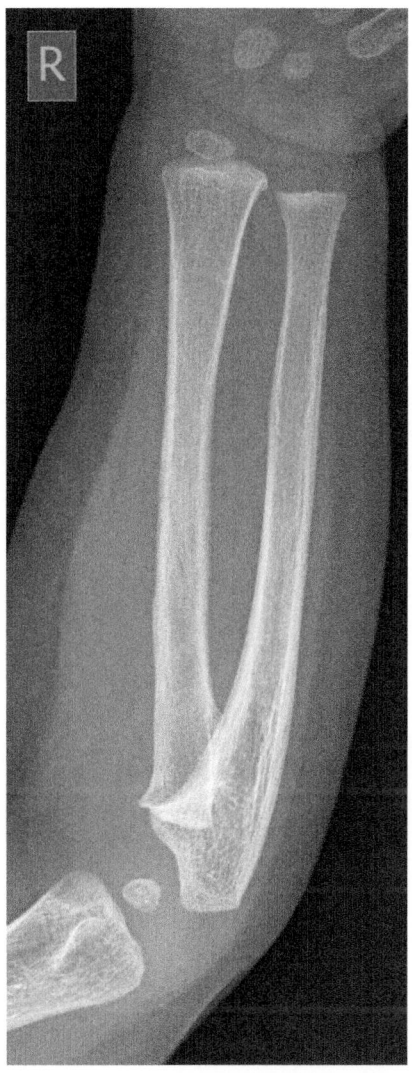

Normal	Abnormal	Diagnosis/Abnormality (only if abnormal)

Image 4

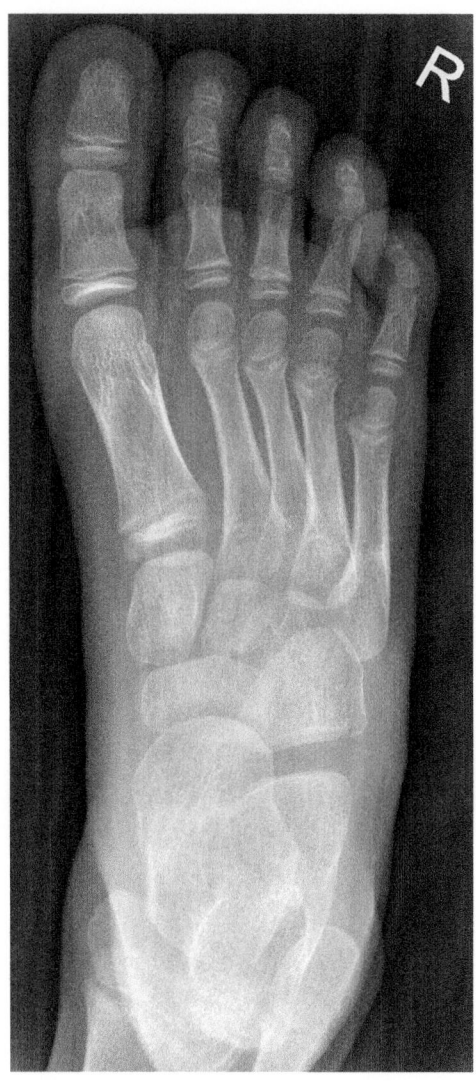

Normal	Abnormal	Diagnosis/Abnormality (only if abnormal)

Image 5

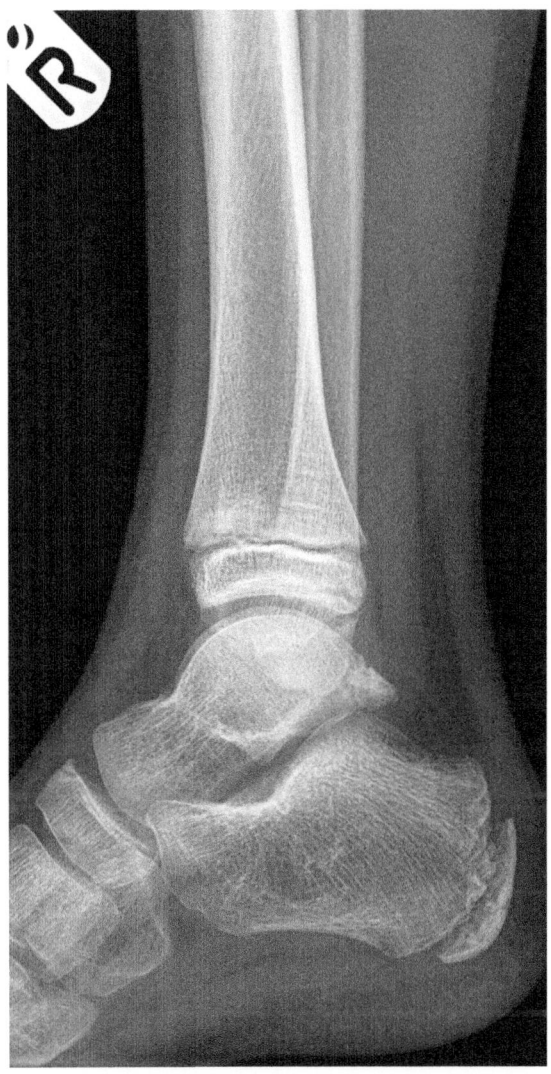

Normal	Abnormal	Diagnosis/Abnormality (only if abnormal)

Image 6

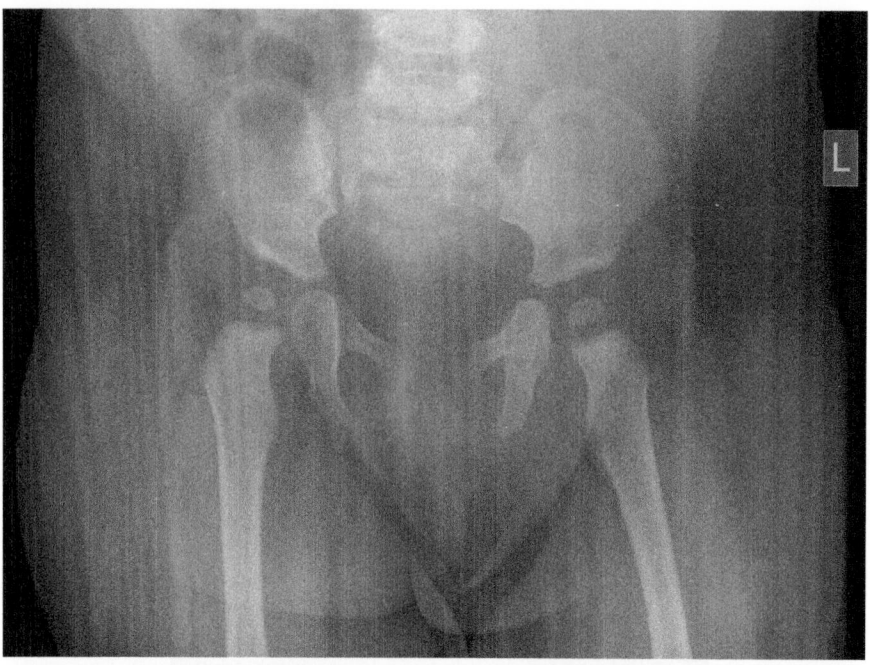

Normal	Abnormal	Diagnosis/Abnormality (only if abnormal)

Image 7

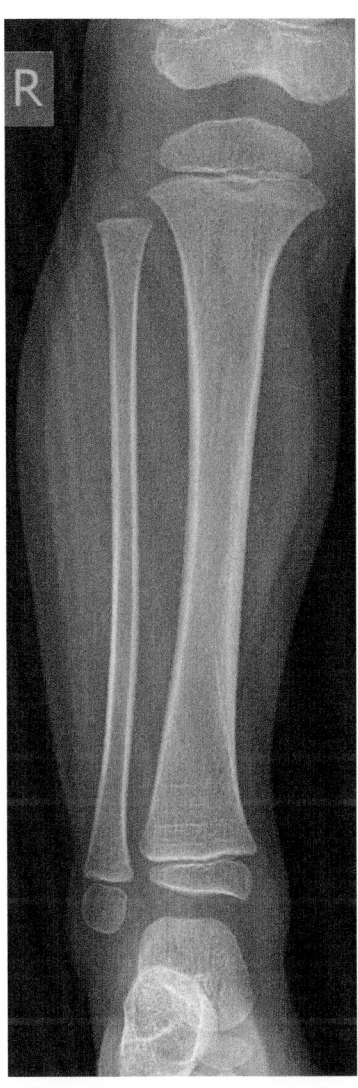

Normal	Abnormal	Diagnosis/Abnormality (only if abnormal)

Image 8

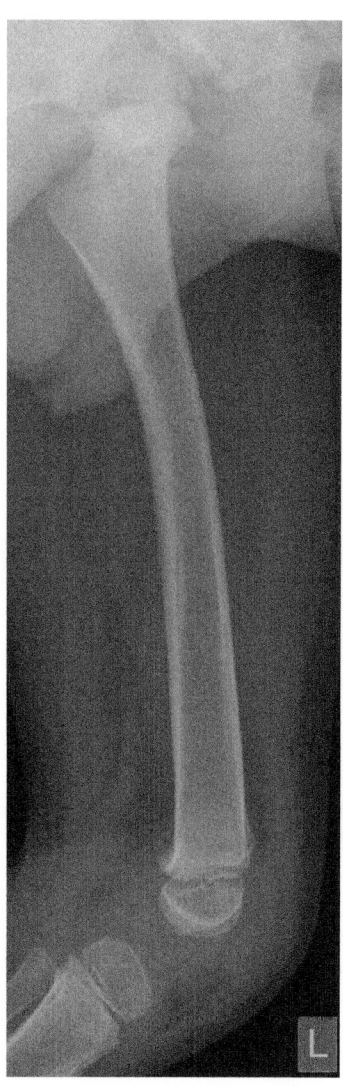

Normal	Abnormal	Diagnosis/Abnormality (only if abnormal)

Image 9

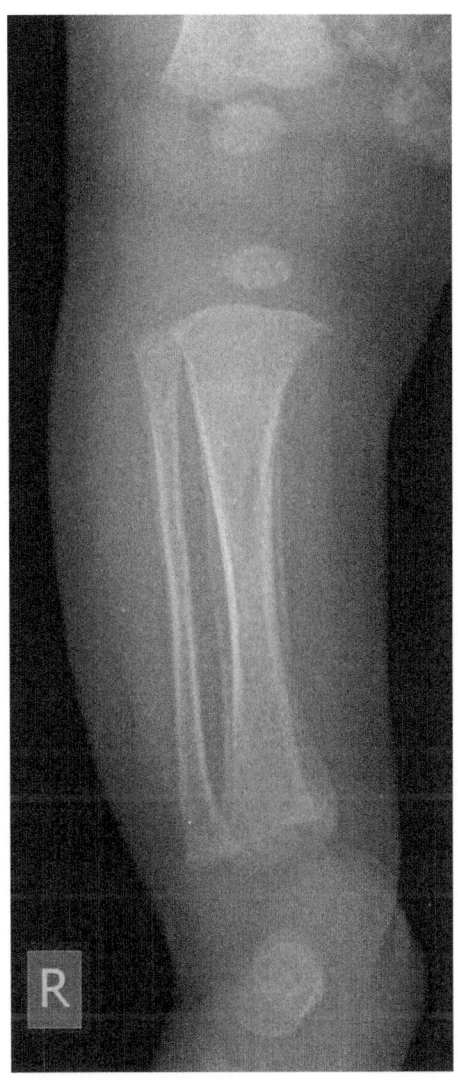

Normal	Abnormal	Diagnosis/Abnormality (only if abnormal)

Image 10

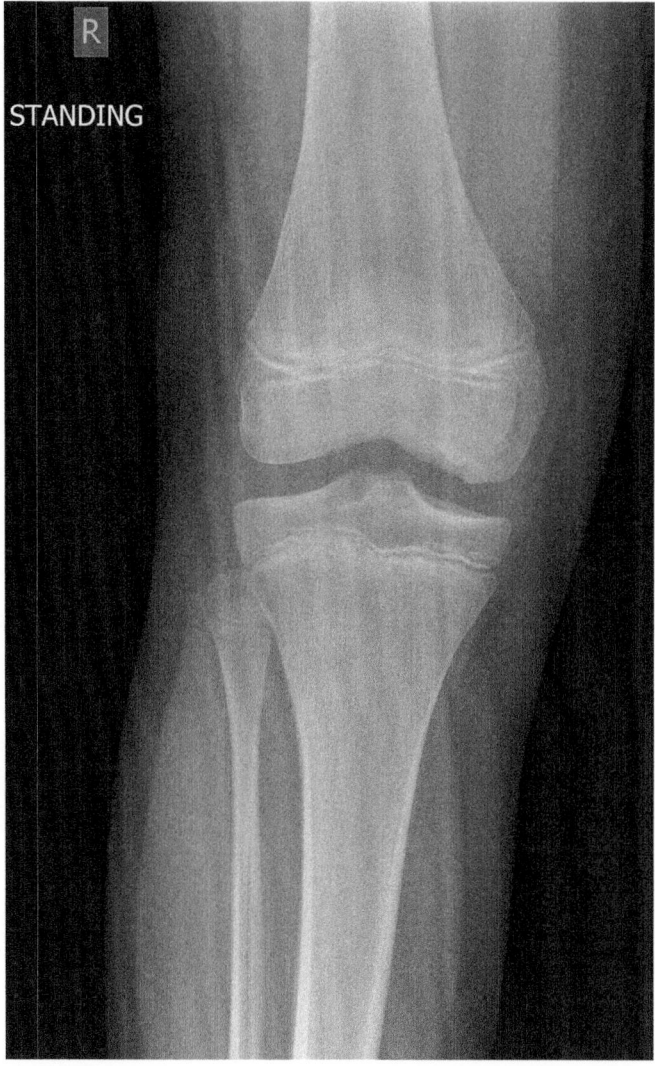

Normal	Abnormal	Diagnosis/Abnormality (only if abnormal)

Image 11

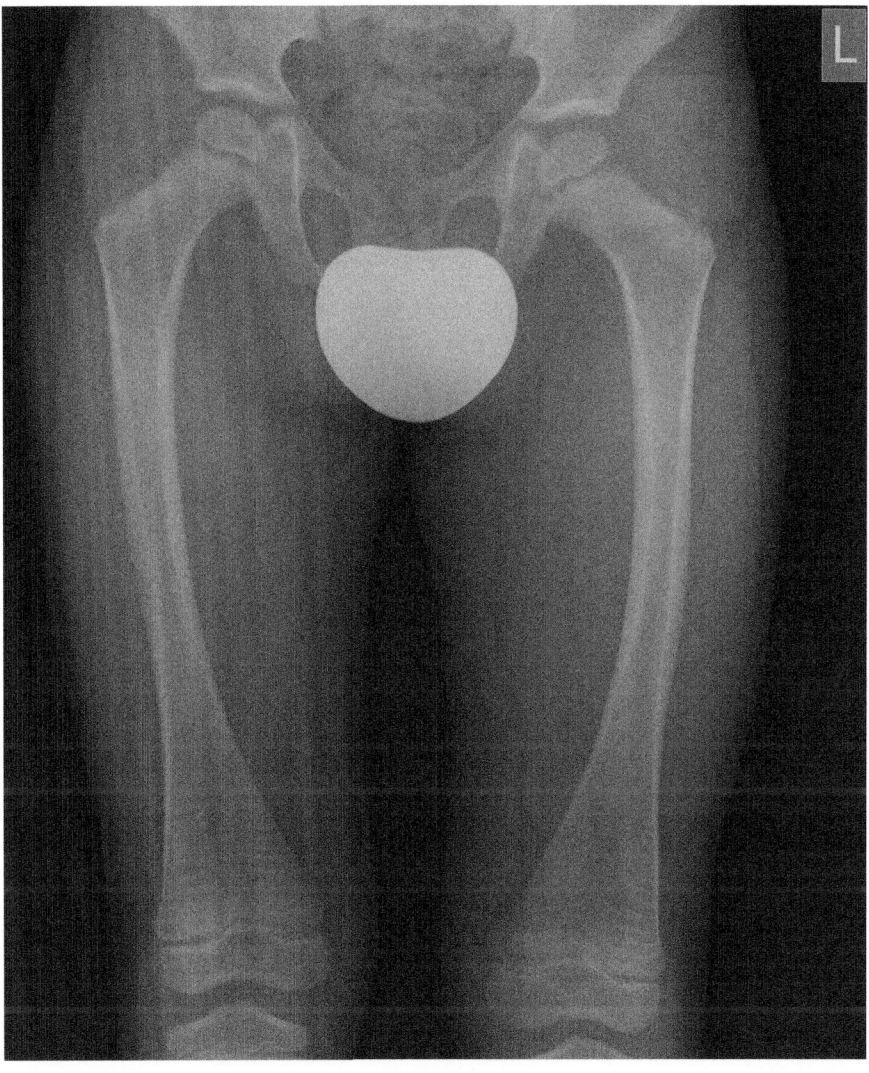

Normal	Abnormal	Diagnosis/Abnormality (only if abnormal)

Image 12

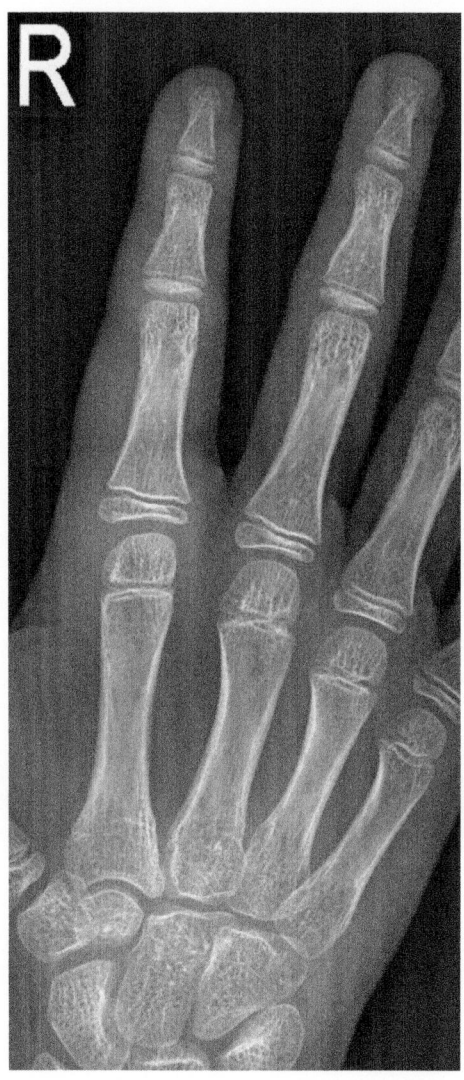

Normal	Abnormal	Diagnosis/Abnormality (only if abnormal)

Image 13

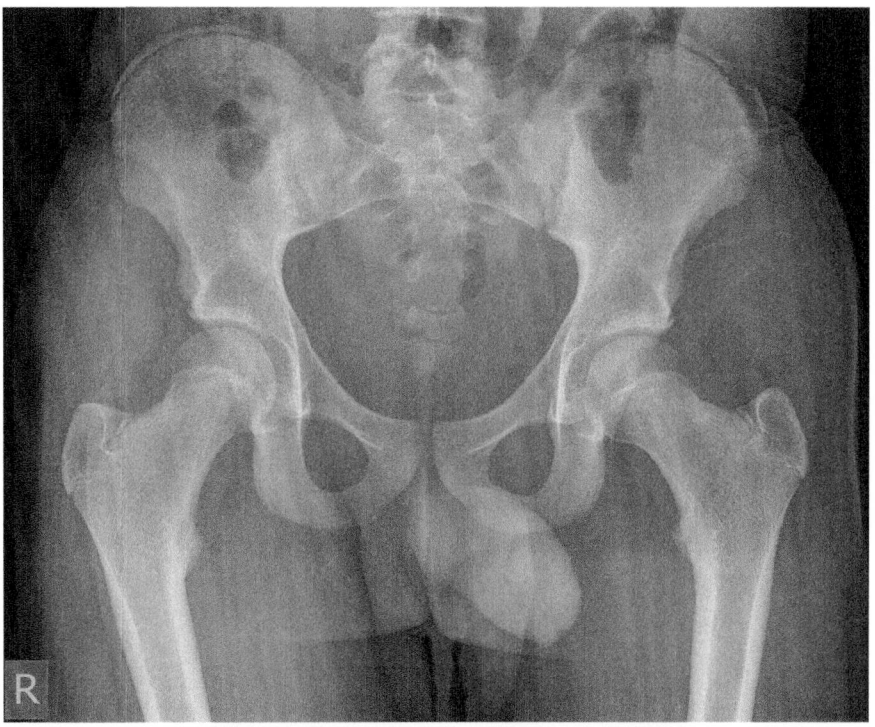

Normal	Abnormal	Diagnosis/Abnormality (only if abnormal)

Image 14

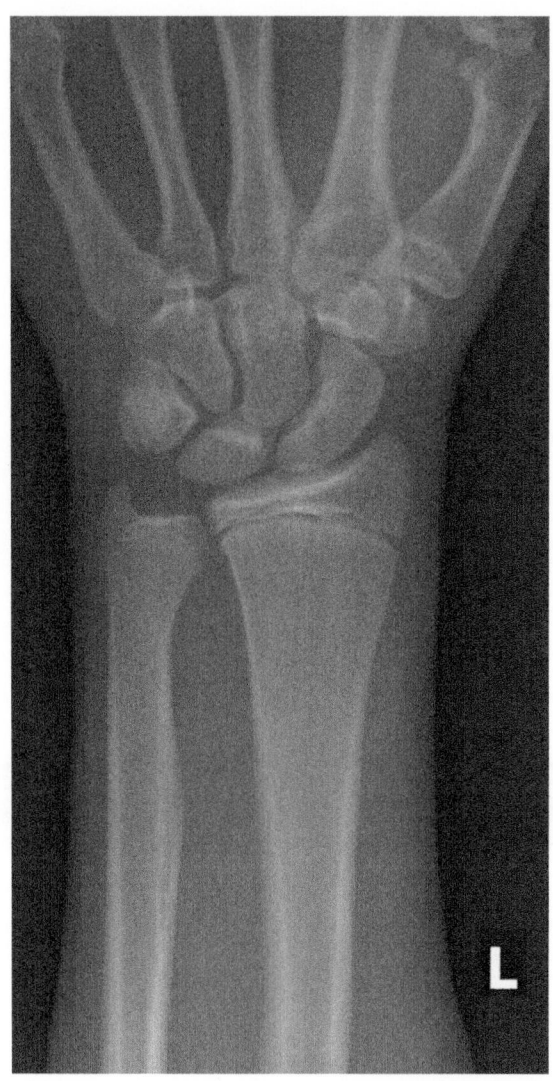

Normal	Abnormal	Diagnosis/Abnormality (only if abnormal)

Image 15

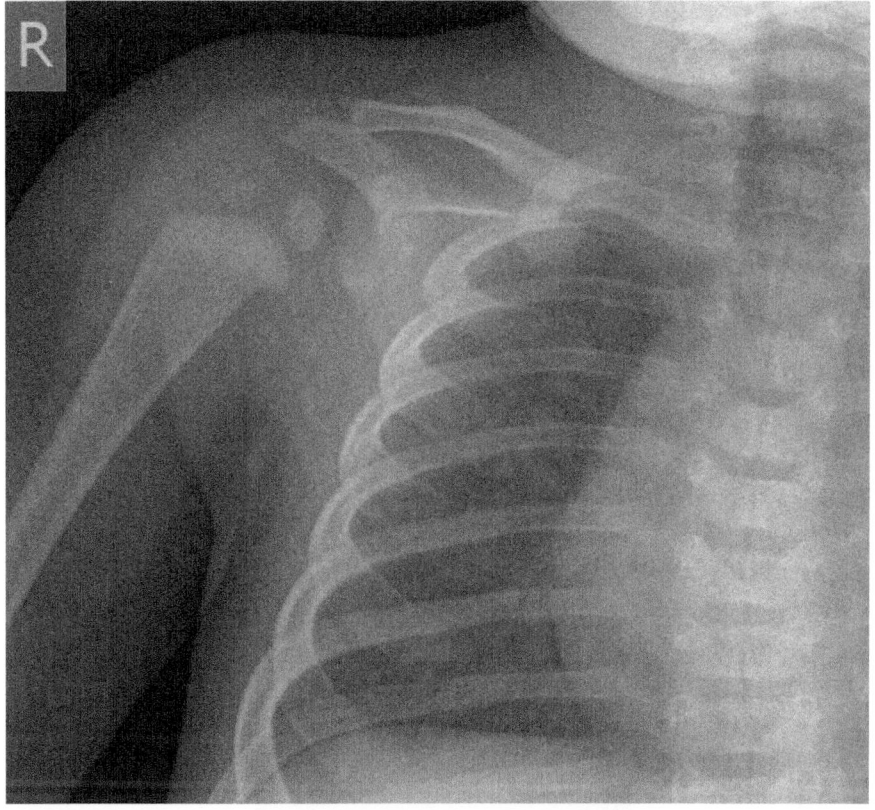

Normal	Abnormal	Diagnosis/Abnormality (only if abnormal)

Image 16

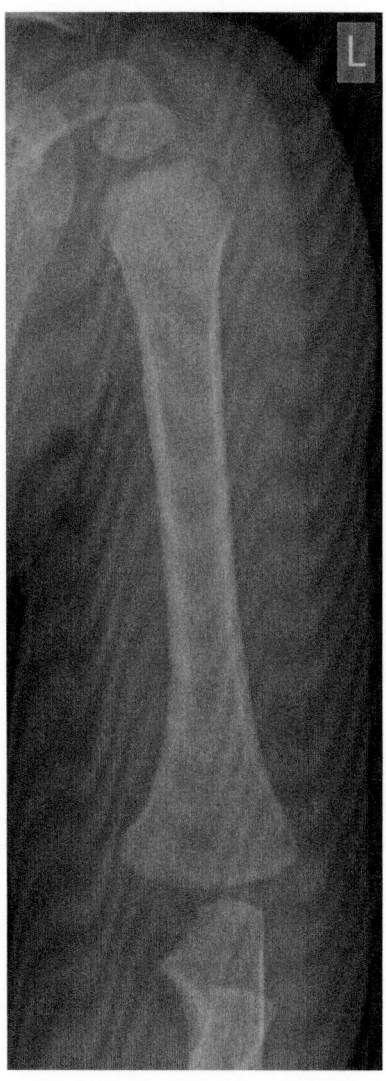

Normal	Abnormal	Diagnosis/Abnormality (only if abnormal)

Image 17

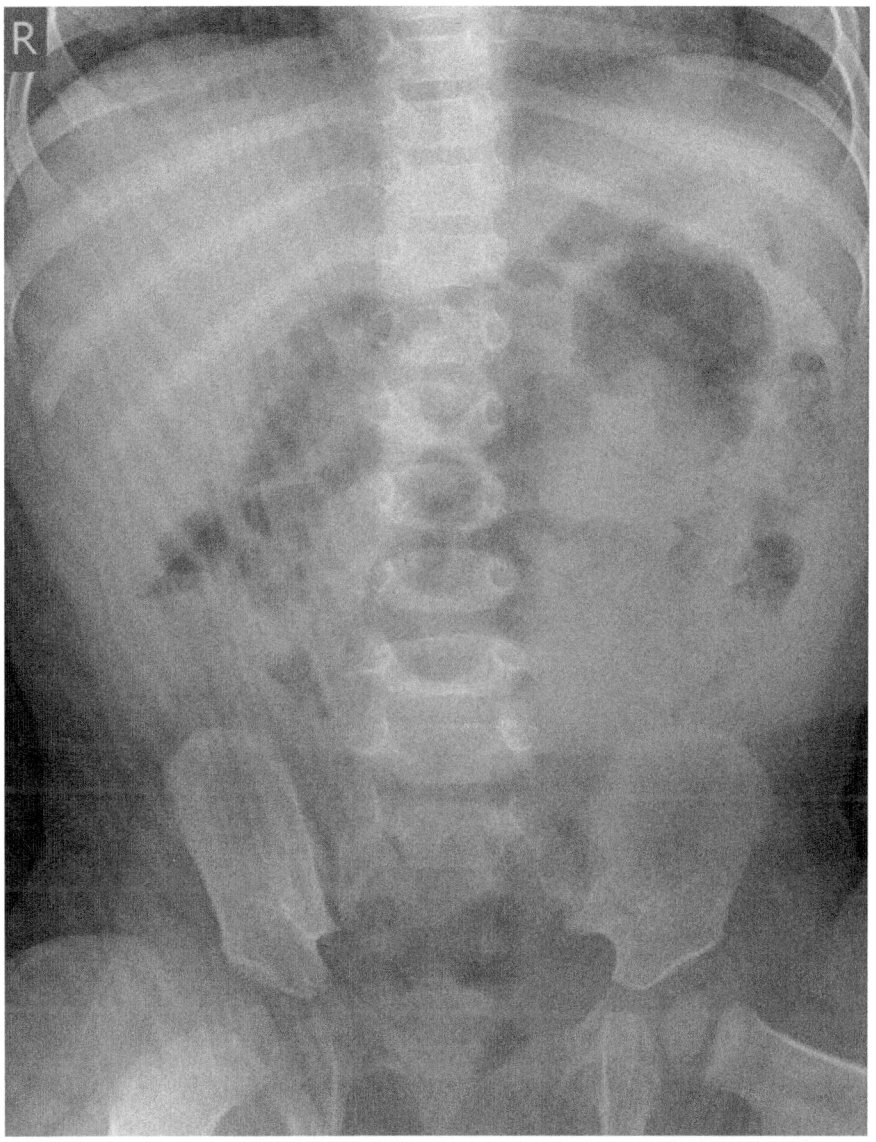

Normal	Abnormal	Diagnosis/Abnormality (only if abnormal)

Image 18

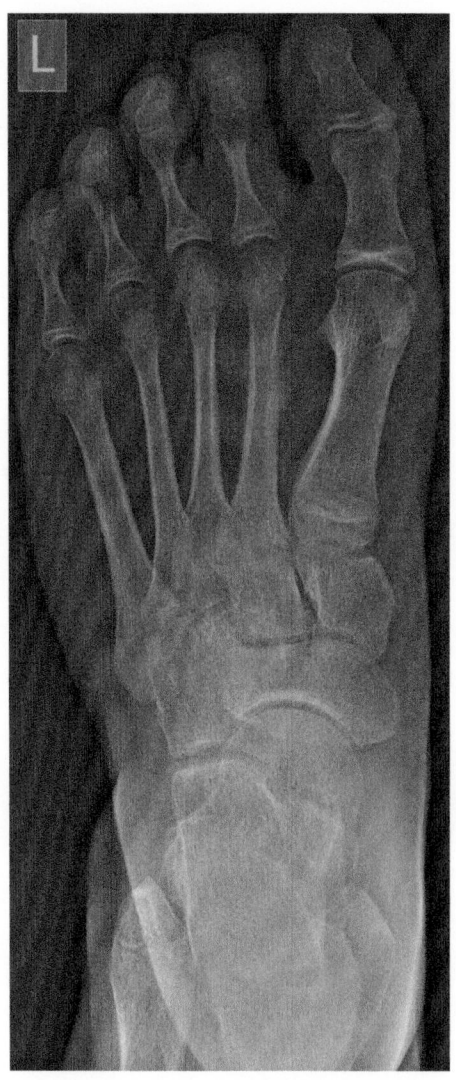

Normal	Abnormal	Diagnosis/Abnormality (only if abnormal)

Image 19

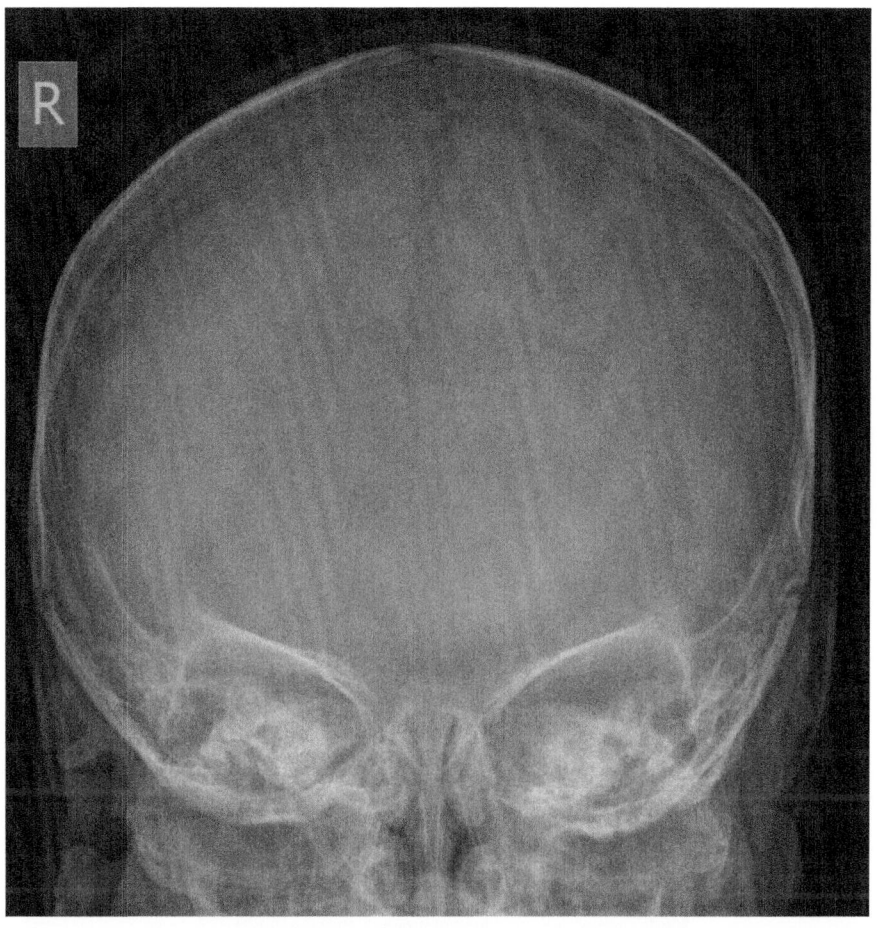

Normal	Abnormal	Diagnosis/Abnormality (only if abnormal)

Image 20

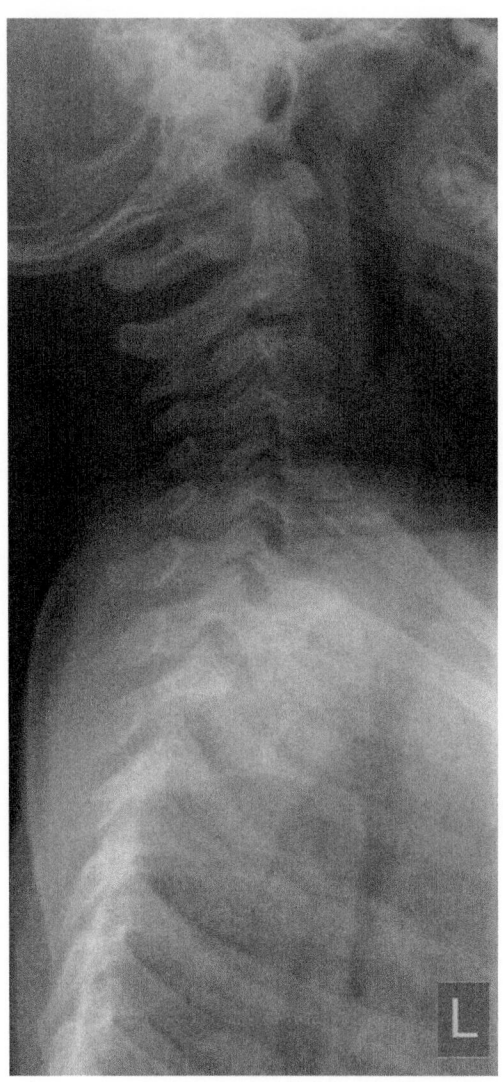

Normal	Abnormal	Diagnosis/Abnormality (only if abnormal)

Image 21

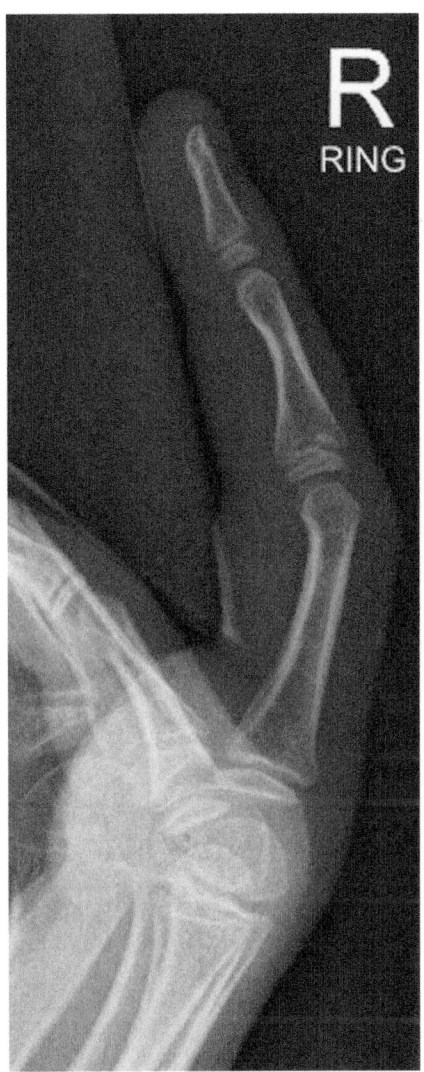

Normal	Abnormal	Diagnosis/Abnormality (only if abnormal)

Image 22

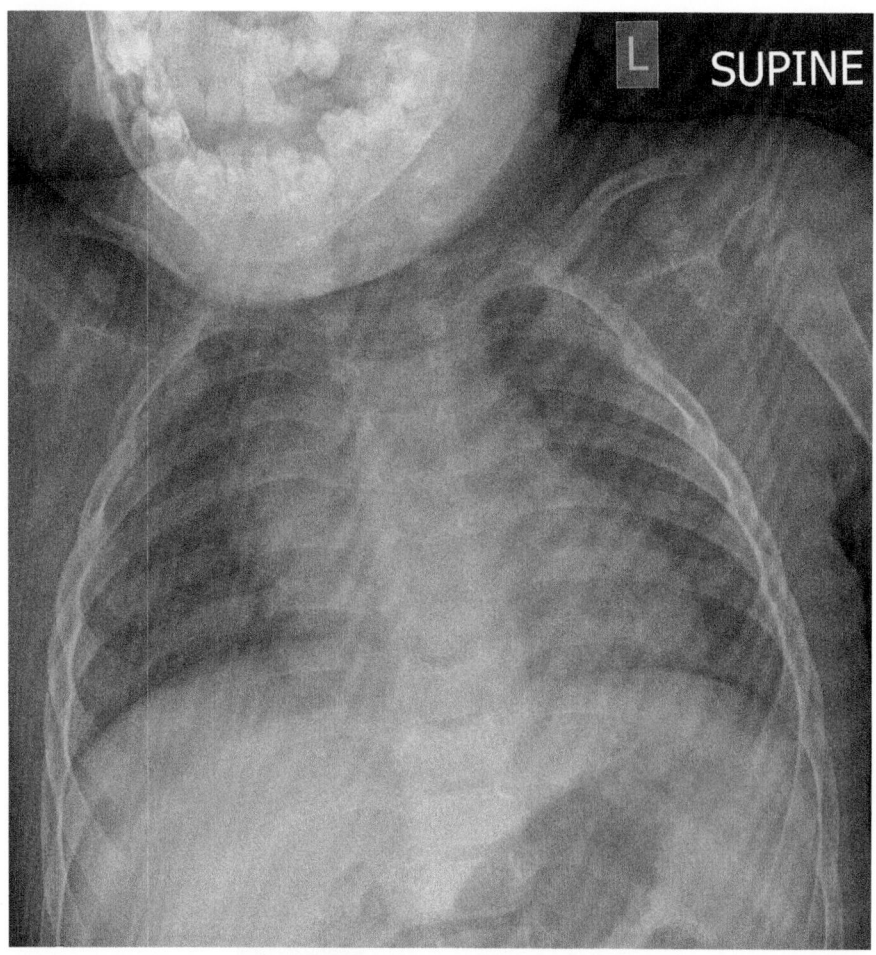

Normal	Abnormal	Diagnosis/Abnormality (only if abnormal)

Image 23

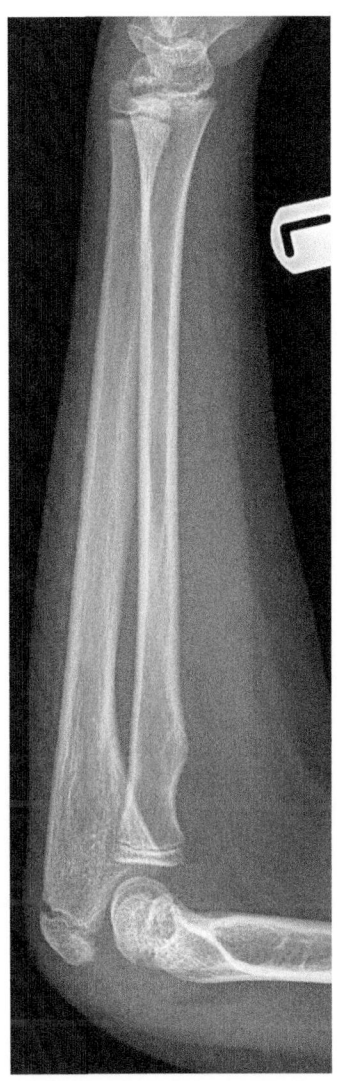

Normal	Abnormal	Diagnosis/Abnormality (only if abnormal)

Image 24

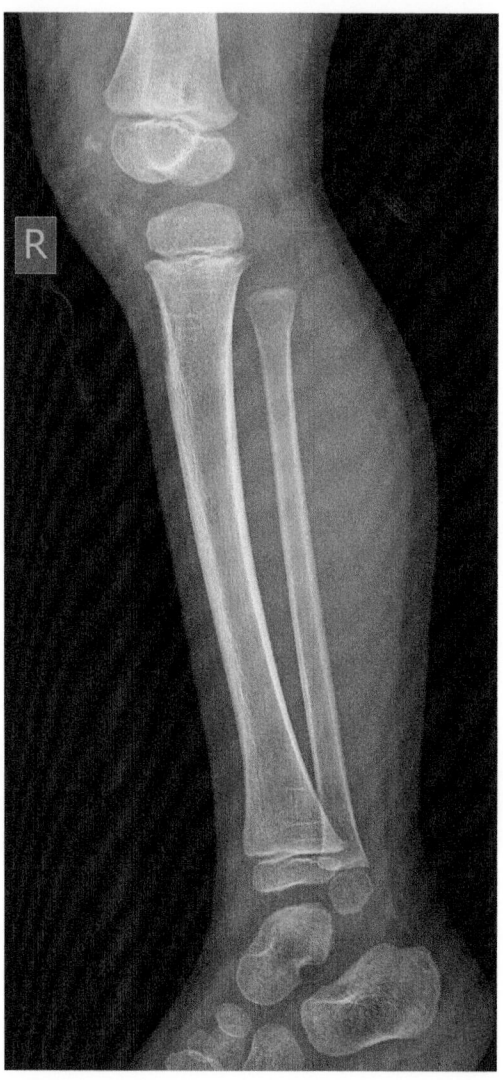

Normal	Abnormal	Diagnosis/Abnormality (only if abnormal)

Image 25

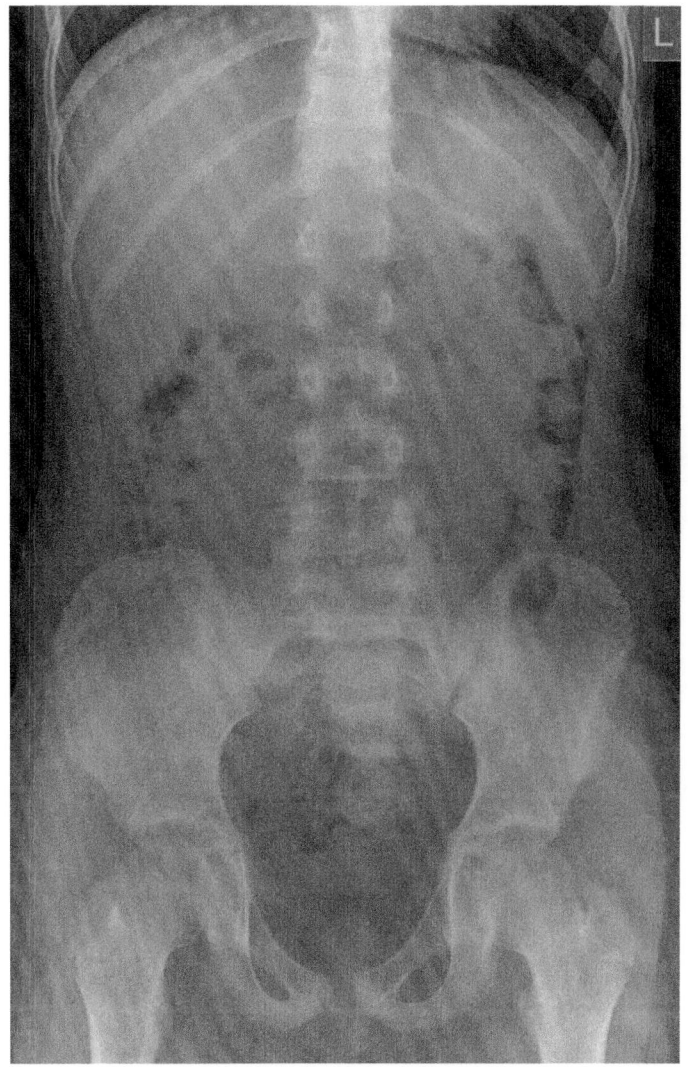

Normal	Abnormal	Diagnosis/Abnormality (only if abnormal)

Image 26

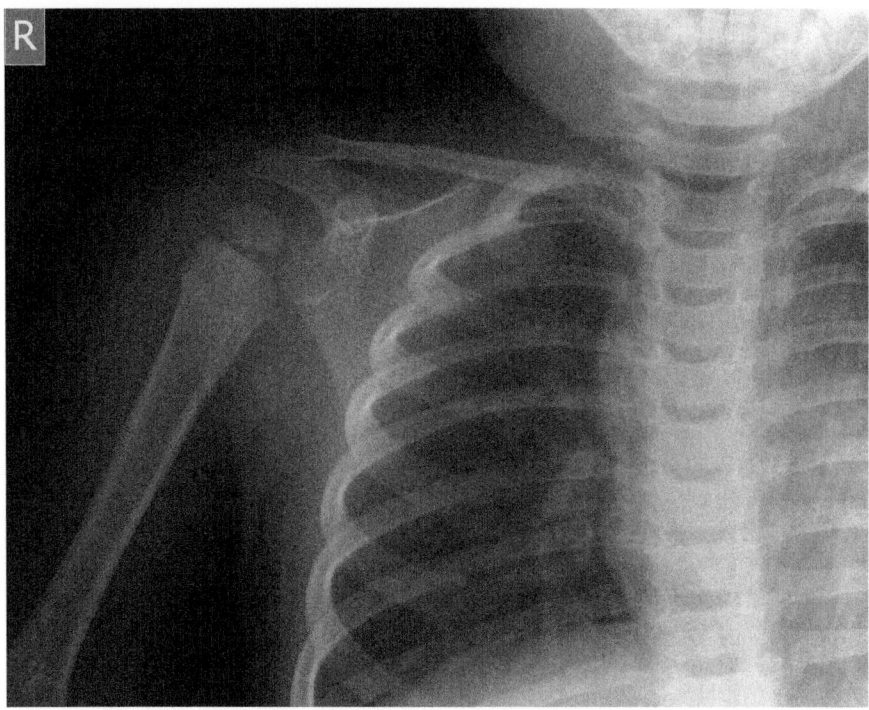

Normal	Abnormal	Diagnosis/Abnormality (only if abnormal)

Image 27

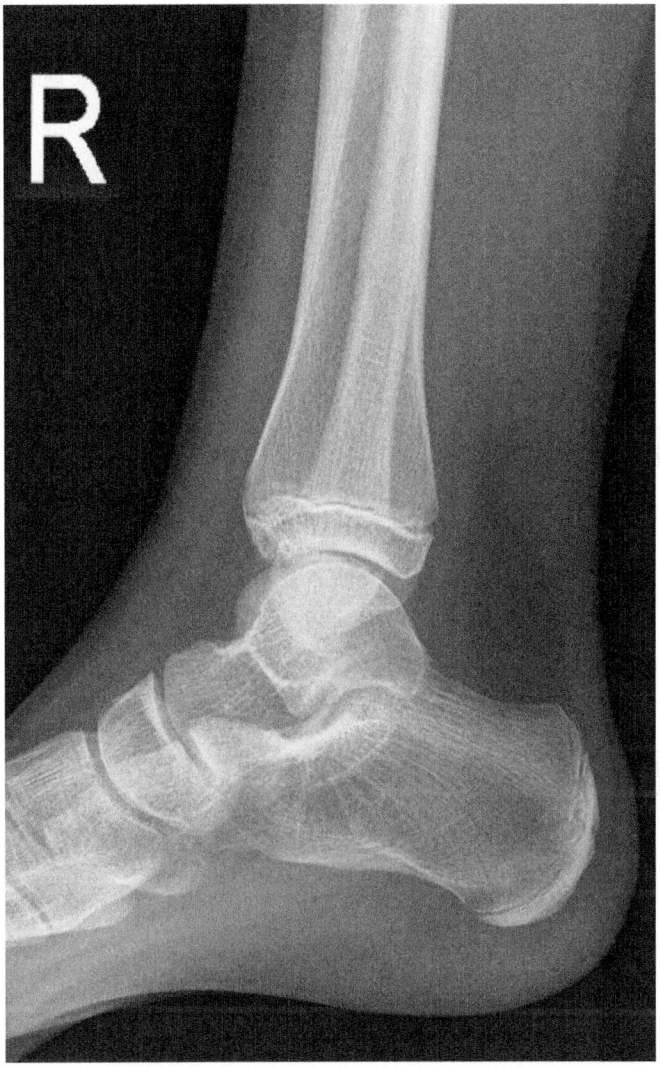

Normal	Abnormal	Diagnosis/Abnormality (only if abnormal)

Image 28

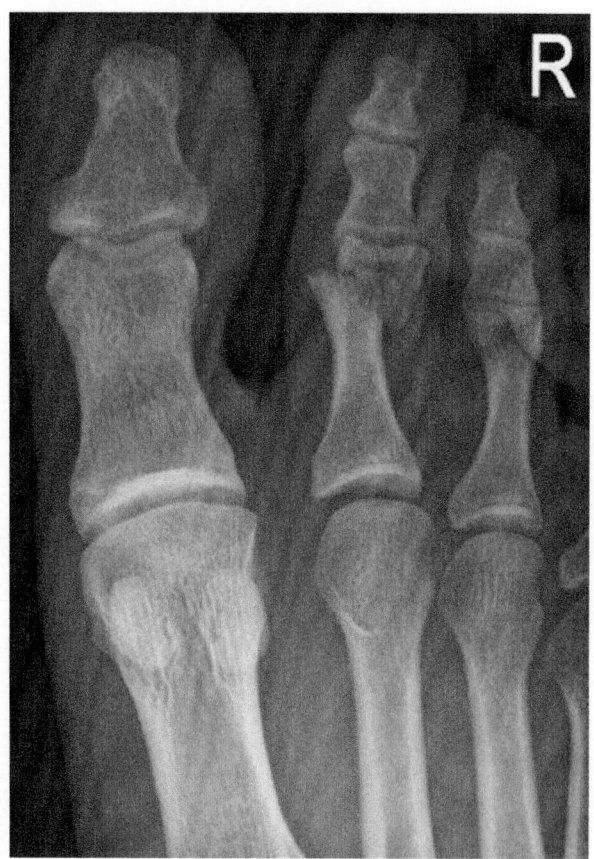

Normal	Abnormal	Diagnosis/Abnormality (only if abnormal)

Image 29

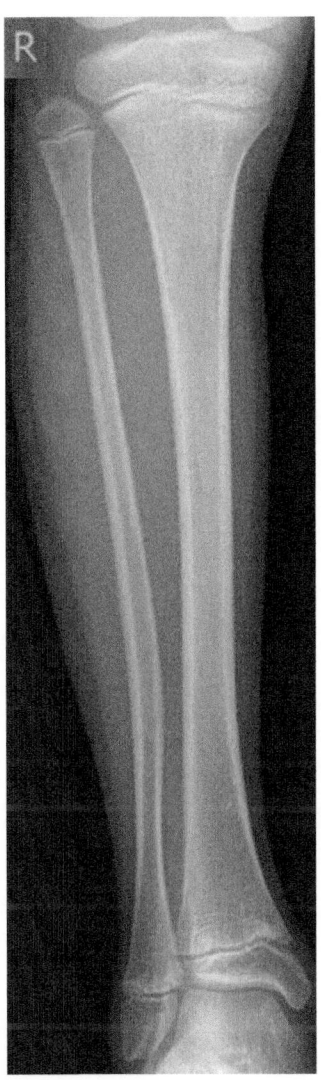

Normal	Abnormal	Diagnosis/Abnormality (only if abnormal)

Image 30

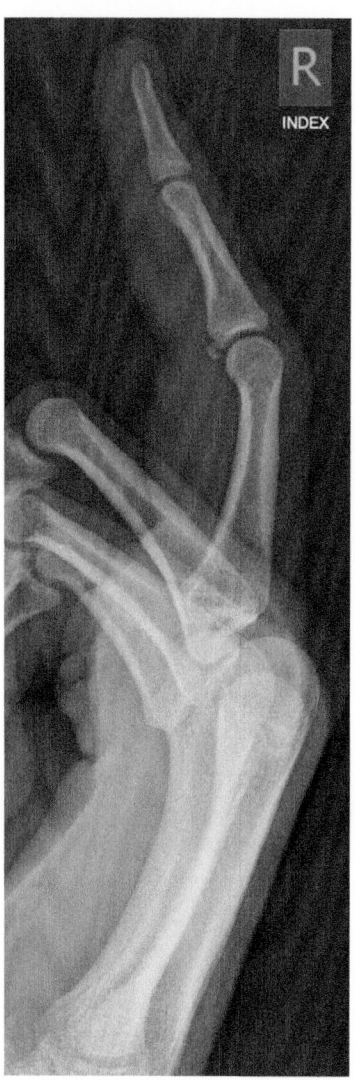

Normal	Abnormal	Diagnosis/Abnormality (only if abnormal)

4.2   Answers

Image	Normal	Abnormal	Diagnosis/abnormality (only if abnormal)
1		✓	Bilateral pneumothoraces
2		✓	# right parietal bone
3	✓		
4		✓	# right cuboid
5	✓		
6		✓	Developmental dysplasia right hip
7	✓		
8	✓		
9		✓	Healing CML and periosteal reaction right tibia and fibula
10		✓	Osteochondral defect right medial distal femoral condyle
11		✓	Zebra/bisphosphonate lines distal femora
12	✓		
13		✓	Avulsion # left iliac crest apophysis
14	✓		
15	✓		
16	✓		
17	✓		
18		✓	Healing # left second metatarsal
19	✓		
20	✓		
21		✓	Buckle # dorsal aspect base right ring finger proximal phalanx
22	✓		
23		✓	Left elbow joint effusion
24	✓		
25	✓		
26		✓	# lateral third right clavicle
27	✓		
28		✓	Oblique # right second toe proximal phalanx
29	✓		
30		✓	Volar plate # base right index finger intermediate phalanx

4.3   Explanations

1. **Bilateral pneumothoraces**
   See explanation for Test 1, Image 10.

2. **# right parietal bone**

4. **# right cuboid**

5. **Normal right ankle radiograph**
   Note the two incidental accessory ossicles, which are not fractures:
   • The os trigonum posterior to the talus which represents a failure of fusion of the lateral tubercle of the posterior talar process.
   • The os supranaviculare at the proximal aspect of the dorsal navicular.

6. **Developmental dysplasia right hip**
   In this radiograph, the right acetabular roof appears shallow when compared to the left. The right proximal femoral ossific nucleus is smaller than the left and appears 'off centre'—the lateral margin of the right ossific nucleus overhangs the lateral most aspect of the acetabular roof indicating a degree of lateral subluxation. This is more formally assessed by drawing a horizontal line along the superior aspects of both tri-radiate cartilages, known as the Hilgenreiner line. This is used as a reference for the Perkin line which is drawn perpendicular to the Hilgenreiner line, alongside the most lateral aspect of the acetabular roof. The proximal femoral ossific nuclei should lie inferomedial to where these two lines intersect, i.e. medial to the Perkin line and inferior to the Hilgenreiner line.

   The Hilgenreiner line is also used as a reference line to calculate the acetabular angle—this is the angle between the Hilgenreiner line and a further line drawn tangential to the acetabular roof. At birth, this angle should measure less than 28°. As the normal hip joints mature, they become progressively shallower and by the age of 1 year the acetabular angle should measure less than 22°. In DDH (and in neuromuscular disorders such as cerebral palsy and some skeletal dysplasias), the acetabular angle will be increased. There are excellent illustrations of these lines provided in the references.

   This radiograph is a subtler example of DDH when compared to the image from Test 2, Image 17. Such findings must be reported to enable a prompt orthopaedic referral and early initiation of treatment.

9. **Healing CML and periosteal reaction right tibia and fibula**
   This is the AP radiograph from the follow-up skeletal survey in the same patient as Test 3, Image 2, which demonstrates distal tibial and fibular metaphyseal fractures/classic metaphyseal lesions (CMLs): this radiograph was performed 14 days after the initial radiograph. This infant was 6 weeks of age at the time of the follow-up skeletal survey.

   This radiograph demonstrates a healing CML and florid healing periosteal reaction reflecting the fact that the periosteum was stripped from the underlying

bone at the time of the initial injury. Depending on whether the periosteum is stripped at the time of injury, CMLs may heal with (as in this case) or without periosteal reaction which may cause difficulties in dating, which in itself is a complex area; however, CMLs usually heal by 4 weeks and always by 6 weeks.

We have included this radiograph as an example of healing periosteal reaction plus a CML. However, remember that periosteal reaction may occur in isolation and be detected on initial/presentation/admission radiographs, in which case the differential diagnosis should include physical abuse, particularly in pre-ambulant infants.

10. **Osteochondral defect right medial distal femoral condyle**
    Osteochondral defects are focal areas of cartilaginous damage adjacent to sub-chondral bone thought to be secondary to repeated microtrauma. This term is used synonymously with *osteochondritis dissecans (OCD)* and is the end result of the separation of an osteochondral fragment which results in the gradual fragmentation of the articular surface, seen in the magnified image below:

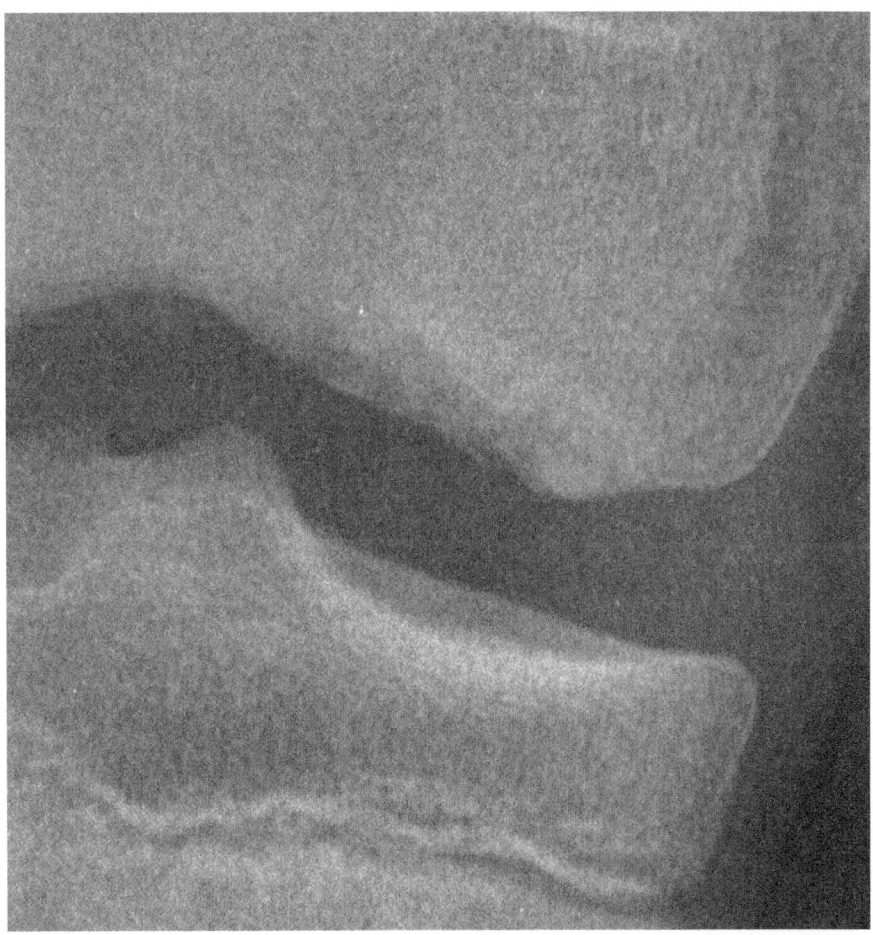

The bony fragment may become an intra-articular loose body. Locations for osteochondral defects include:
- Femoral condyle (most common)
- Talar dome
- Capitellum of the humerus

MRI is the test of choice and is essential in determining management.

11. **Zebra/bisphosphonate lines distal femora**
These sclerotic lines alternating with the less dense native bone in the distal femoral metaphyses are known as 'zebra' or 'bisphosphonate lines'. In this case, the underlying condition is osteogenesis imperfecta (OI), a group of congenital disorders of collagen type 1 production affecting bone and connective tissue.

The sclerotic lines represent new bone formation during repeated episodes of cyclical bisphosphonate therapy. Bisphosphonates work by inhibiting osteoclast function and excessive doses may lead to iatrogenic osteopetrosis; note the flaring of the distal femoral metaphyses in this case, reminiscent of the Erlenmeyer flask deformity of osteopetrosis. If you are considering a diagnosis of OI, look for associated features, e.g. acute/healing fractures, osteopenia, Wormian bones, and platybasia.

The differential for sclerotic metaphyseal lines includes:
- Growth arrest/resumption lines: seen after periods of 'metabolic stress', i.e. acute illness, where growth arrests and then resumes when the acute stressor has resolved
- Bisphosphonate therapy (as in this case)
- Rickets: particularly those on prolonged treatment in the case of vitamin D dependent rickets
- Osteopetrosis
- Chemotherapy
- Chronic anaemia: seen in sickle cell disease and thalassemia
- Treated leukaemia

13. **Avulsion # left iliac crest apophysis**
Careful inspection reveals the avulsion fracture of the left iliac crest apophysis. Apophyseal avulsion injuries are common findings on pelvic/hip radiographs when performed for pain in sporty/active children. In the paediatric population, the tendons are stronger than the apophyses, such that a strong muscular contraction will result in an apophyseal avulsion fracture rather than a sprain or tear of the tendon.

Bony structure—Tendinous attachment (from proximal to distal):
- Iliac crest—Abdominal muscles
- Anterior superior iliac spine (ASIS)—Sartorius and tensor fascia latae
- Anterior inferior iliac spine (AIIS)—Rectus femoris
- Greater trochanter—Gluteus medius and minimus

- Lesser trochanter—Iliopsoas
- Pubic symphysis—Adductors
- Ischial tuberosity—Hamstrings

Tip for the viva:
- This is common exam fodder: *the above pairings should be learnt rote.*

18. **Healing # left second metatarsal**
Periosteal new bone formation may take up to 14 days to be detected on radiographs.

21. **Buckle # dorsal aspect base right ring finger proximal phalanx**

22. **Normal chest radiograph**
This radiograph is normal. The prominence of the superior mediastinum is consistent with thymus and is normal.

23. **Left elbow joint effusion**
See explanation for Test 1, Image 11.

24. **Normal right tibia/fibula radiograph**
The ossification anterior to the left distal femur is the patella ossification centre. The patella can have variable ossification at all ages and can appear fragmented on occasion. See the explanation for Test 2, Image 8.

26. **# lateral third right clavicle**

28. **Oblique # right second toe proximal phalanx**

30. **Volar plate # base right index finger intermediate phalanx**
These avulsion fractures result from hyperextension injuries resulting in an intra-articular fracture of the volar plate of the proximal interphalangeal joint. Fractures which involve a significant portion of the articular surface can result in joint instability because a greater portion of stabilising collateral ligaments are attached to the avulsed fragment.

Further Reading

Image 5

Jones J et al (2018) Os trigonum. https://radiopaedia.org/articles/os-trigonum. Accessed April 2018

Image 9

Please see the Test 2, Image 14 references regarding the imaging of suspected physical abuse in infants and young children

Image 10

Bell D, Gaillard F et al (2018) Osteochondritis dissecans. https://radiopaedia.org/articles/osteo-chondritis-dissecans. Accessed April 2018

Kan JH (2018) Osteochondral abnormalities: pitfalls, injuries, and osteochondritis dissecans. http://www.arrs.org/shoparrs/products/s11p_sample.pdf. Accessed July 2018

Sharma R, Gaillard F et al (2018) Osteochondral defect. https://radiopaedia.org/articles/osteo-chondral-defect. Accessed April 2018.

Thapa MM, Chaturvedi A, Iyer RS et al (2012) MRI of pediatric patients: part 2, normal variants and abnormalities of the knee. AJR Am J Roentgenol. 198(5):W456–W465

Image 11

Al Muderis M, Azzopardi T, Cundy P (2007) Zebra lines of pamidronate therapy in children. J Bone Joint Surg Am. 89(7):1511–1516

Bell DJ, Morgan MA et al (2018) Growth arrest lines. https://radiopaedia.org/articles/growth-arrest-lines. Accessed April 2018

Thurston M, Jones J et al (2018) Alternating radiolucent and radiodense metaphyseal lines. https://radiopaedia.org/articles/alternating-radiolucent-and-radiodense-metaphyseal-lines. Accessed April 2018

Image 13

Aiyer A, Moore D (2018) Pelvis fractures – pediatric. https://www.orthobullets.com/pediat-rics/3000/pelvis-fractures%2D%2Dpediatric. Accessed July 2018

Bomer J, Holscher H et al (2018) Hip pathology in children. http://www.radiologyassistant.nl/en/p557dccf34fb1a/hip-pathology-in-children.html. Accessed April 2018

Stevens MA, El-Khoury GY, Kathol MH et al (1999) Imaging features of avulsion injuries. Radiographics. 19(3):655–672

Image 27

Niknejad MT et al (2018) Os subfibulare. https://radiopaedia.org/articles/os-subfibulare. Accessed April 2018

Image 30

Lujikx T, Hsu C-T et al (2018) Volar plate avulsion injury. https://radiopaedia.org/articles/volar-plate-avulsion-injury. Accessed April 2018

Test 5

5

5.1 Images

Image 1

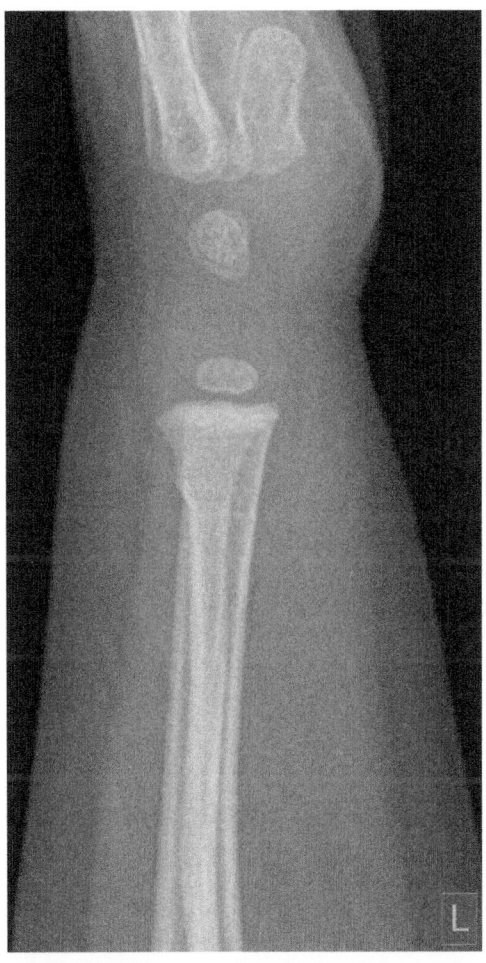

Normal	Abnormal	Diagnosis/Abnormality (only if abnormal)

© Springer Nature Switzerland AG 2019
M. Paddock, A. C. Offiah, *Paediatric Radiology Rapid Reporting for FRCR Part 2B*,
https://doi.org/10.1007/978-3-030-01965-5_5

Image 2

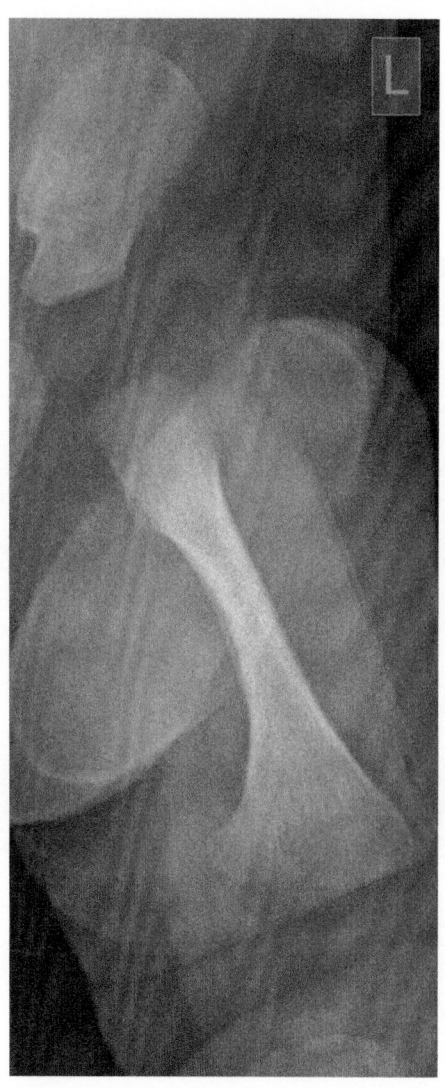

Normal	Abnormal	Diagnosis/Abnormality (only if abnormal)

Image 3

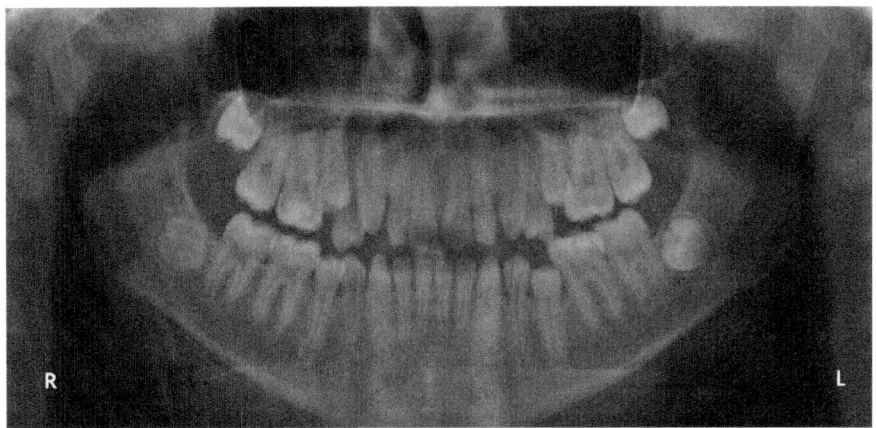

Normal	Abnormal	Diagnosis/Abnormality (only if abnormal)

Image 4

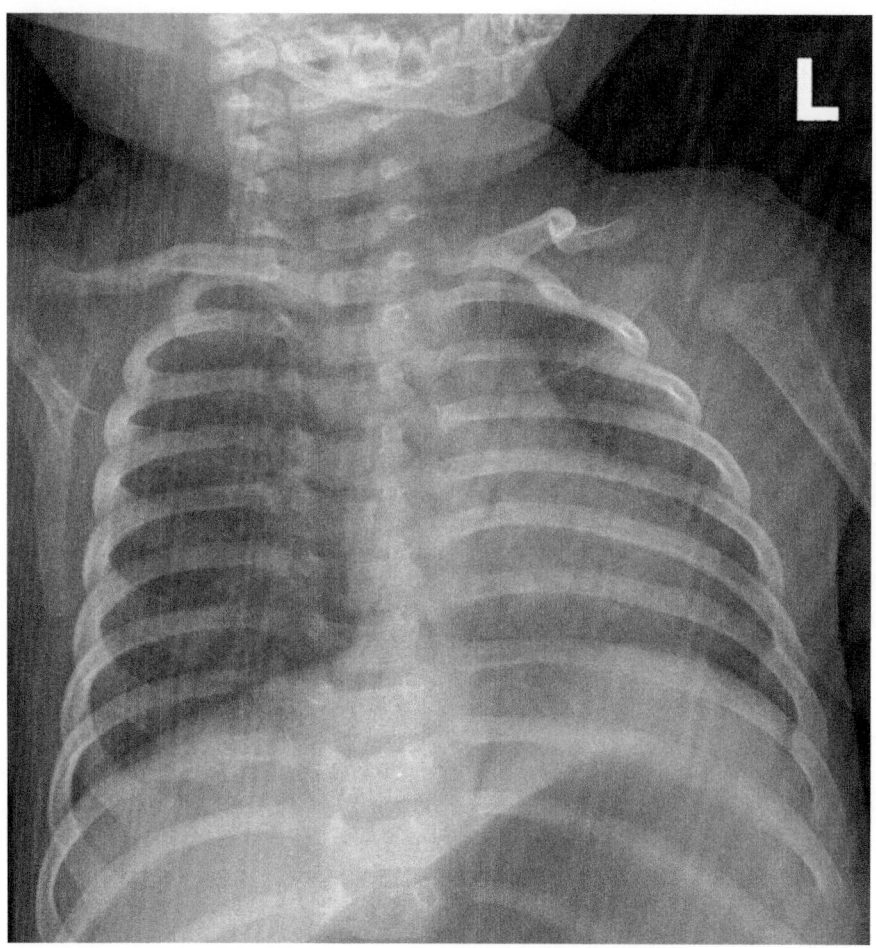

Normal	Abnormal	Diagnosis/Abnormality (only if abnormal)

Image 5

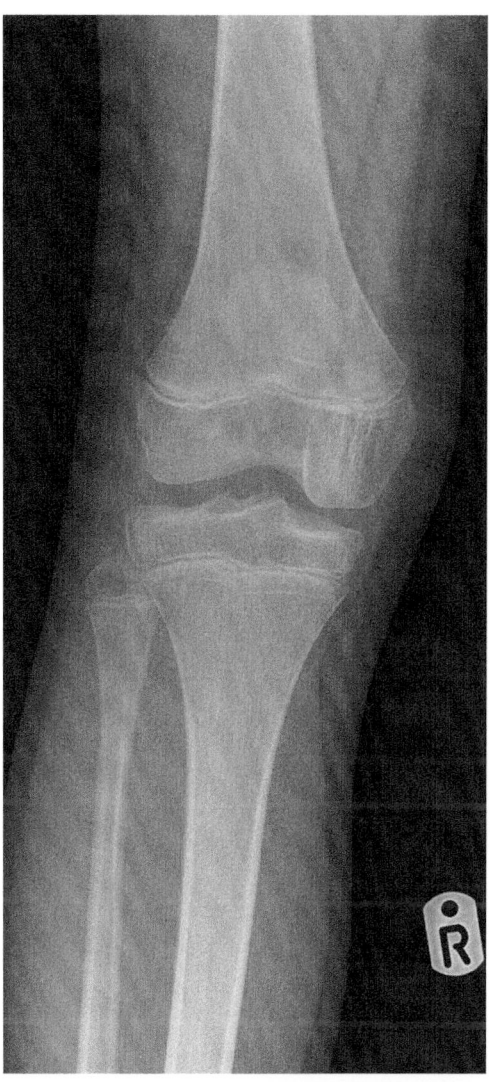

Normal	Abnormal	Diagnosis/Abnormality (only if abnormal)

Image 6

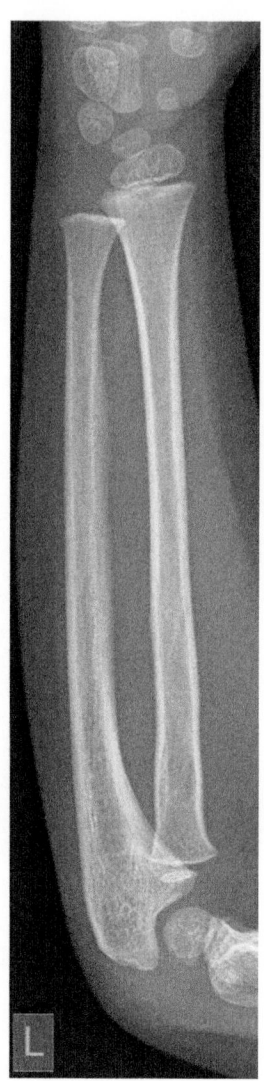

Normal	Abnormal	Diagnosis/Abnormality (only if abnormal)

Image 7

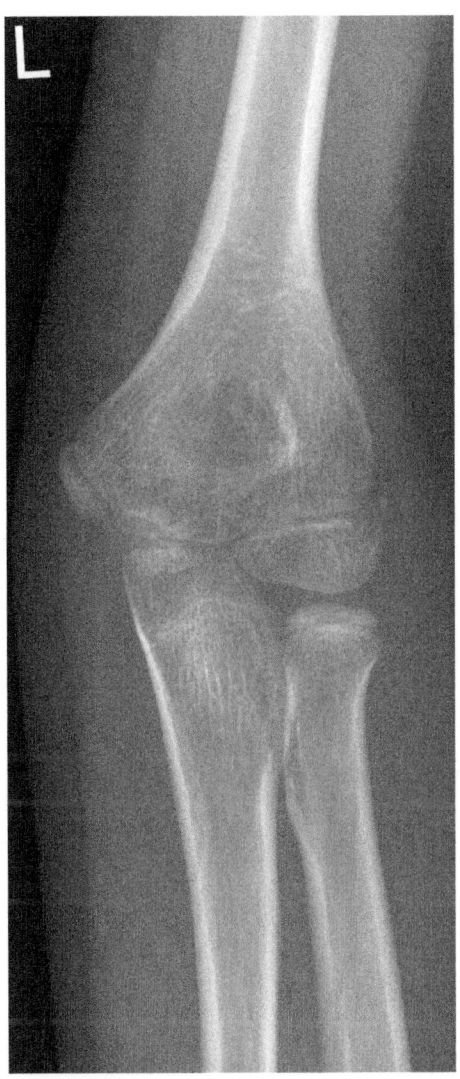

Normal	Abnormal	Diagnosis/Abnormality (only if abnormal)

Image 8

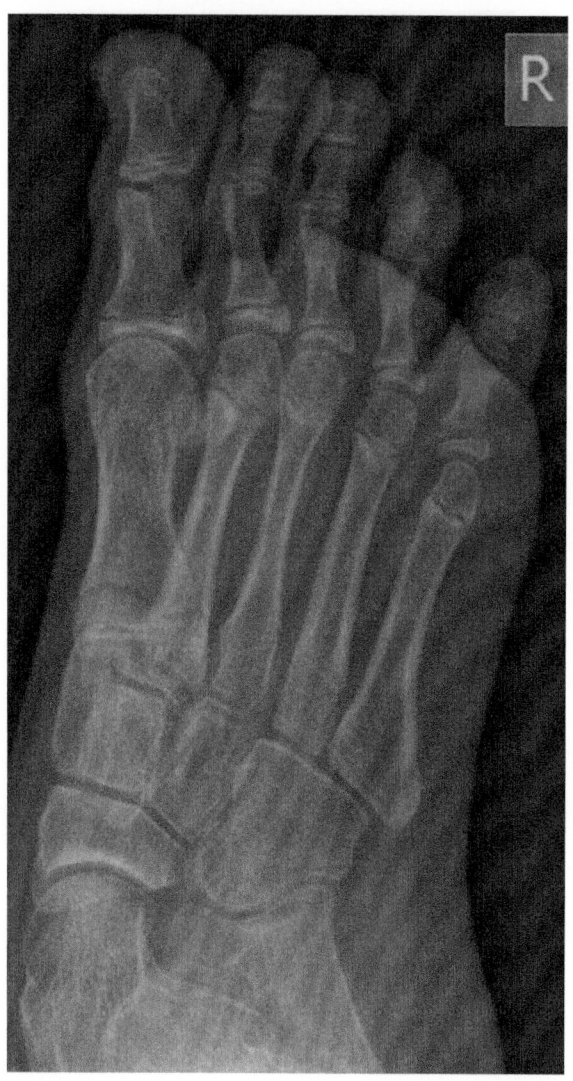

Normal	Abnormal	Diagnosis/Abnormality (only if abnormal)

Image 9

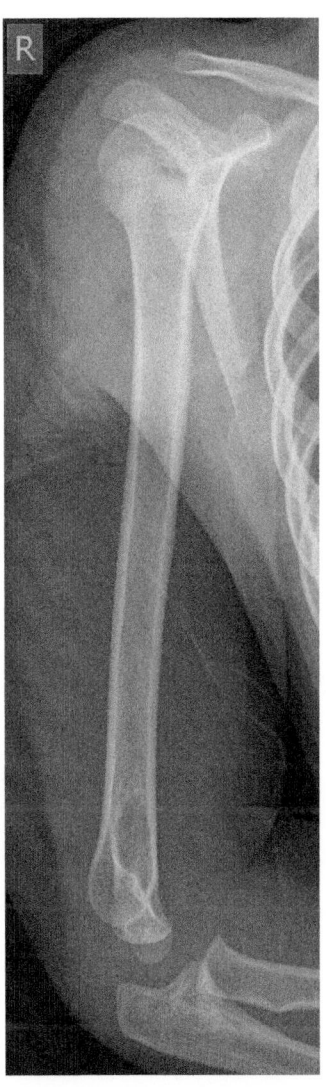

Normal	Abnormal	Diagnosis/Abnormality (only if abnormal)

Image 10

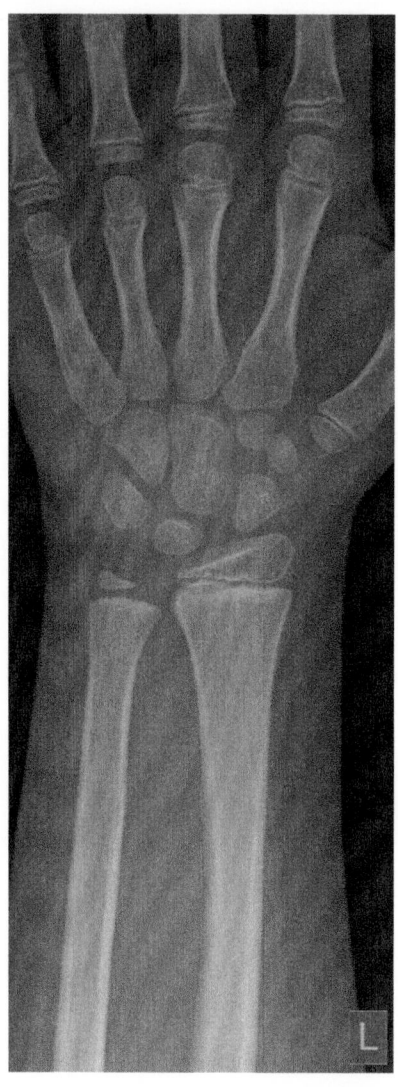

Normal	Abnormal	Diagnosis/Abnormality (only if abnormal)

Image 11

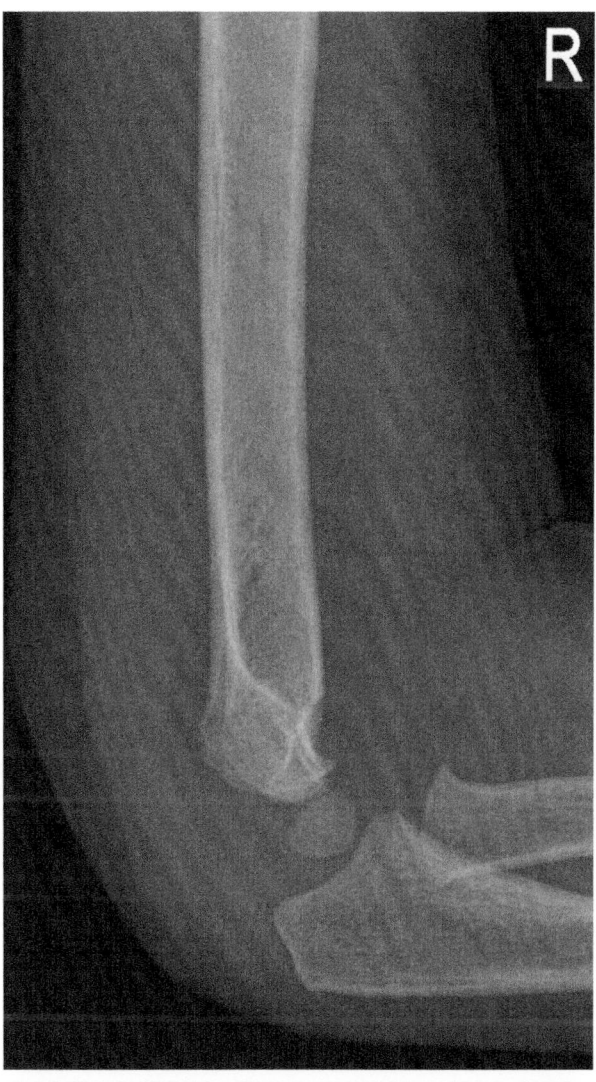

Normal	Abnormal	Diagnosis/Abnormality (only if abnormal)

Image 12

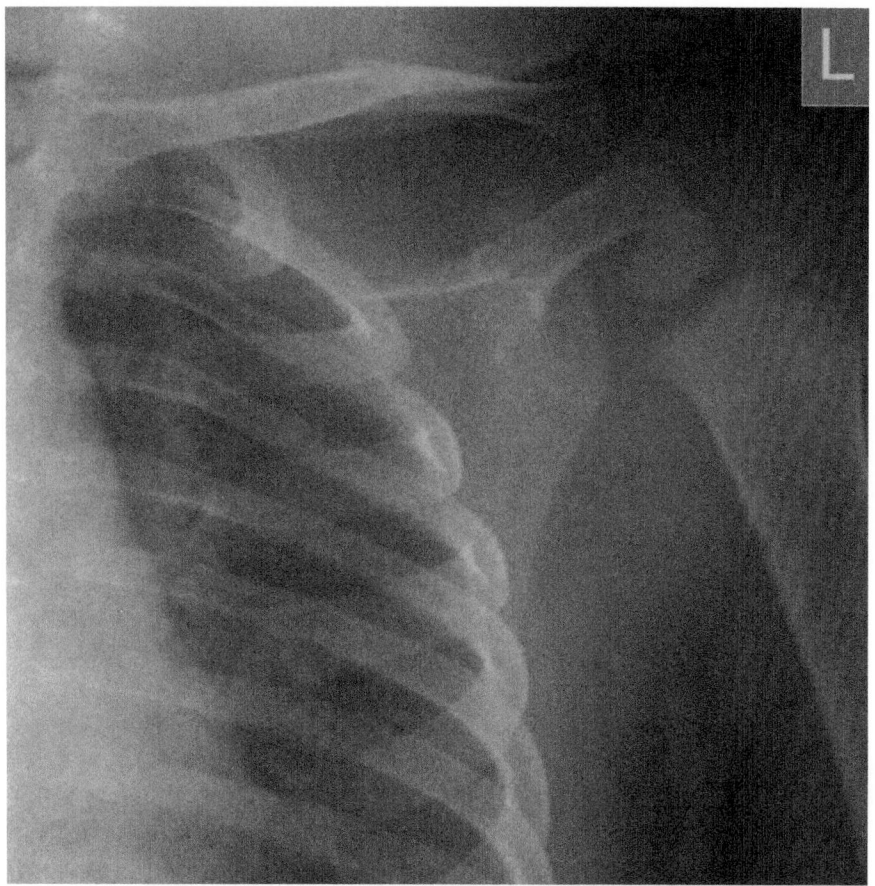

Normal	Abnormal	Diagnosis/Abnormality (only if abnormal)

Image 13

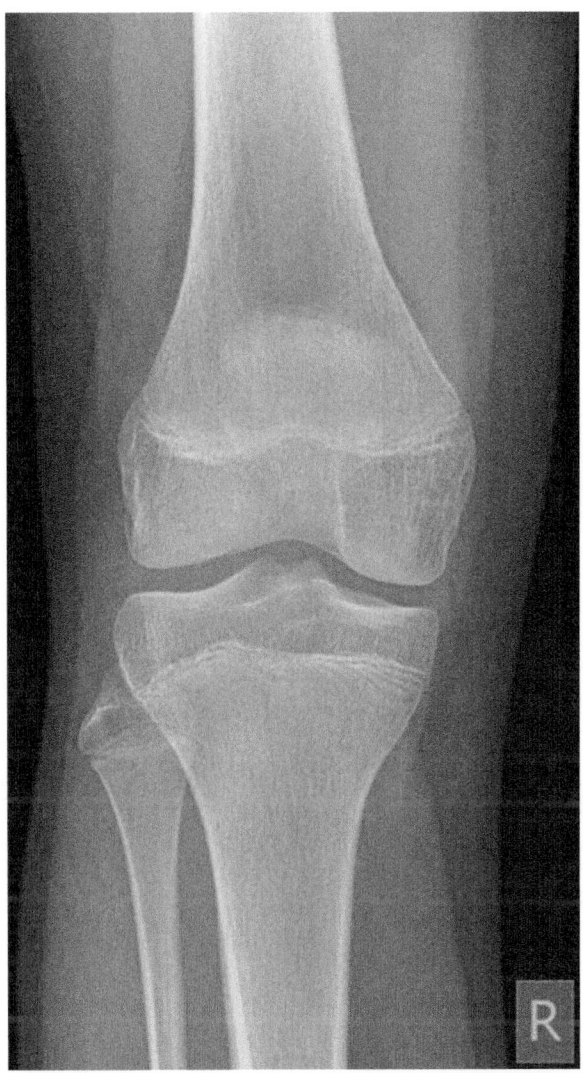

Normal	Abnormal	Diagnosis/Abnormality (only if abnormal)

Image 14

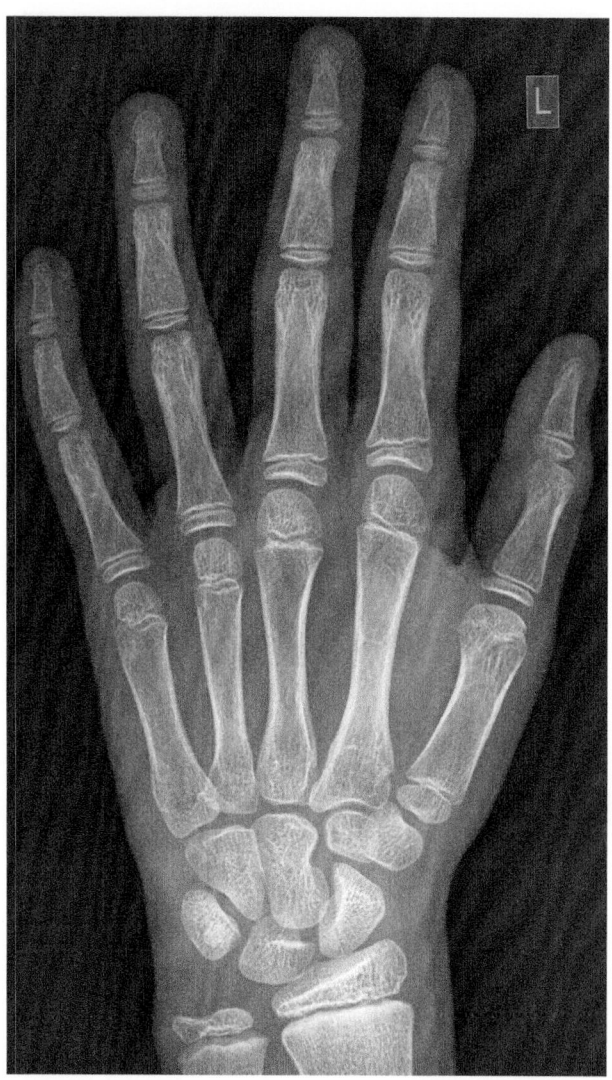

Normal	Abnormal	Diagnosis/Abnormality (only if abnormal)

Image 15

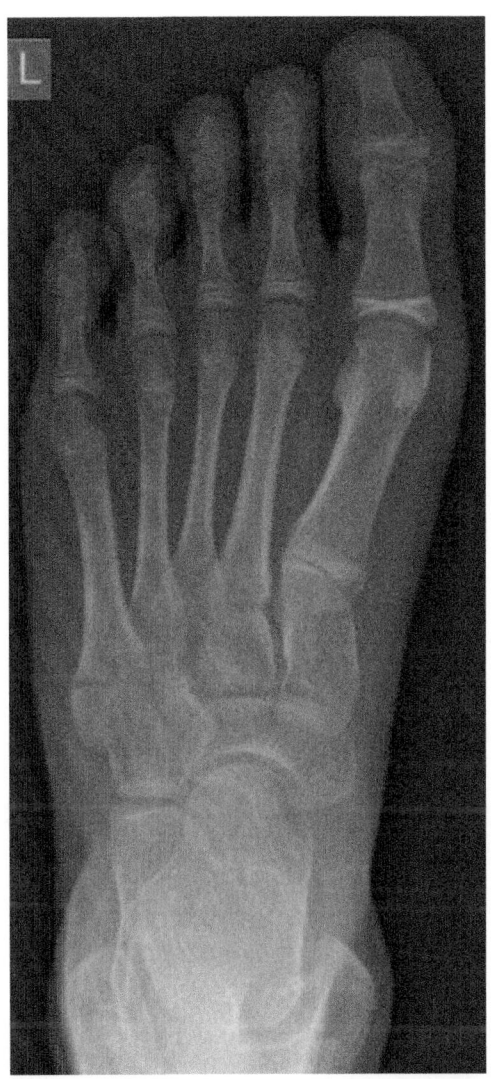

Normal	Abnormal	Diagnosis/Abnormality (only if abnormal)

Image 16

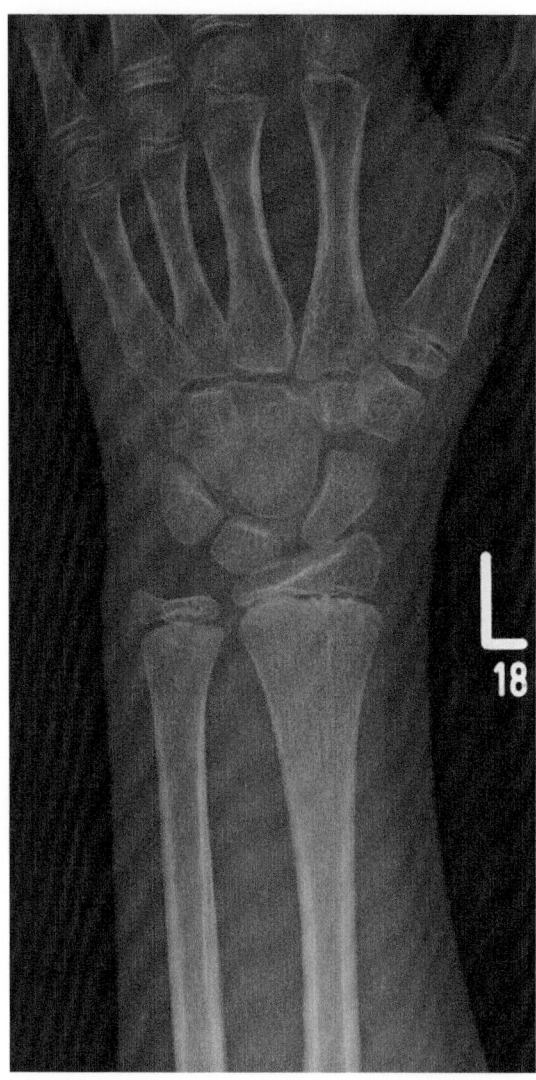

Normal	Abnormal	Diagnosis/Abnormality (only if abnormal)

Image 17

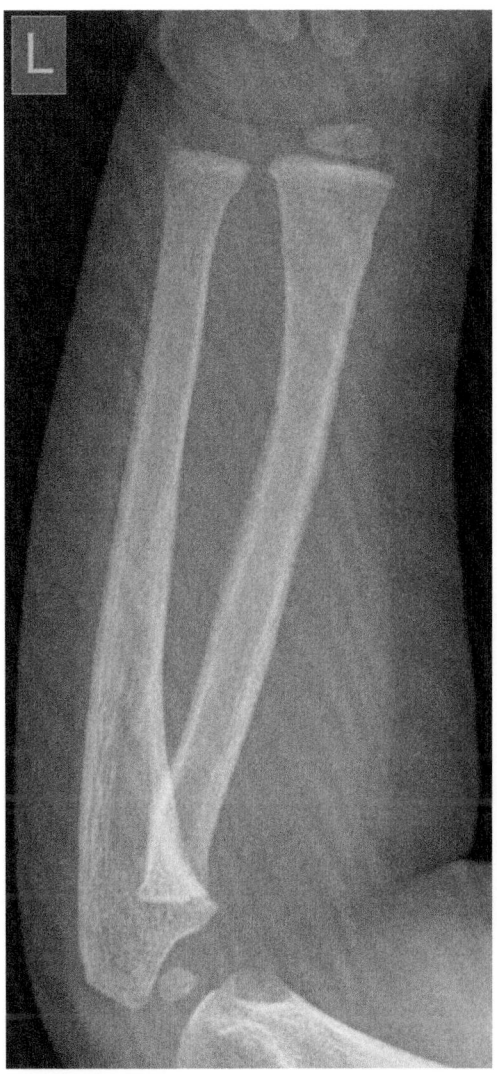

Normal	Abnormal	Diagnosis/Abnormality (only if abnormal)

Image 18

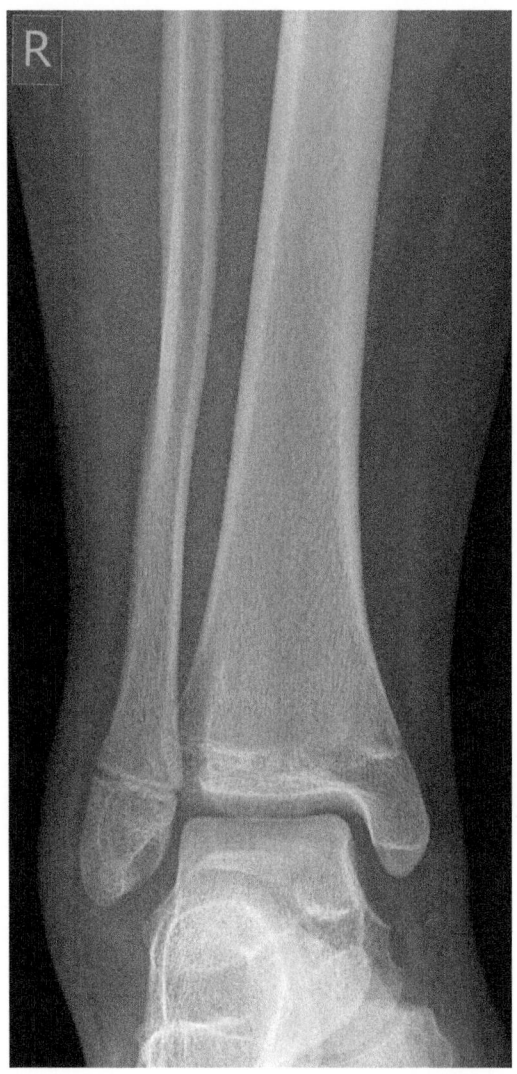

Normal	Abnormal	Diagnosis/Abnormality (only if abnormal)

Image 19

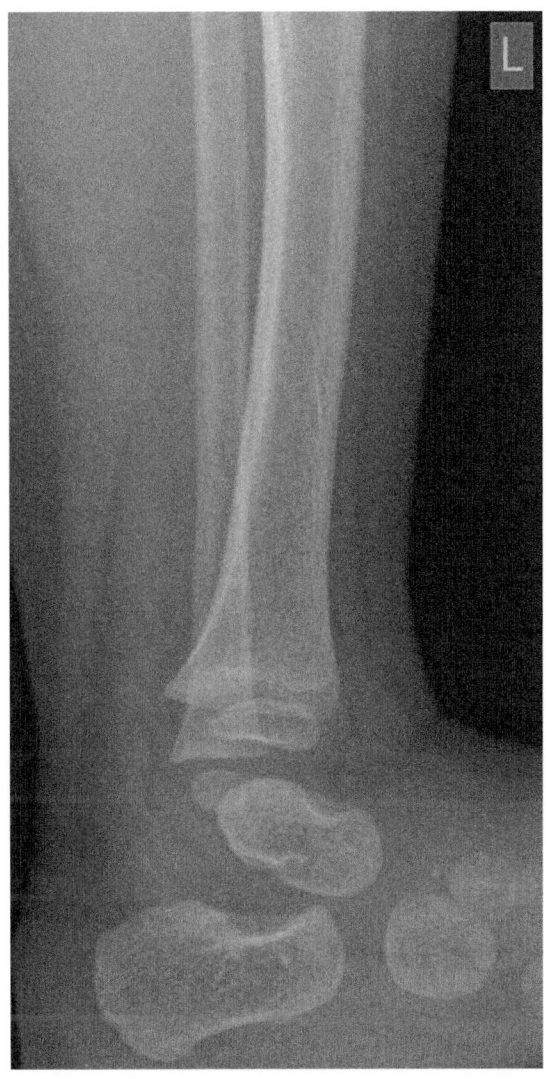

Normal	Abnormal	Diagnosis/Abnormality (only if abnormal)

Image 20

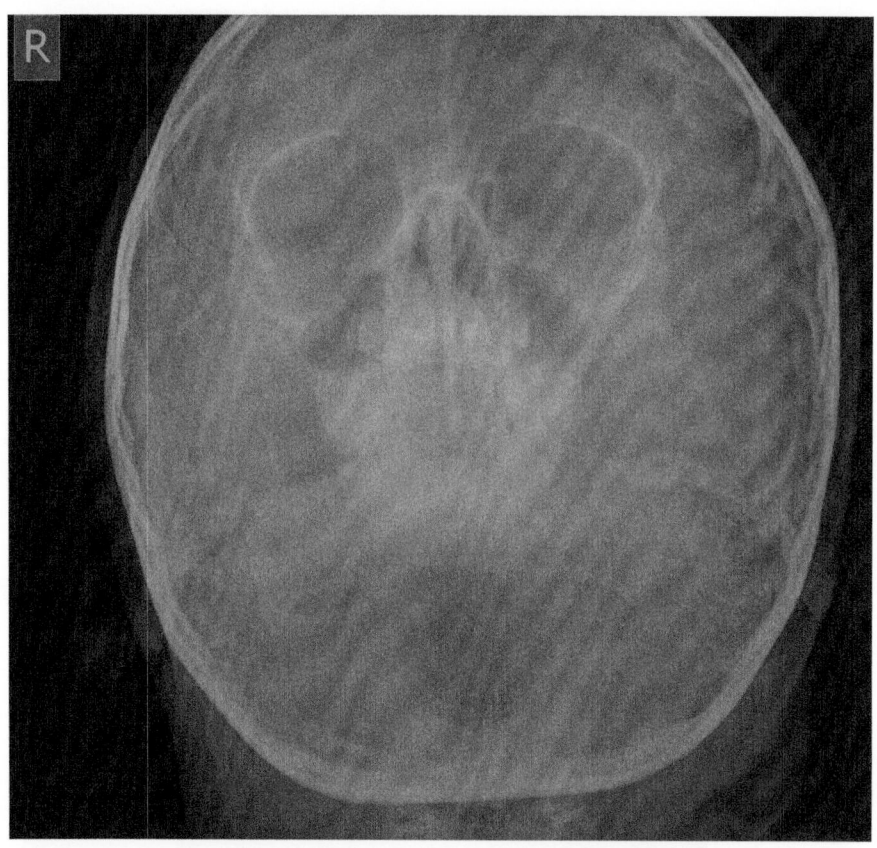

Normal	Abnormal	Diagnosis/Abnormality (only if abnormal)

Image 21

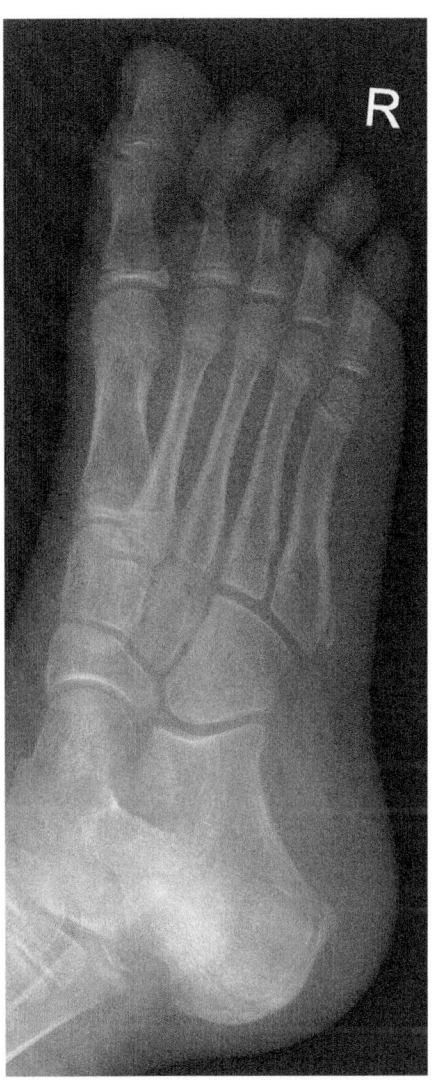

Normal	Abnormal	Diagnosis/Abnormality (only if abnormal)

Image 22

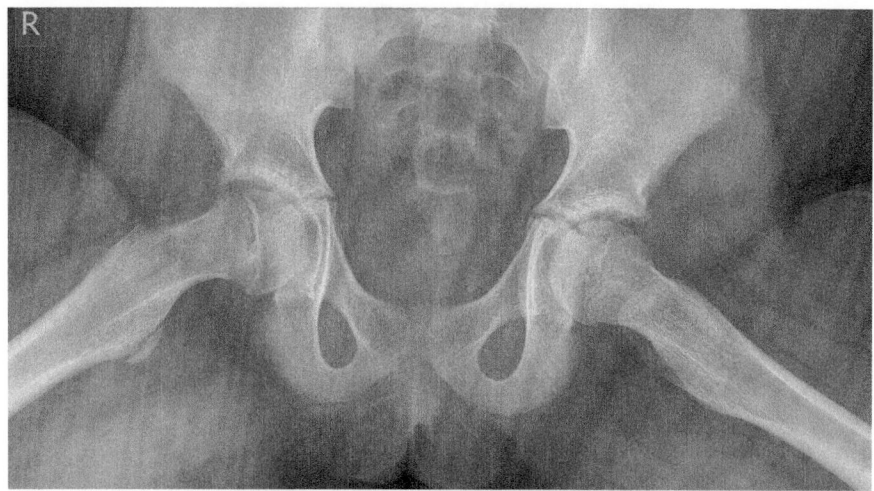

Normal	Abnormal	Diagnosis/Abnormality (only if abnormal)

Image 23

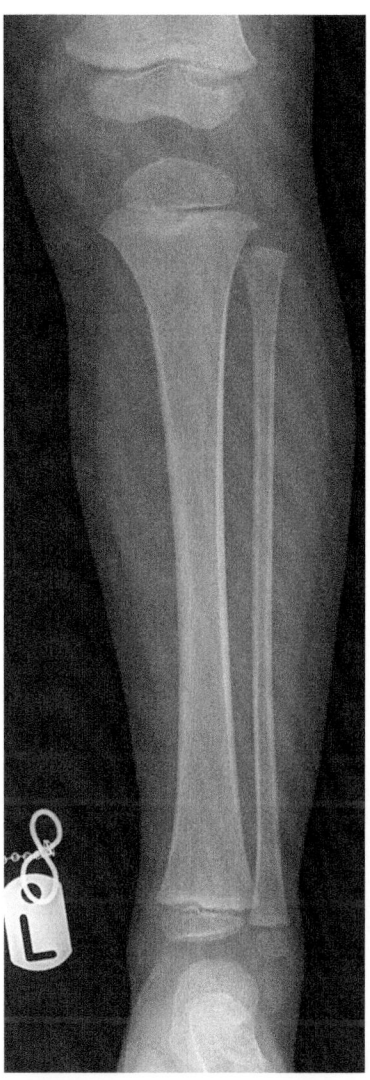

Normal	Abnormal	Diagnosis/Abnormality (only if abnormal)

Image 24

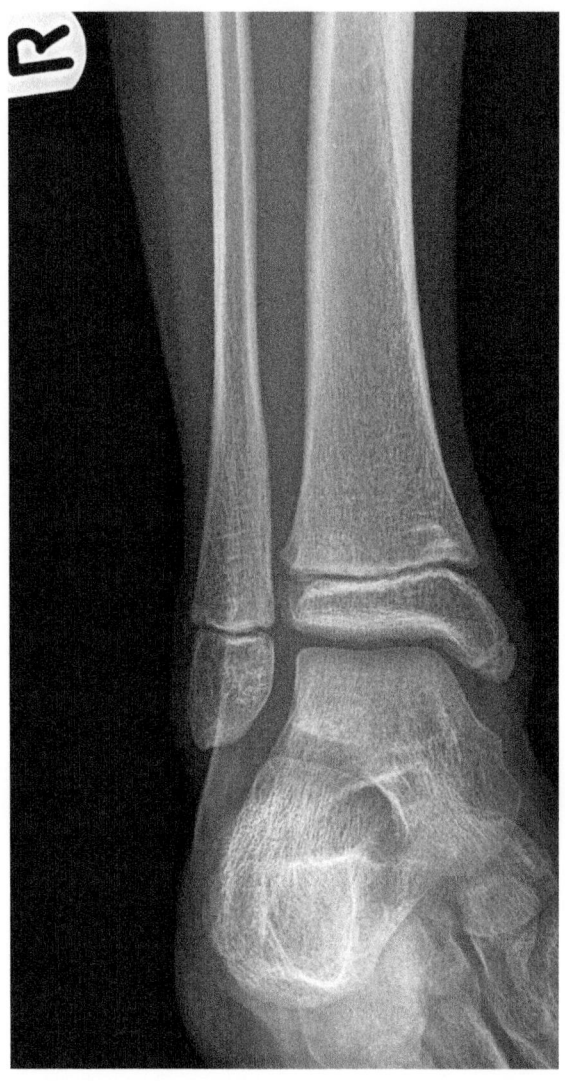

Normal	Abnormal	Diagnosis/Abnormality (only if abnormal)

Image 25

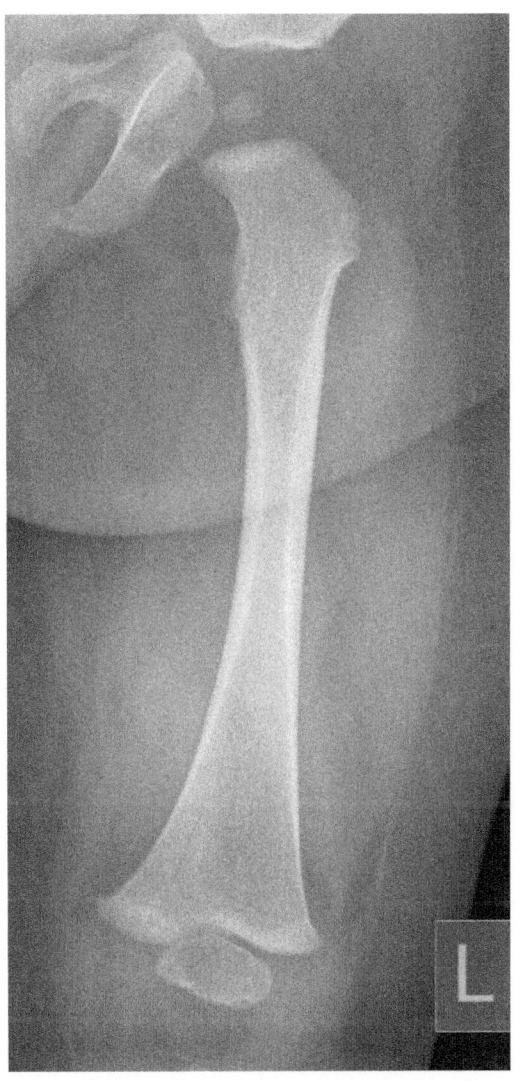

Normal	Abnormal	Diagnosis/Abnormality (only if abnormal)

Image 26

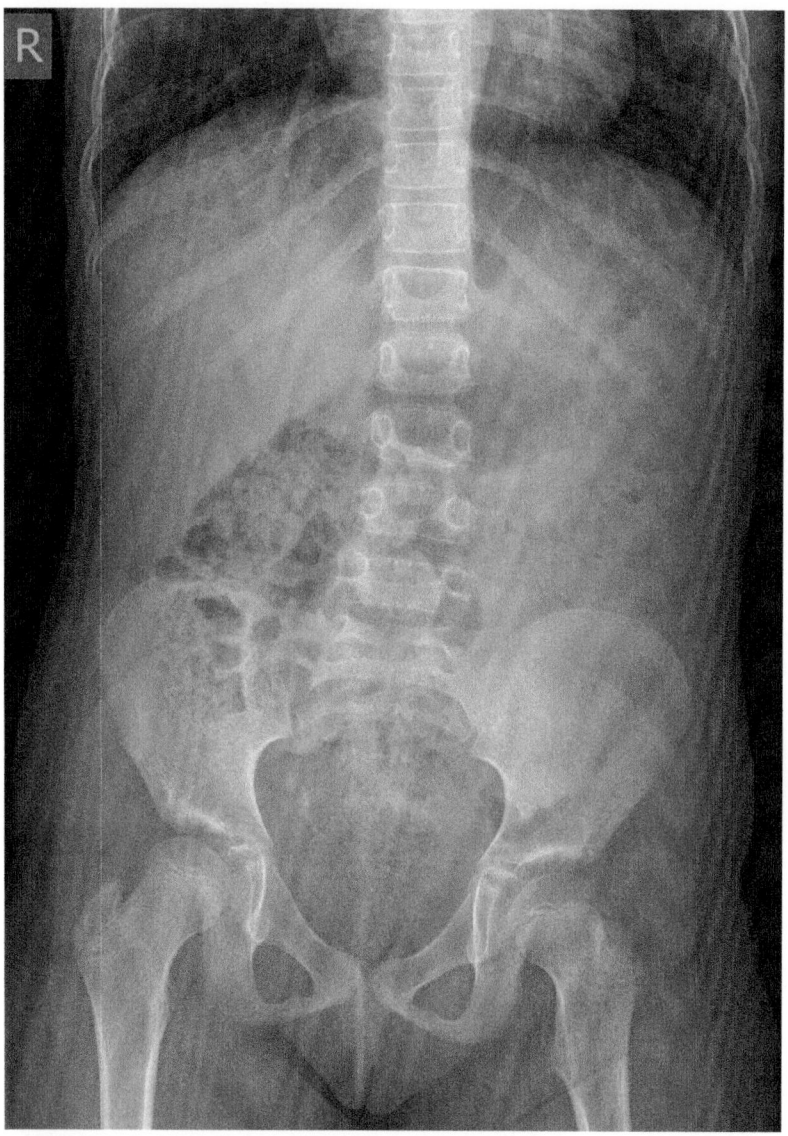

Normal	Abnormal	Diagnosis/Abnormality (only if abnormal)

Image 27

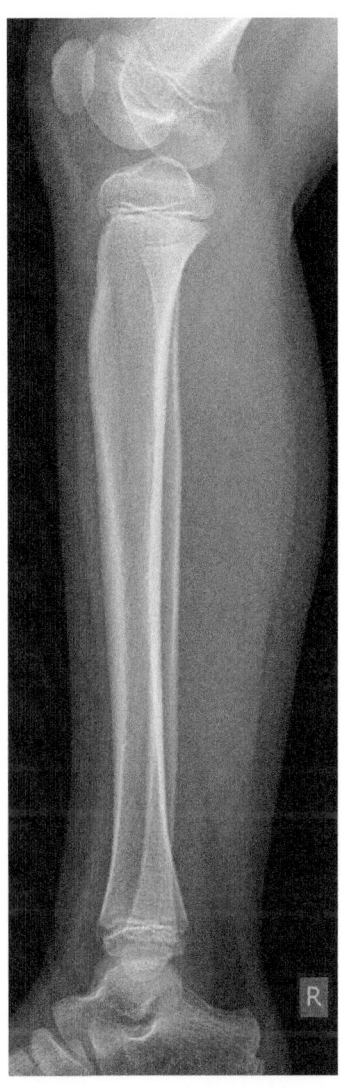

Normal	Abnormal	Diagnosis/Abnormality (only if abnormal)

Image 28

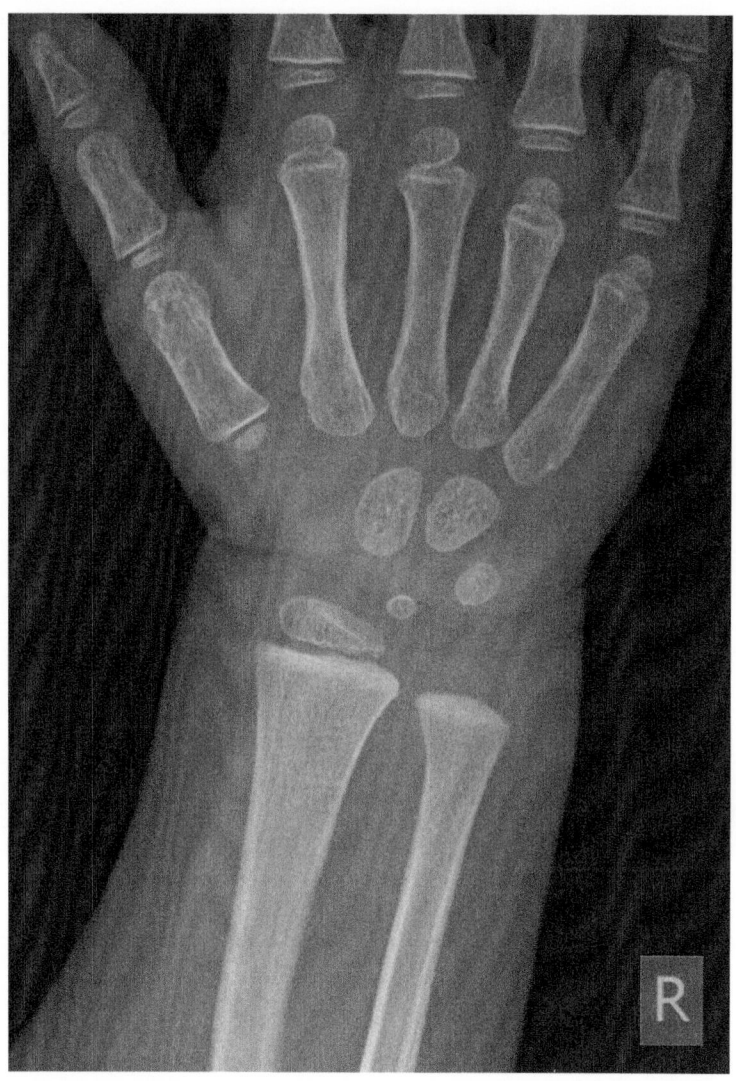

Normal	Abnormal	Diagnosis/Abnormality (only if abnormal)

Image 29

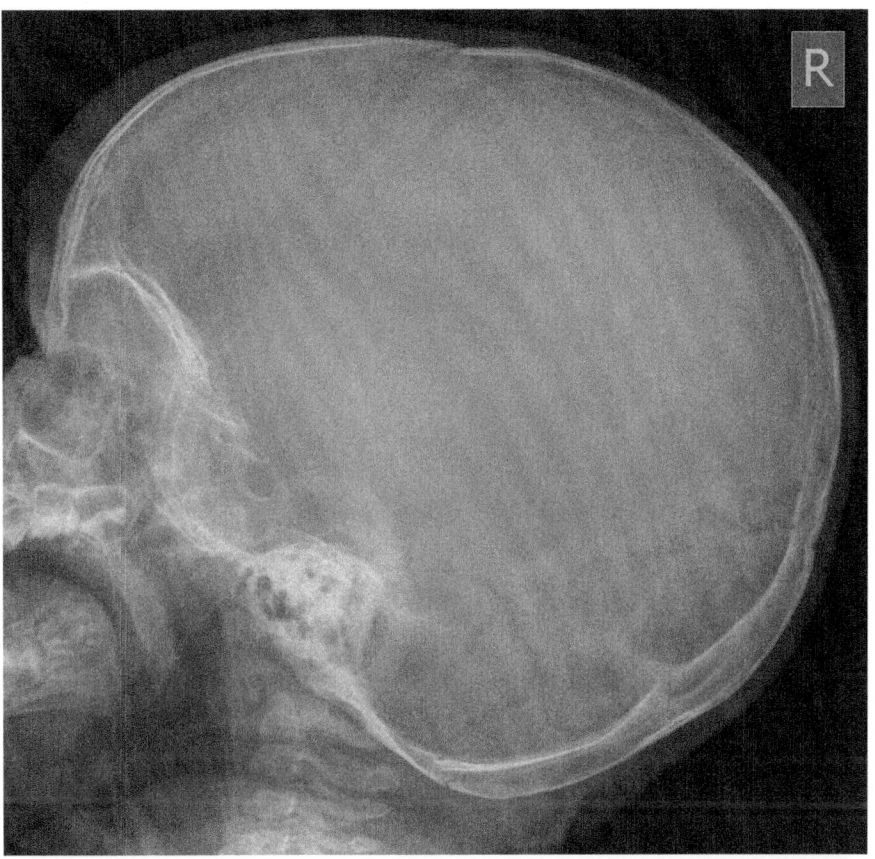

Normal	Abnormal	Diagnosis/Abnormality (only if abnormal)

Image 30

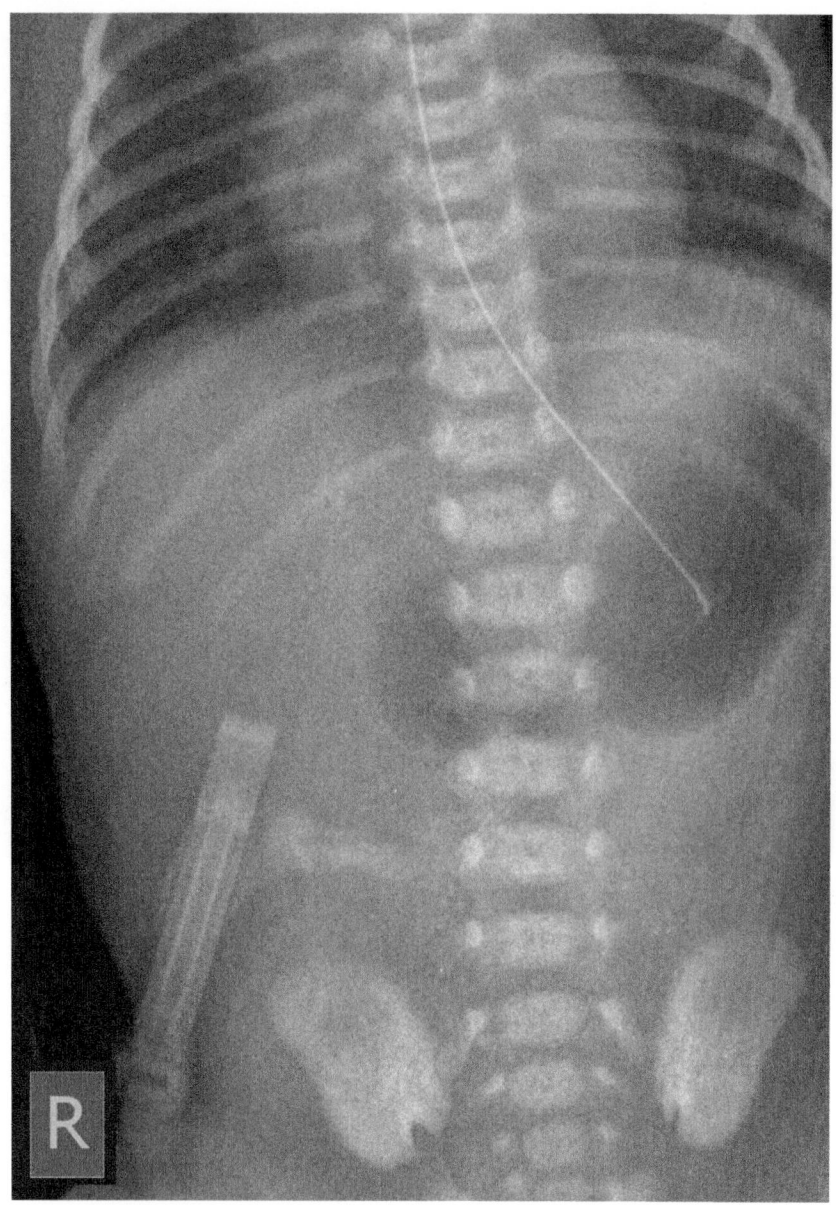

Normal	Abnormal	Diagnosis/Abnormality (only if abnormal)

5.2 Answers

Image	Normal	Abnormal	Diagnosis/abnormality (only if abnormal)
1		✓	Buckle # left distal radius
2	✓		
3	✓		
4		✓	Healing # right ninth posterior rib
5		✓	Fibrous cortical defect right distal medial femur
6	✓		
7	✓		
8		✓	Salter-Harris 2 # base right little toe proximal phalanx
9	✓		
10	✓		
11		✓	Right supracondylar #
12		✓	# left midshaft clavicle
13	✓		
14	✓		
15		✓	# base left fifth metatarsal
16	✓		
17		✓	Buckle #s left distal radius and ulna
18		✓	Salter-Harris 1 # right distal fibula
19	✓		
20		✓	Right frontal bone #
21	✓		
22		✓	Right slipped upper femoral epiphysis
23	✓		
24	✓		
25	✓		
26		✓	Multiple right distal ureteric calculi (Steinstrasse)
27	✓		
28	✓		
29	✓		
30		✓	Double bubble sign/duodenal atresia

5.3   Explanations

1. **Buckle # left distal radius**

2. **Normal physiological periosteal reaction**
   This radiograph is normal. Physiological periosteal reaction in the newborn is a common radiographic finding and can be seen in up to one-third of infants, usually between 1 and 4 months of age. The radiographic findings are typified by a 'benign' pattern of symmetrical periosteal reaction along the diaphyses, but *not* the metaphyses of long bones (the femora, tibiae, and humeri and less commonly radius and ulna).
   Periosteal reaction can range from benign to aggressive:
   Solid/unilamellar < multilamellated/'onion skin' < spiculated/'sun burst' < Codman's triangle.
   There is a differential when periosteal reaction has been identified depending on the clinical context:
   - Prostaglandin E therapy: in those infants who have a duct-dependent lesion (i.e. a congenital cardiac disorder or lesion which requires the patent ductus arteriosus [PDA] to remain open for survival), prostaglandin therapy is used to maintain PDA patency, usually until definitive surgical correction. The periosteal reaction may be diffuse, and there is usually a history of extended use and admission to a neonatal intensive/special care unit to support this radiographic finding.
   - **TORCH** infections: these are infections which are acquired either transplacentally or at birth. The mnemonic stands for: **T**oxoplasmosis; **O**thers (HIV and syphilis); **R**ubella; **C**ytomegalovirus (CMV); **H**erpes simplex.
     An important finding which may be seen in congenital rubella, syphilis, and CMV is irregularity, fraying, and longitudinally aligned linear bands of metaphyseal sclerosis known as 'celery stalk metaphysis'.
     A pathognomonic radiographic sign of congenital syphilis is the 'Wimberger sign' which refers to focal bilateral metaphyseal destruction of the medial aspect of the proximal tibia. However, this must not be confused with the 'Wimberger *ring* sign' which refers to dense sclerosis/calcification around an epiphysis, which itself (the centre) is relatively radiolucent, and is thought to result from bleeding and is seen in scurvy (hypovitaminosis C).
   - Suspected physical abuse/inflicted injury
   - Caffey disease: also known as infantile cortical hyperostosis, is usually a self-limiting disorder characterised by periostitis and soft tissue inflammation. Infants can present within the first few months of life with systemic features such as fever, irritability, erythema, and tender soft tissue swelling. The flat bones are typically affected, with the mandible constituting the majority of cases (75–80%). When long bones are involved, the ulnae are more commonly affected. The radiographic findings are typified by dense subperiosteal

new bone formation, subperiosteal cortical hyperostosis, sclerosis, and associated soft tissue swelling. If not self-limiting, long-term sequelae may result in remodelling, asymmetry, or synostosis of adjacent bones.

- Metastases: commonly from neuroblastoma but may be seen in lymphoma and/or leukaemia.

4. **Healing # right ninth posterior rib**
   Note the expanded callus consistent with a healing fracture, better visualised in the magnified image below:

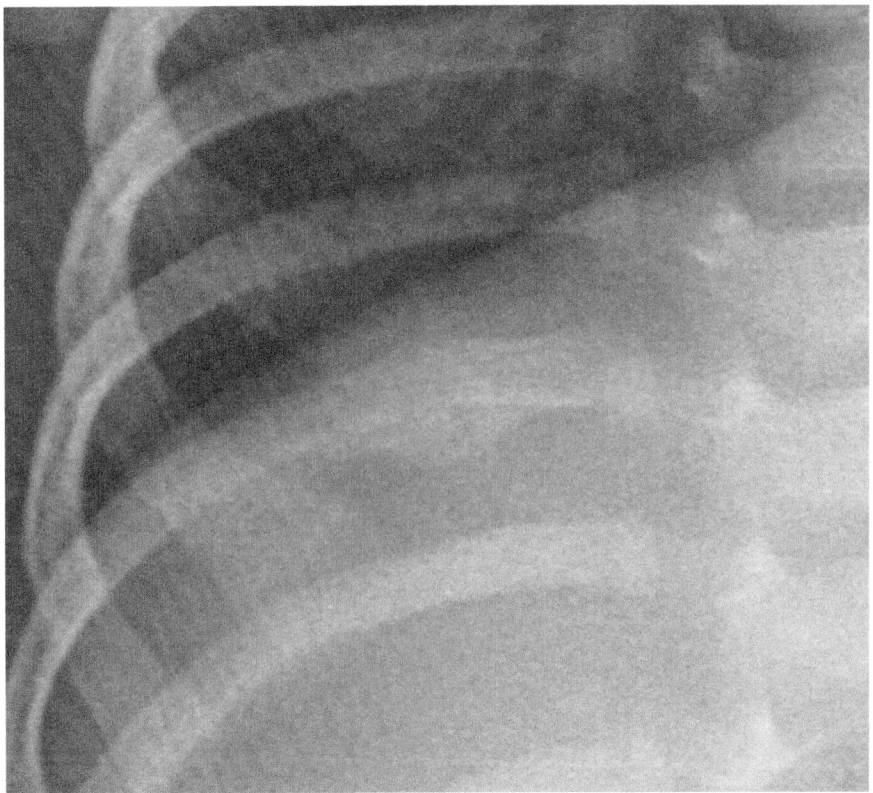

We emphasise that every rib (and indeed, every bony structure) must be scrutinised on every paediatric chest radiograph, not only in the examination but in clinical practice, also. Physical abuse in infants and young children is insidious and may present at any time—radiologists must be vigilant: acute/healing fractures may be detected on radiographs performed for another/unrelated indication and the radiologist may be the first to raise the suspicion of inflicted injury. This 4-month-old male was presented to the ED with unexplained bruising to his flanks.

Tip for the viva:
- Remember that the follow-up skeletal survey is a vital part of the imaging investigation for suspected physical abuse and is performed 11–14 days following the initial skeletal survey. Acute rib fractures may be missed on initial imaging and are more easily identified on follow-up radiographs as healing callus develops. Acute fractures are missed on radiographs because they are often incomplete, usually minimally displaced, and may be difficult to differentiate from bronchial and vascular markings.

5. **Fibrous cortical defect right distal medial femur**
   Fibrous cortical defects (FCDs) are benign, lucent, 'do not touch' lesions which are common: there is a male predilection. The appearances are characterised by lucent lesions confined to the cortex with a thin rim of sclerosis and no involvement of the underlying medullary cavity. There is no associated periosteal reaction. Given their ubiquity and benignity, further imaging is not required (and discouraged). See the FCD in the magnified image below:

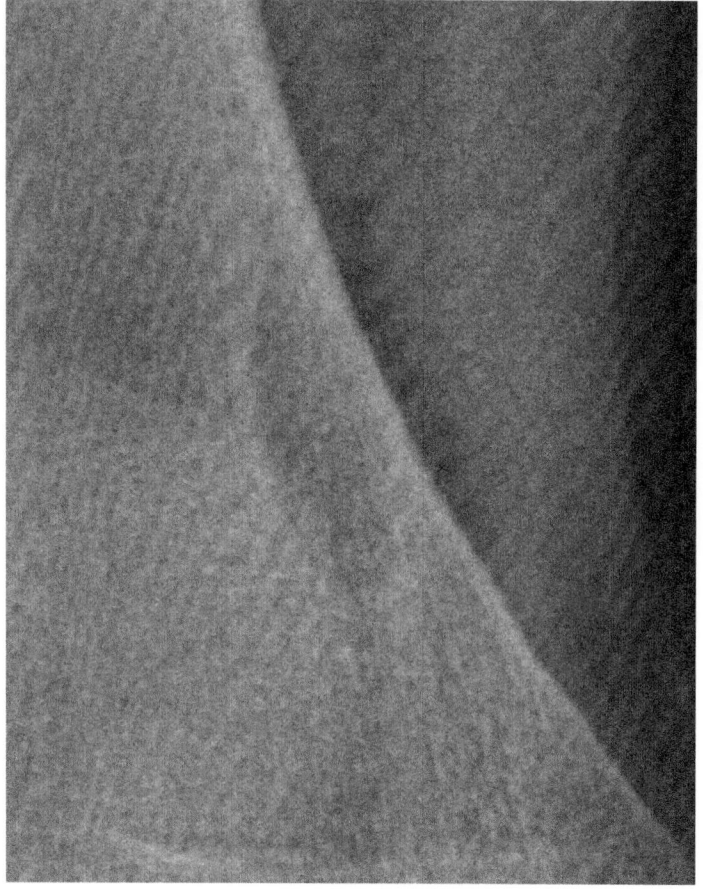

   Non-ossifying fibromas (NOF) are histologically similar to FCDs but by definition measure greater than 3 cm (FCDs measure less than 3 cm).

6. **Normal left forearm radiograph**

   This radiograph is normal. The rectangular 'bump' along the ulnar aspect of the distal ulna represents the subperiosteal bone collar, which is found at the end of long bones and is a normal finding.

7. **Normal left elbow**

   This radiograph is normal. The small osseous fragment adjacent to the lateral aspect of the capitellum is the normal ossification centre of the lateral epicondyle. There is no associated soft tissue swelling and the surrounding muscle-fat planes are preserved. The lucency in the left radial tuberosity is normal and is the site of insertion of the left biceps brachii tendon. Note the not yet completely ossified trochlear epiphysis which is a little fragmented but is also normal.

8. **Salter-Harris 2 # base right little toe proximal phalanx**

11. **Right supracondylar fracture**

   See the explanation for Test 1, Image 11.

12. **# left midshaft clavicle**

15. **# base left fifth metatarsal**

   See the explanation for Test 1, Image 7. There is an acute transversely orientated fracture through the base of the left fifth metatarsal with adjacent soft tissue swelling.

16. **Normal left wrist radiograph**

   The focus of ossification projected over the joint space between the left triquetrum and hamate is the ossification centre for the left pisiform bone.

17. **Buckle #s left distal radius and ulna**

18. **Salter-Harris 1 # right distal fibula**

   See the explanation for Test 1, Image 30 where the Salter-Harris classification is described. Note the lateral widening of the right distal fibular physis with overlying soft tissue swelling. These fractures must not be overlooked; often the key finding is the disproportionate amount of soft tissue swelling overlying a widened physis (compare the right distal fibular and tibial physes).

20. **Right frontal bone #**

   It is important that you are able to differentiate normal suture lines from fractures. Note the right frontal bone fracture projected over the superomedial aspect of the right orbit seen in the magnified image below:

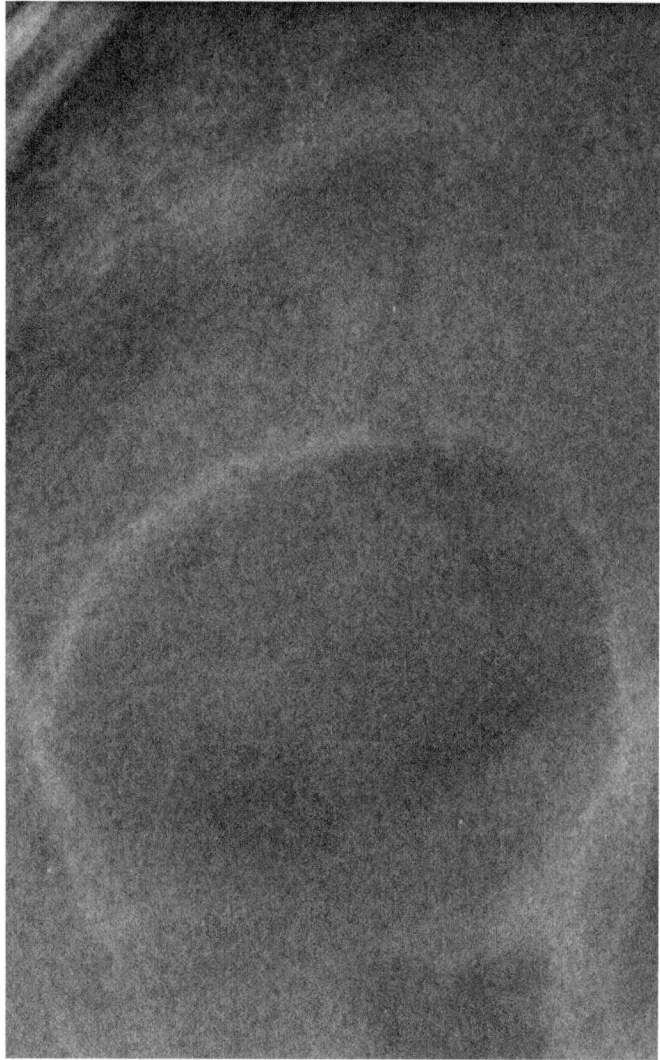

22. **Right slipped upper femoral epiphysis**
   See the explanation for Test 2, Image 12.

26. **Multiple right distal ureteric calculi (Steinstrasse)**
   The abnormality in this radiograph is subtle but again reinforces the point that
   one must adopt a systematic approach when interpreting any radiograph. Once
   you have seen the abnormality, as magnified in the image below, the asymmetry
   between both sides of the pelvis cannot be ignored:

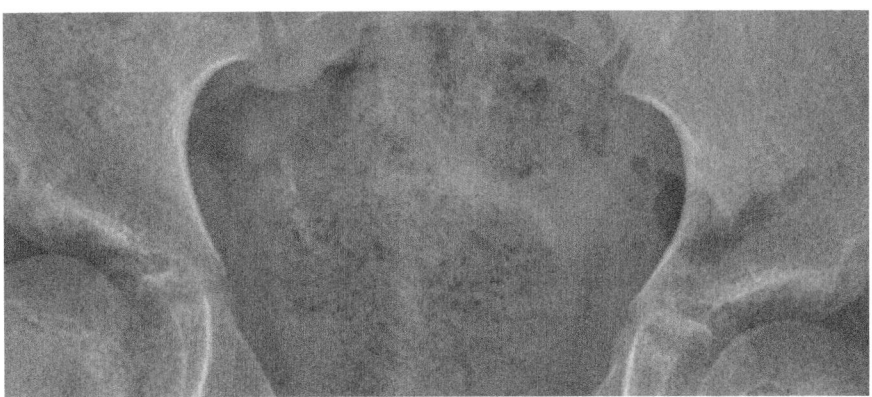

The term 'Steinstrasse', literally German for *stone street*, describes a column of calculi that blocks the ureter; however, the term is generally used in the context of distal ureteric obstruction as a complication following extracorporeal shock wave lithotripsy (EWSL).

29. **Normal skull radiograph**

This radiograph is normal. The intrasural bones seen in the lambdoid sutures are normal.

The differential diagnosis for multiple Wormian bones (more than 10) includes:

- **P**yknodysostosis
- **O**steogenesis imperfecta
- **R**ickets
- **K**inky hairy syndrome (also known as Menkes disease)
- **C**leidocranial dysplasia
- **H**ypothyroidism; **H**ypophosphatasia
- **O**topalatodigital syndrome
- **P**rimary acro-osteolysis (also known as Hajdu-Cheney); **P**achydermoperiostosis
- **S**yndrome of Down's (Trisomy 21)

30. **Double bubble sign/duodenal atresia**

This radiograph shows the classic 'double bubble sign' of duodenal atresia: the stomach and first part of the duodenum are distended, and gas filled, with an absence of distal gas indicating complete atresia (i.e. a blind ending duodenum). This is thought to result from failure of recanalisation of the bowel lumen (which is a solid tube in fetal life) which should occur around the end of the first trimester.

Affected patients present with vomiting and abdominal distension secondary to duodenal obstruction. If the atretic segment is distal to the ampulla of Vater, there will be bilious vomiting; if the atresia is proximal to the ampulla, the vomiting will be non-bilious.

Duodenal atresia is associated with other conditions:

- Down syndrome (Trisomy 21): approximately 30% of those infants with duodenal atresia may have Down syndrome; conversely approximately 3% of those with Down syndrome may have duodenal atresia.
- VACTERL syndrome: which constitutes the following constellation of congenital abnormalities:
  - **V**ertebral anomalies: these may comprise of hemivertebrae, butterfly vertebrae, or block vertebrae; caudal regression; and/or spina bifida.
  - **A**norectal anomalies: includes the spectrum of anal atresia which can range from a membranous separation or complete congenital absence. Following clinical evaluation by surgical colleagues, a lower GI contrast examination may be required to delineate the anatomy and evaluate the presence of fistula (e.g. recto-vesical). Anal atresia is itself associated with duodenal atresia.
  - **C**ardiac anomalies: examination with echocardiography is indicated in this clinical context to exclude a structural defect.
  - **T**racheo-oesophageal fistula (TOF, in the UK) ± oesophageal atresia (OA): the history is typically that of antenatal polyhydramnios and failure to pass a nasogastric tube (NGT) at birth. Radiographs will show the distal portion of the NGT coiled in the proximal oesophageal pouch. This is then usually replaced with a Replogle tube (a double lumen tube which [in contrast to an NGT] has a number of side holes). The Replogle tube rests in the proximal oesophageal pouch to simultaneously irrigate and aspirate secretions/debris. There are five types of TOF with which you should be familiar. The most common type (type A, 85%) comprises of a proximal OA with a distal TOF. The presence of gas in the stomach and bowel on radiography indicates that a distal fistula is present and is useful to remember in the examination setting.
  - **R**enal anomalies: These may include the spectrum of cystic renal disease (autosomal recessive polycystic kidney disease [ARPKD], multicystic dysplastic kidney [MCDK]), pre-tumorous (nephroblastomatosis), and tumorous conditions (mesoblastic nephroma, multilocular cystic nephroma), obstructive renal disease (congenital pelviureteric junction [PUJ] obstruction), positional abnormalities (e.g. crossed fused renal ectopia), and renal dys/agenesis.
  - **R**adial ray anomalies: these are characterised by unilateral or bilateral absence (aplasia/hypoplasia) of varying portions of the radius and thumb.
  - **L**imb anomalies: usually polydactyly.
- Other intestinal atresias:
  - Jejunal
  - Ileal
  - Anal: as described above.
- Annular pancreas: this is a developmental/embryonic abnormality in which the pancreas encases the duodenum which may lead to duodenal obstruction.

Note that a complete or severely obstructing duodenal web can also give the 'double bubble' radiographic appearance; often the web will occur in the second part of the duodenum. If the web is partial/not completely obstructing, there will usually be some distal gas visualised. A 'triple bubble sign' may be seen in jejunal atresia—the atresia can be anywhere from the ligament of Treitz (the duodenojejunal [DJ] flexure) to the jejunoileal junction. Additionally, there may be more than one atretic jejunal segment.

Tip for the viva:
• Most paediatric surgical centres will have a pathway for evaluating infants with suspected VACTERL syndrome. Discuss this with your local paediatric radiologists and surgeons.

Further Reading

Image 2

Bell DJ et al (2018) Celery stalk metaphysis. https://radiopaedia.org/articles/celery-stalk-metaph-ysis. Accessed April 2018

Kwon DS, Spevak MR, Flecther K, Kleinman PK (2002) Physiologic subperiosteal new bone for-mation: prevalence, distribution and thickness in neonates and infants. AJR Am J Roentgenol 179(4):985–988

St-Amant M et al (2018a) Wimberger sign. https://radiopaedia.org/articles/wimberger-sign-1. Accessed April 2018

St-Amant M et al (2018b) Wimberger ring sign. https://radiopaedia.org/articles/wimberger-ring-sign-1. Accessed April 2018

University of Virginia (2018) Newborn periosteal reaction. https://www.med-ed.virginia.edu/courses/rad/peds/ms_webpages/ms6cnewperrxn.html. Accessed April 2018

University of Washington (2018) Periosteal reaction. https://rad.washington.edu/about-us/aca-demic-sections/musculoskeletal-radiology/teaching-materials/online-musculoskeletal-radiol-ogy-book/periosteal-reaction/. Accessed August 2018

van der Woude JH, Smithuis R (2010) Bone tumor – systemic approach and differential diagnosis. http://www.radiologyassistant.nl/en/p494e15cbf0d8d/bone-tumor-systematic-approach-and-differential-diagnosis.html#i4b331f308764e. Accessed April 2018

Image 4

Please see the Test 2, Image 14 references regarding the imaging of suspected physical abuse in infants and young children

Image 5

Blaz M, Palczewski P, Swiatkowski J, Golebiowski M (2011) Cortical fibrous defects and non-ossifying fibromas in children and young adults: The analysis of radiological features in 28 cases and a review of literature. Pol J Radiol. 76(4):32–39

Levine SM, Lambiase RE, Petchprapa CN (2003) Cortical lesions of the tibia: characteristic appearances at conventional radiography. Radiographics. 23(1):157–177

Weeakkody Y, Gaillard F et al (2018) Fibrous cortical defect. https://radiopaedia.org/articles/fibrous-cortical-defect. Accessed May 2018

Image 26

Bickle I, Sorrentino S et al (2018) Steinstrasse. https://radiopaedia.org/articles/steinstrasse. Accessed May 2018

Sayed MA, el-Taher AM, Aboul-Ella HA, Shaker SE (2001) Steinstrasse after extracorporeal shockwave lithotripsy: aetiology, prevention and management. BJU Int. 88(7):675–678

Image 29

Gaillard F et al (2018) Wormian bones (mnemonic). https://radiopaedia.org/articles/wormian-bones-mnemonic. Accessed July 2018

Marti B, Sirinelli D, Maurin L, Carpentier E (2013) Wormian bones in a general population. Diagn Interv Imaging. 94(4):428–432

Image 30

Bell DJ, Gaillard F et al (2018) Congenital tracheo-oesophageal fistula. https://radiopaedia.org/articles/congenital-tracheo-oesophageal-fistula. Accessed May 2018

Gaillard F et al (2018a) Double bubble sign (duodenum). https://radiopaedia.org/articles/double-bubble-sign-duodenum. Accessed May 2018

Gaillard F et al (2018b) VACTERL association. https://radiopaedia.org/articles/vacterl-association-1. Accessed May 2018

Goel A, Jones J et al (2018) Duodenal atresia. https://radiopaedia.org/articles/duodenal-atresia. Accessed May 2018

Glick Y, Bickle I et al (2018) Triple bubble sign. https://radiopaedia.org/articles/triple-bubble-sign. Accessed May 2018

Hamidi H, Jones J et al (2018). Anal atresia. https://radiopaedia.org/articles/anal-atresia. Accessed May 2018

Hacking C, Jha P et al (2018) Annual pancreas. https://radiopaedia.org/articles/annular-pancreas

Kang O et al (2018) Congenital renal anomalies. https://radiopaedia.org/articles/congenital-renal-anomalies. Accessed May 2018

Vergult S, Hoogeboom AJ, Bijlsma EK et al (2013) Complex genetics of radial ray deficiencies: screening of a cohort of 54 patients. Genet Med 15(3):195–202

Weerakkody Y, Salam H et al (2018) Jejunal atresia. https://radiopaedia.org/articles/jejunal-atresia. Accessed May 2018

6.1   Images

Image 1

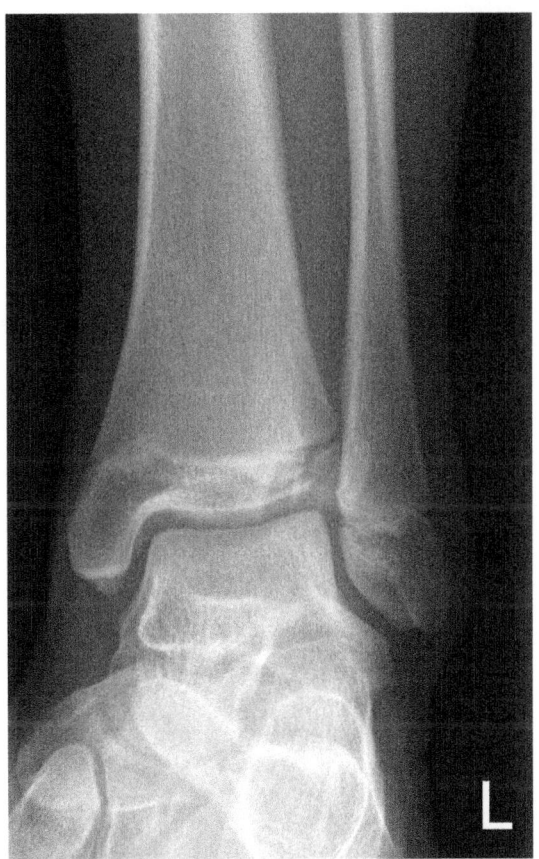

Normal	Abnormal	Diagnosis/Abnormality (only if abnormal)

Image 2

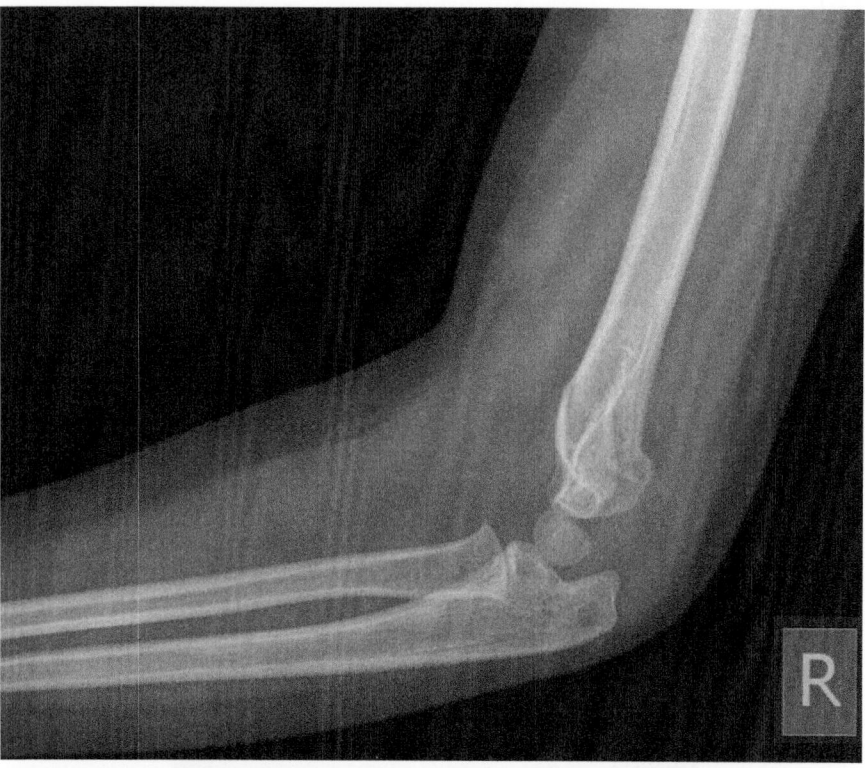

Normal	Abnormal	Diagnosis/Abnormality (only if abnormal)

Image 3

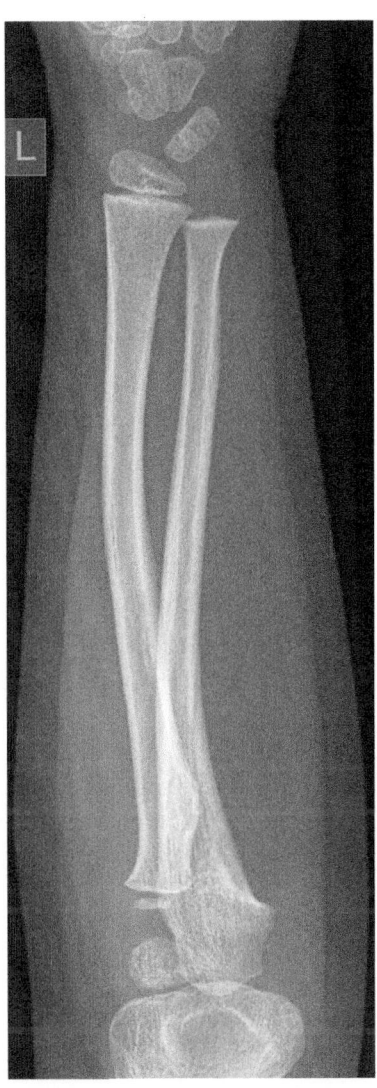

Normal	Abnormal	Diagnosis/Abnormality (only if abnormal)

Image 4

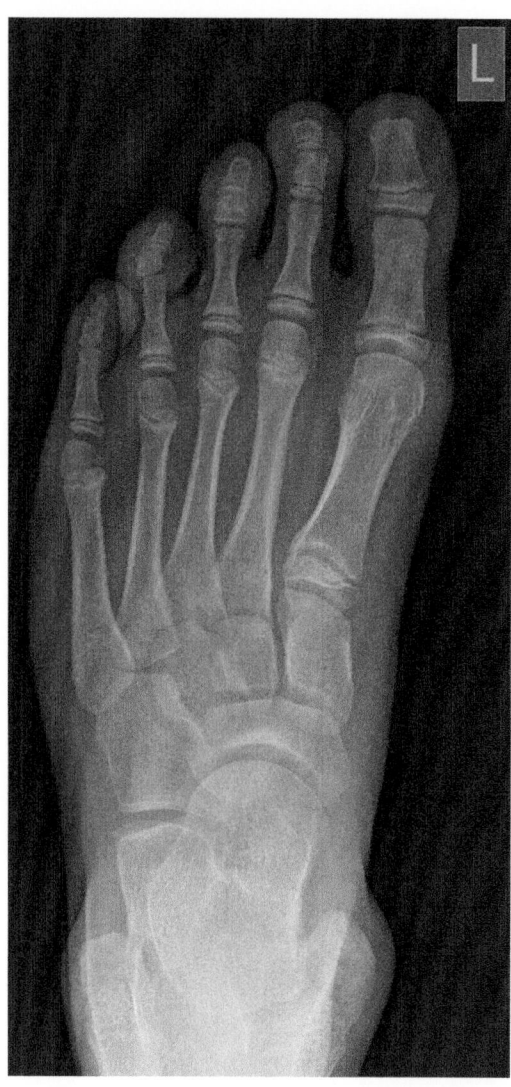

Normal	Abnormal	Diagnosis/Abnormality (only if abnormal)

Image 5

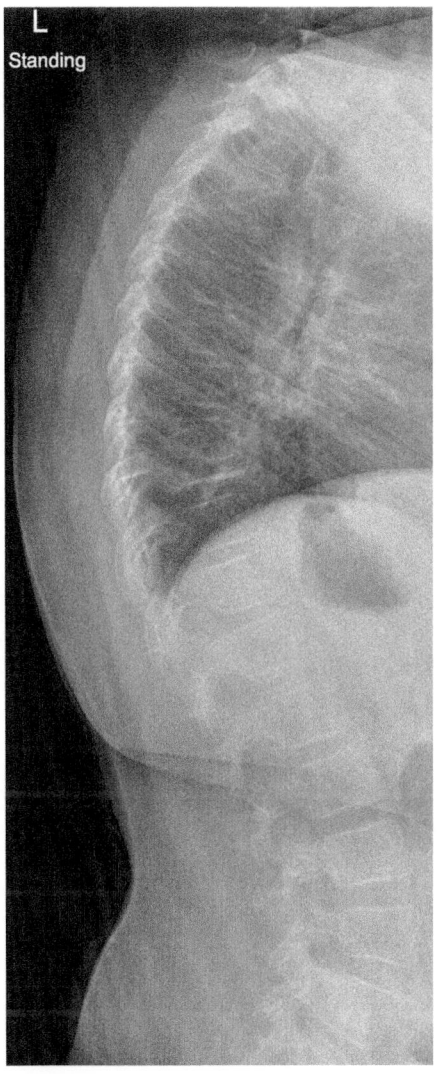

Normal	Abnormal	Diagnosis/Abnormality (only if abnormal)

Image 6

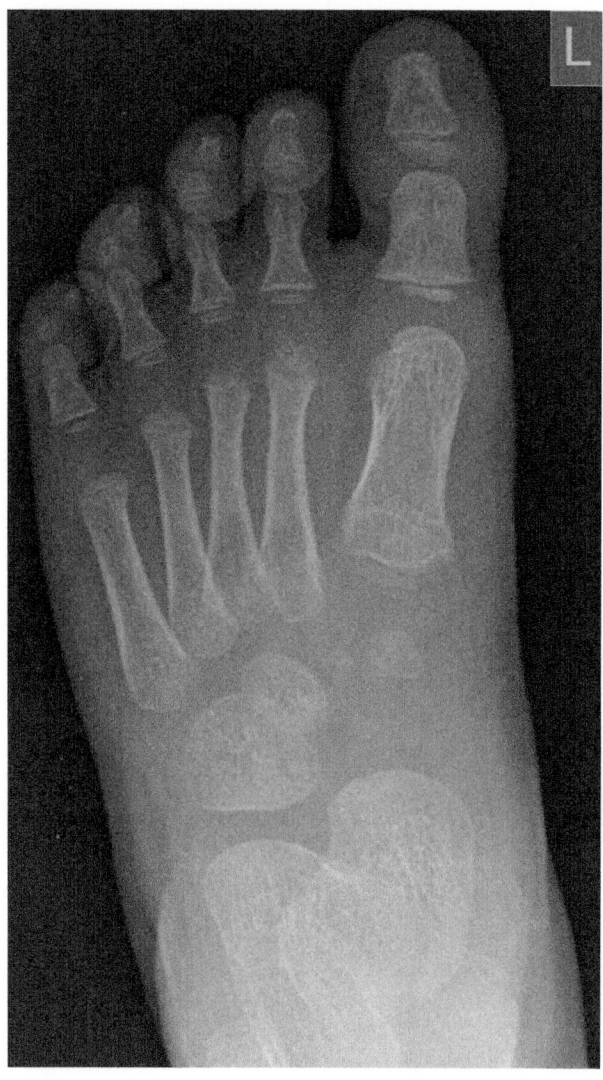

Normal	Abnormal	Diagnosis/Abnormality (only if abnormal)

Image 7

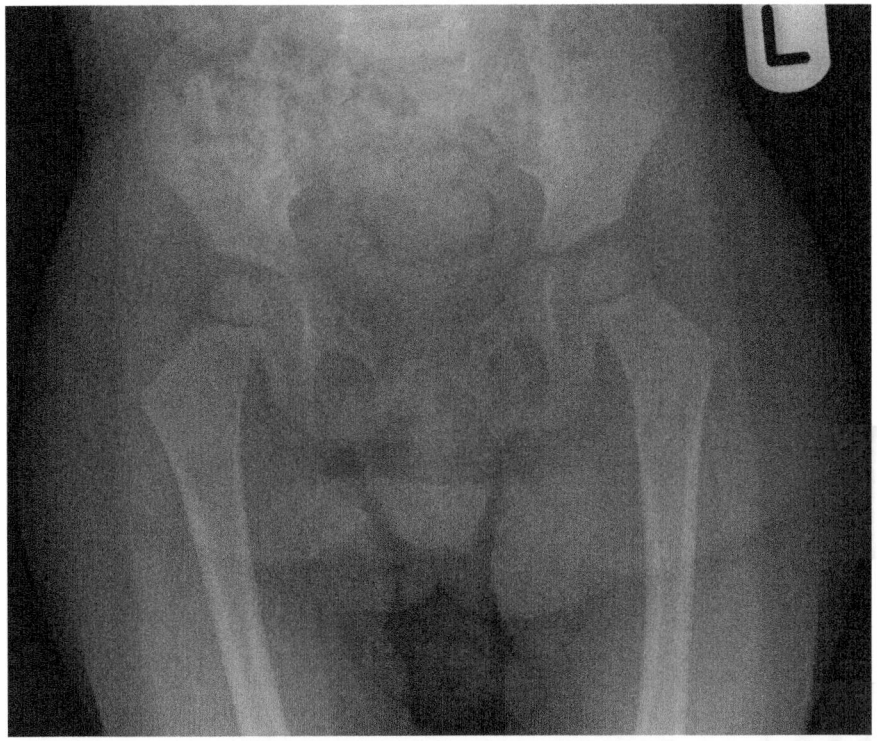

Normal	Abnormal	Diagnosis/Abnormality (only if abnormal)

Image 8

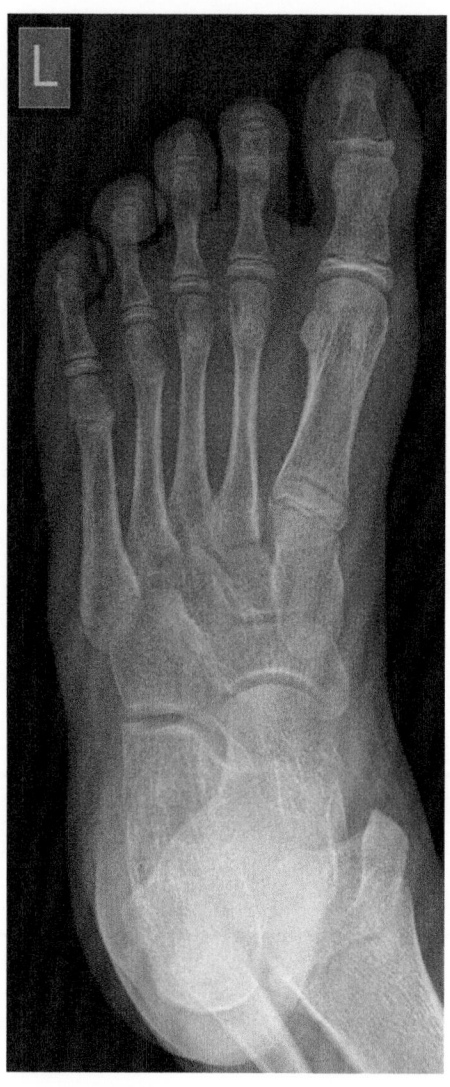

Normal	Abnormal	Diagnosis/Abnormality (only if abnormal)

Image 9

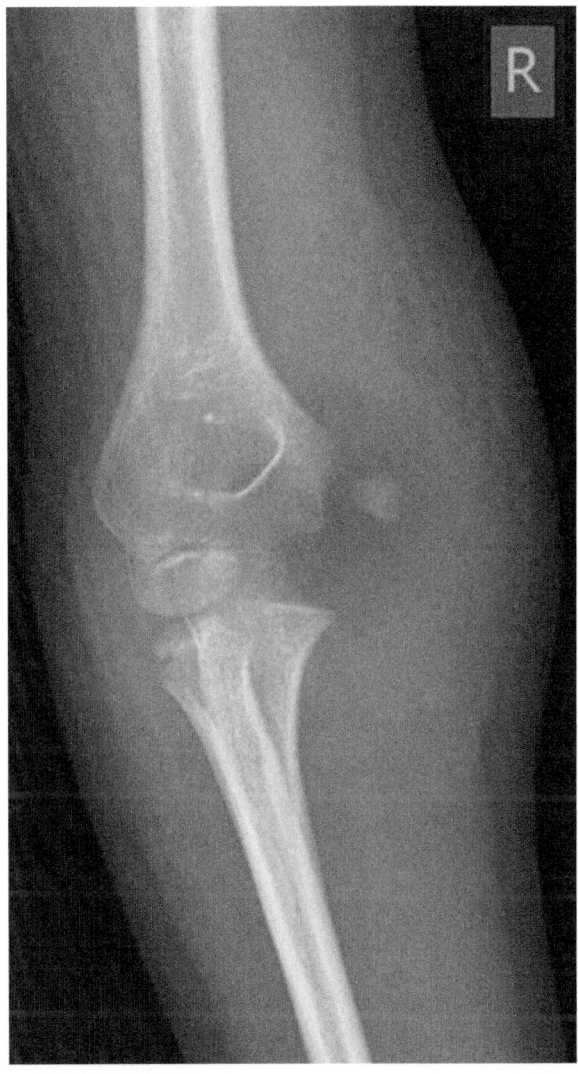

Normal	Abnormal	Diagnosis/Abnormality (only if abnormal)

Image 10

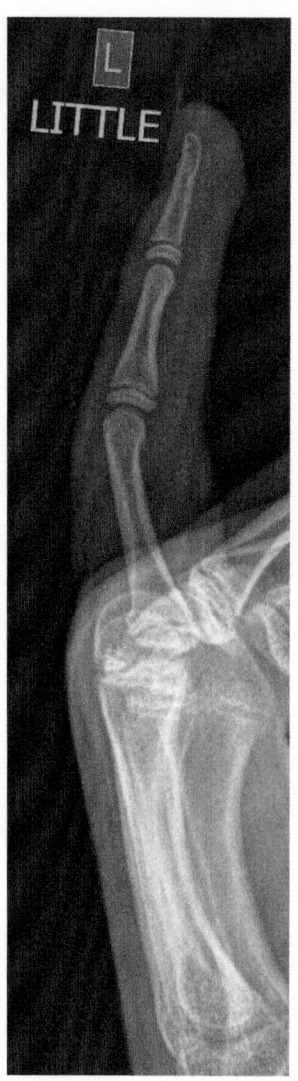

Normal	Abnormal	Diagnosis/Abnormality (only if abnormal)

Image 11

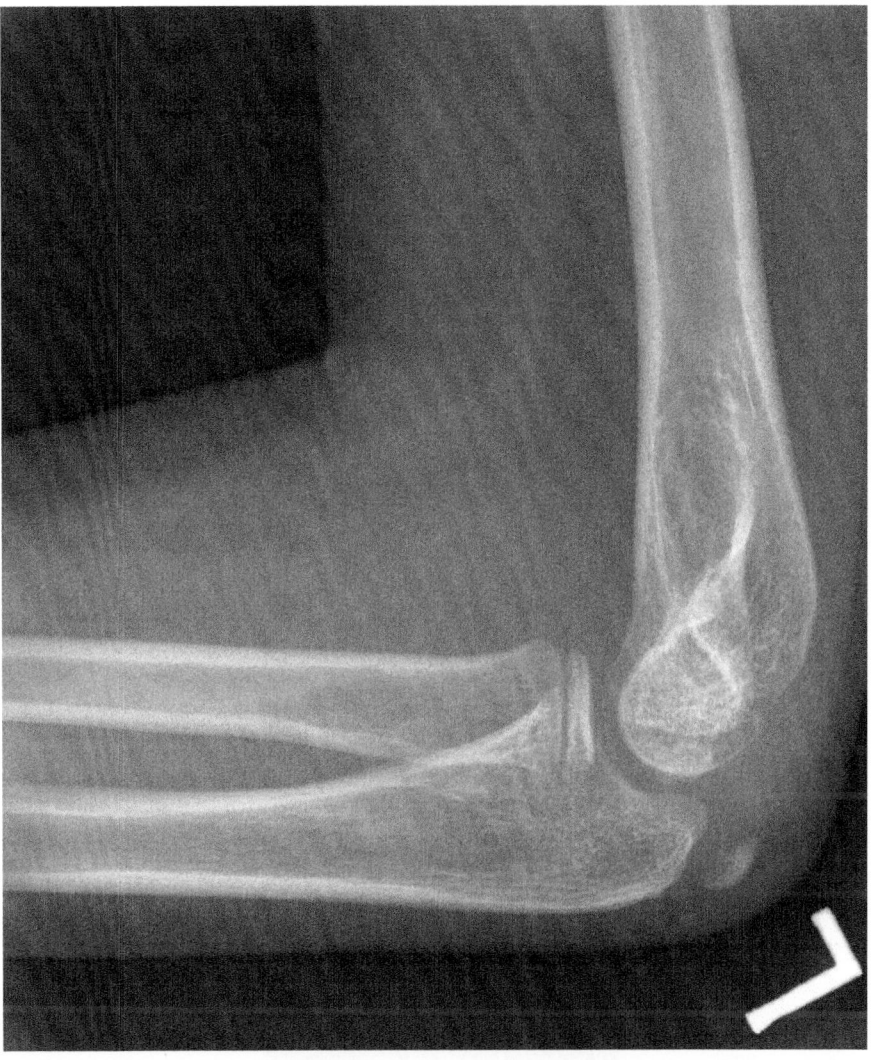

Normal	Abnormal	Diagnosis/Abnormality (only if abnormal)

Image 12

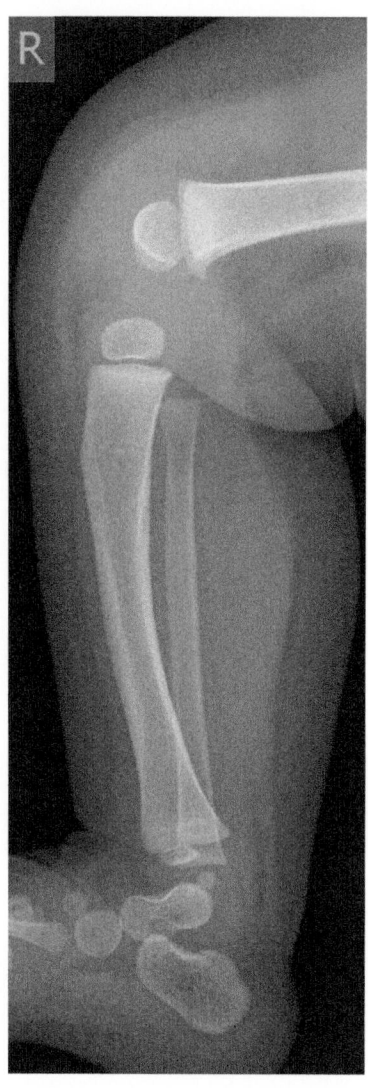

Normal	Abnormal	Diagnosis/Abnormality (only if abnormal)

Image 13

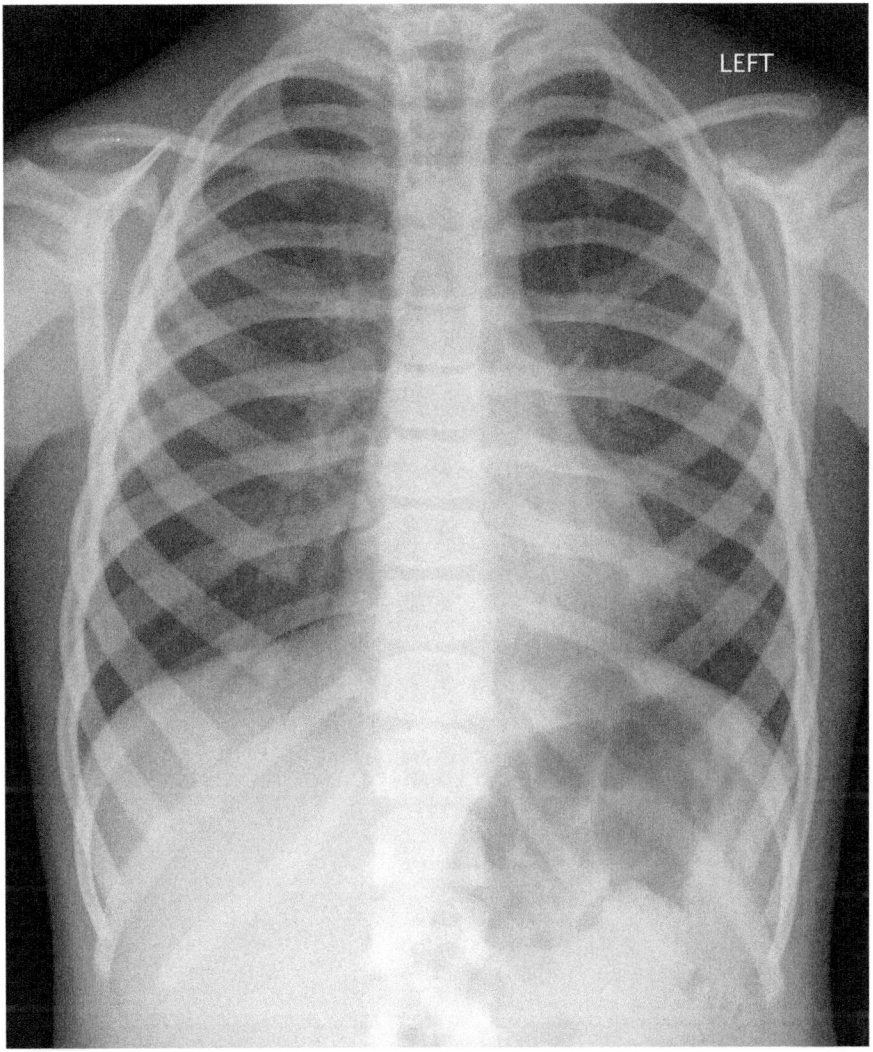

Normal	Abnormal	Diagnosis/Abnormality (only if abnormal)

Image 14

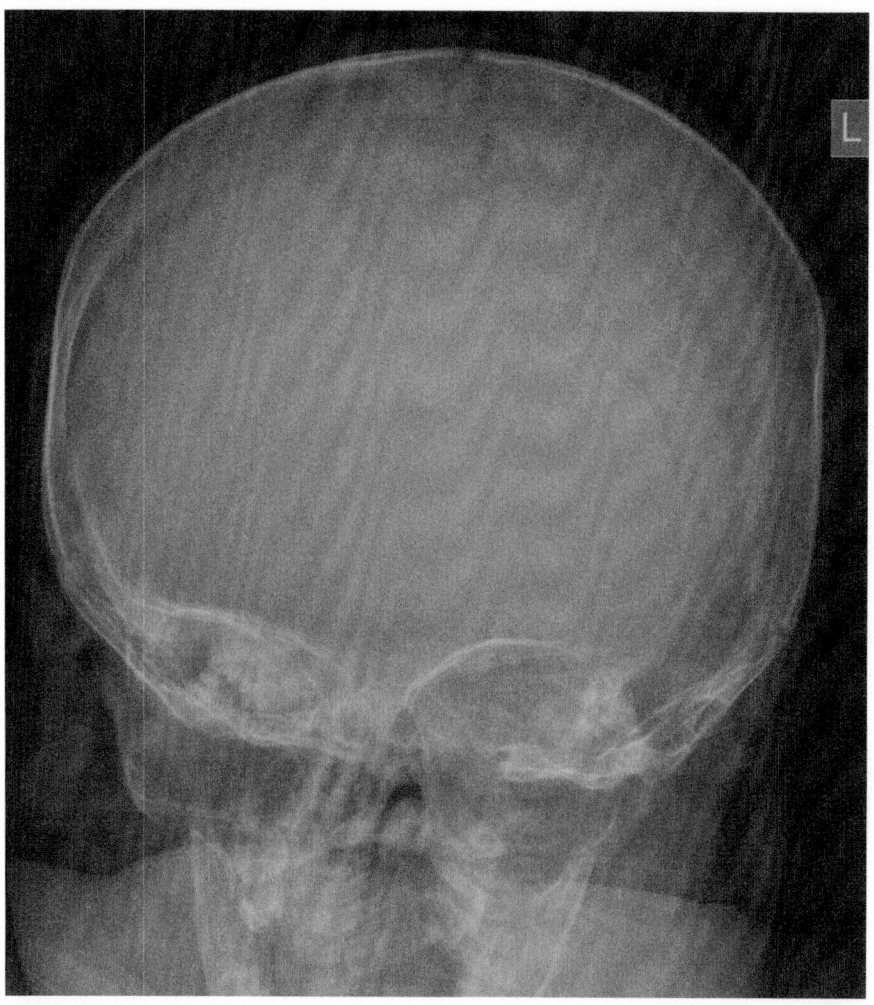

Normal	Abnormal	Diagnosis/Abnormality (only if abnormal)

Image 15

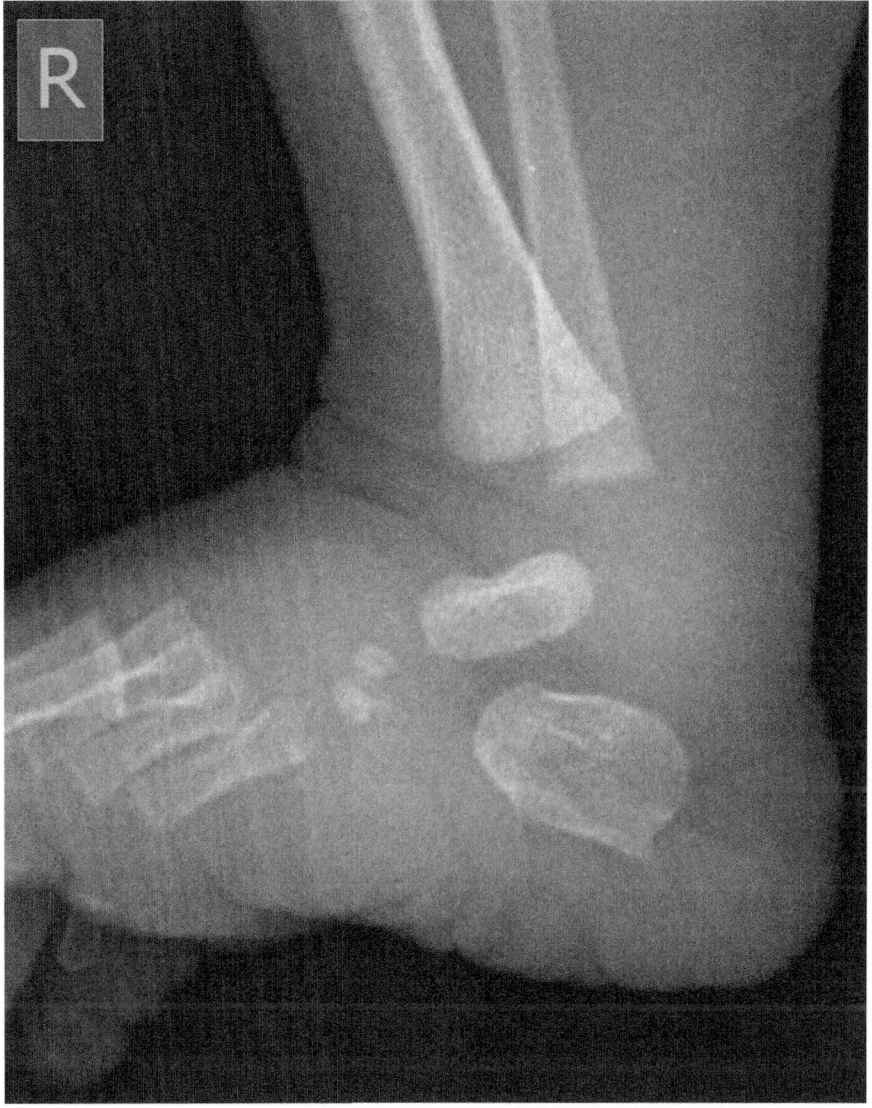

Normal	Abnormal	Diagnosis/Abnormality (only if abnormal)

Image 16

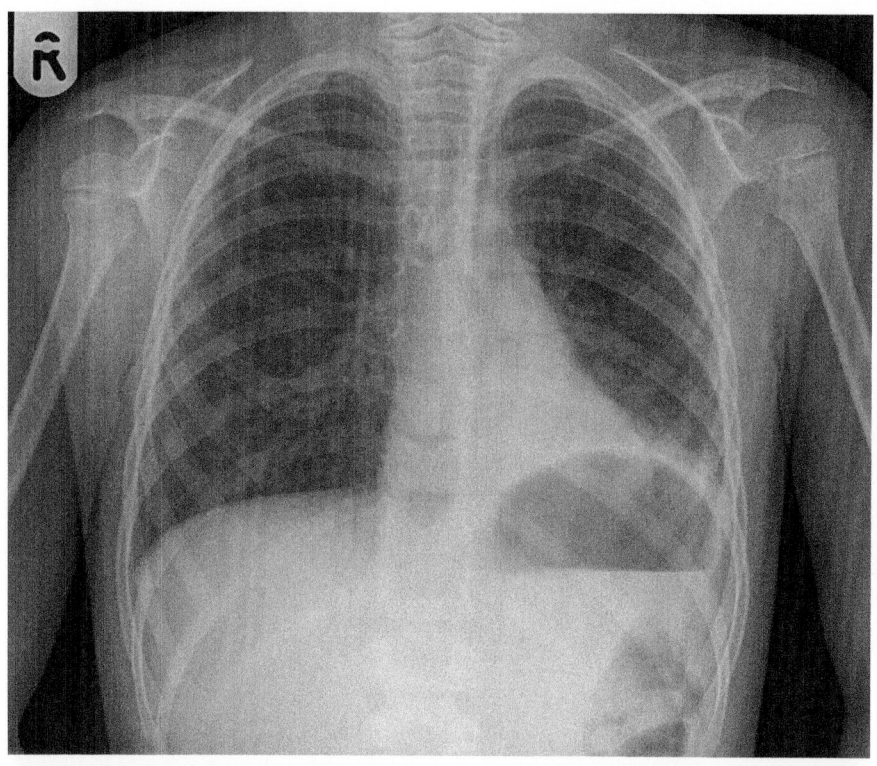

Normal	Abnormal	Diagnosis/Abnormality (only if abnormal)

Image 17

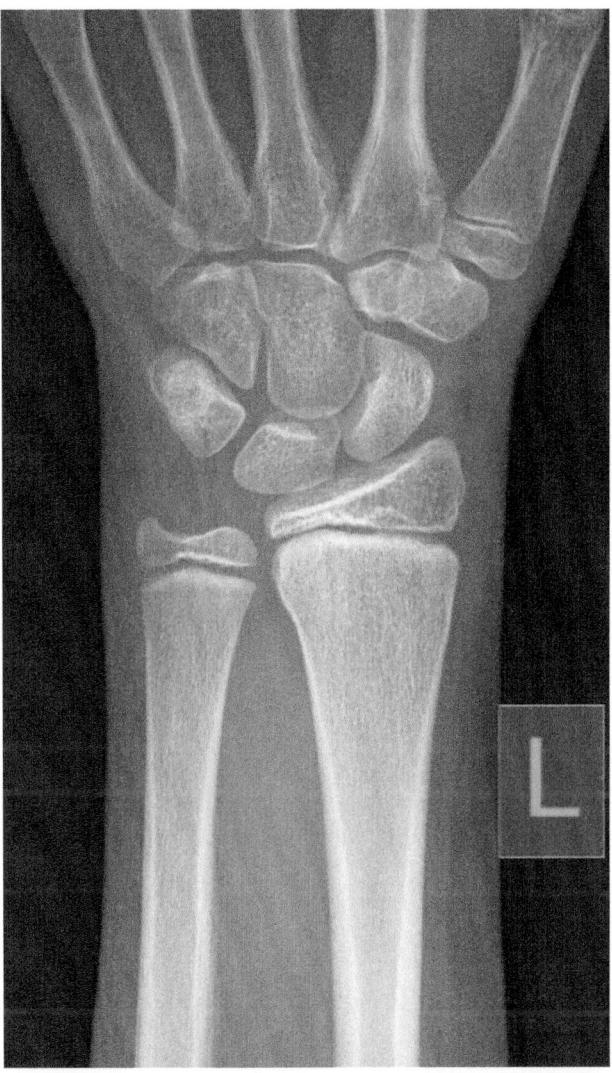

Normal	Abnormal	Diagnosis/Abnormality (only if abnormal)

Image 18

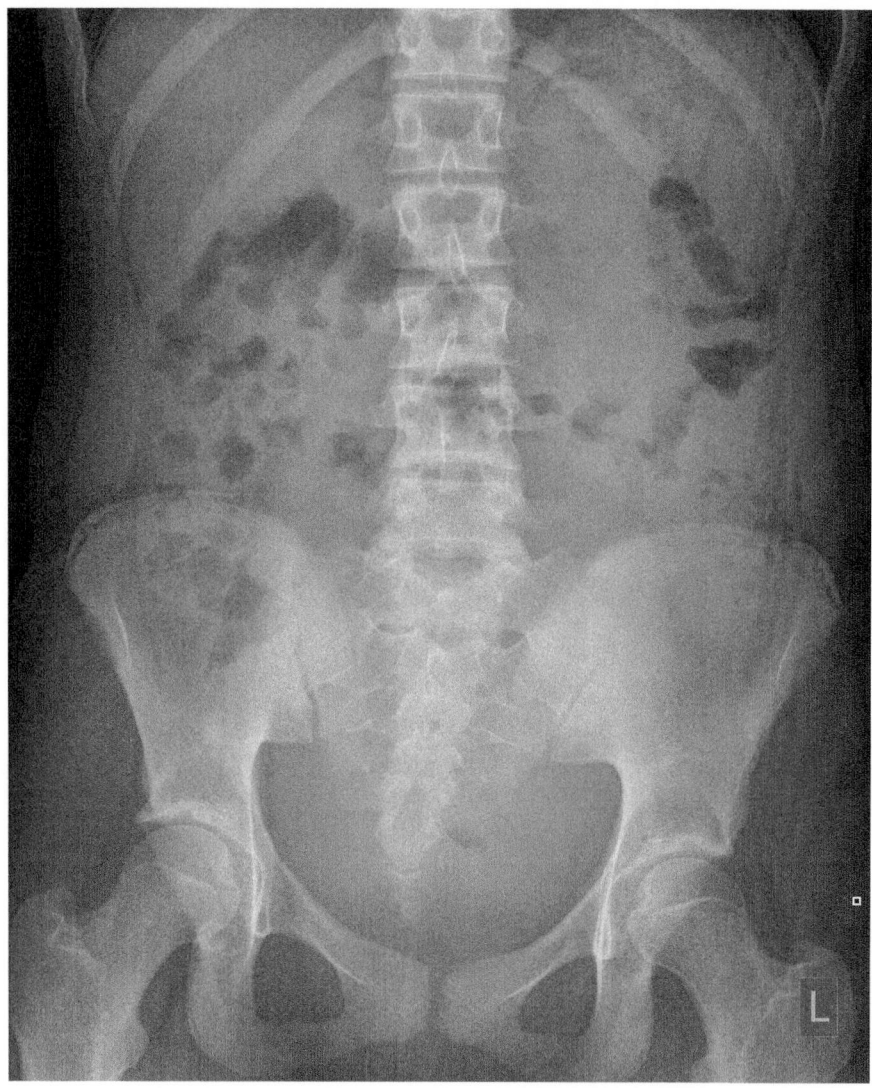

Normal	Abnormal	Diagnosis/Abnormality (only if abnormal)

Image 19

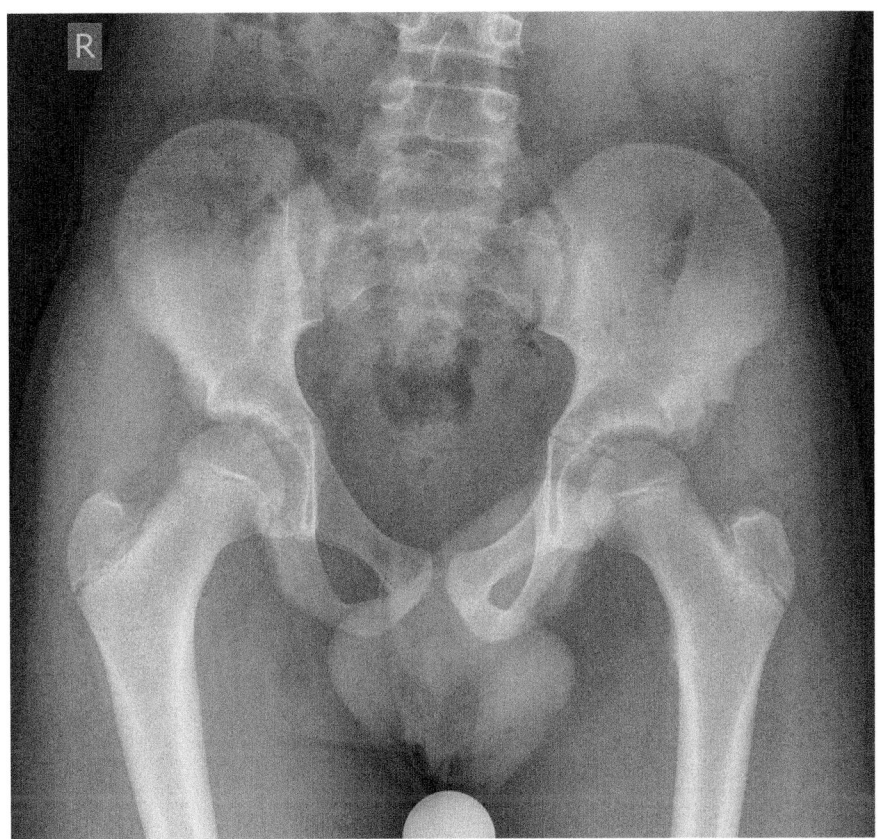

Normal	Abnormal	Diagnosis/Abnormality (only if abnormal)

Image 20

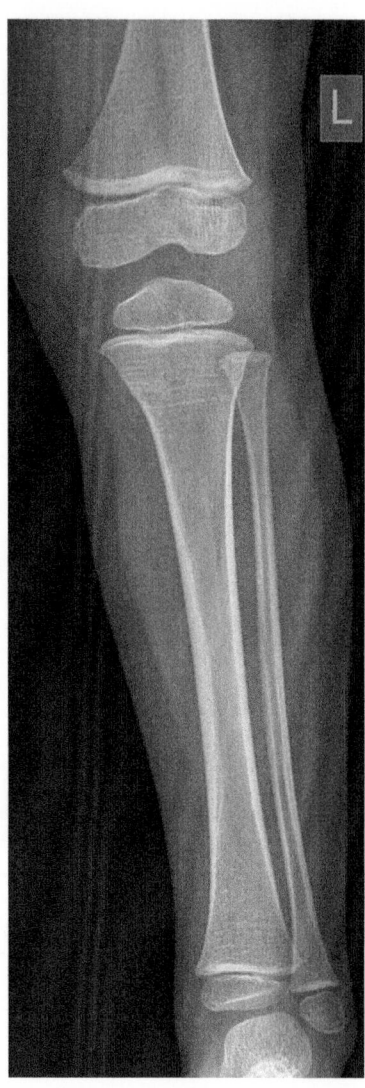

Normal	Abnormal	Diagnosis/Abnormality (only if abnormal)

Image 21

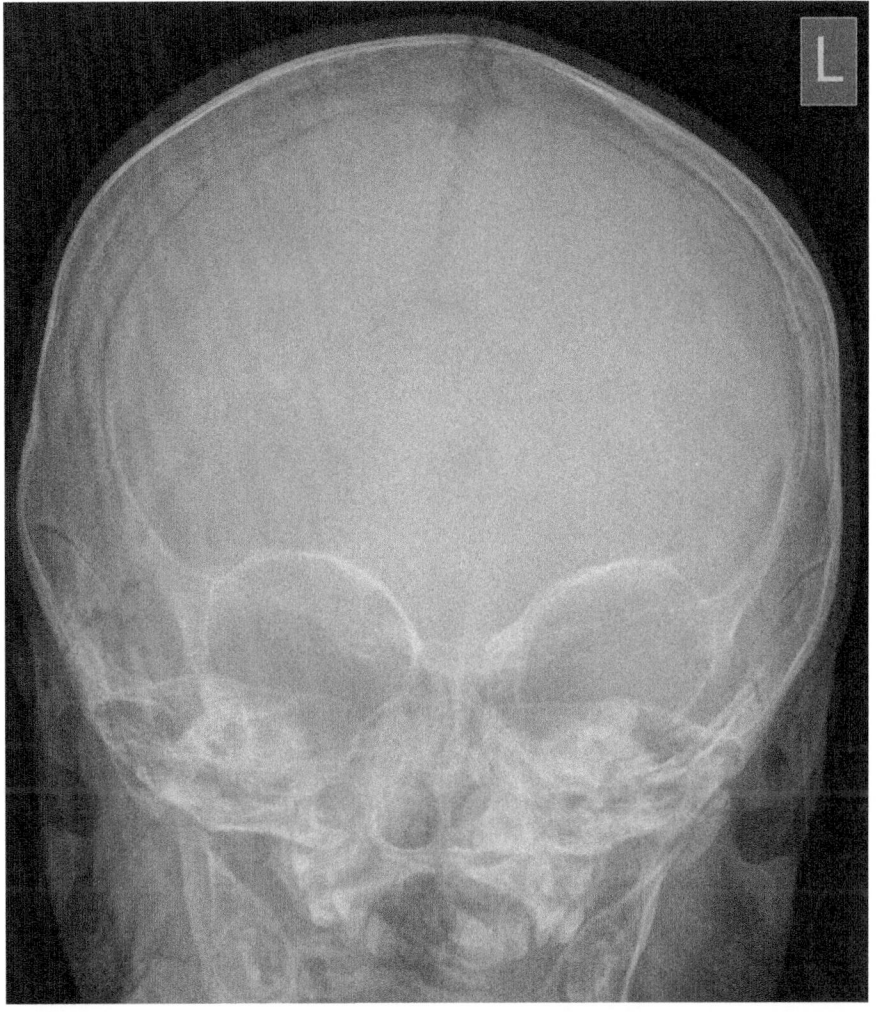

Normal	Abnormal	Diagnosis/Abnormality (only if abnormal)

Image 22

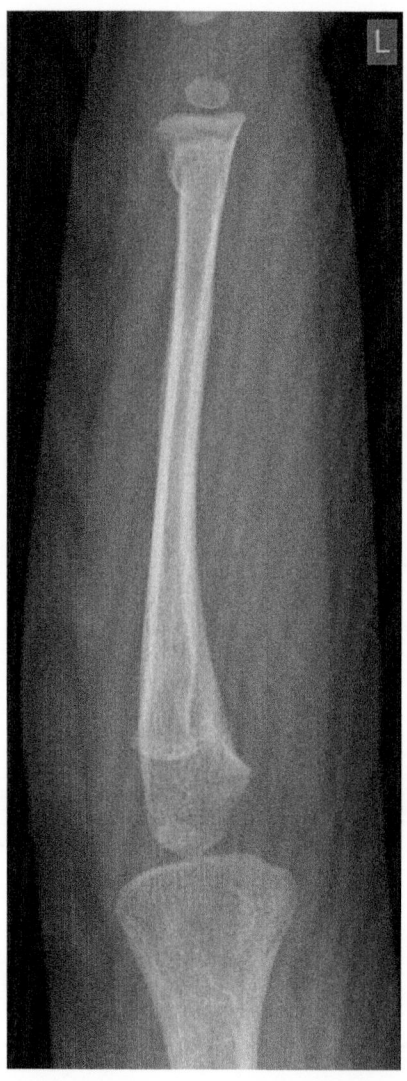

Normal	Abnormal	Diagnosis/Abnormality (only if abnormal)

Image 23

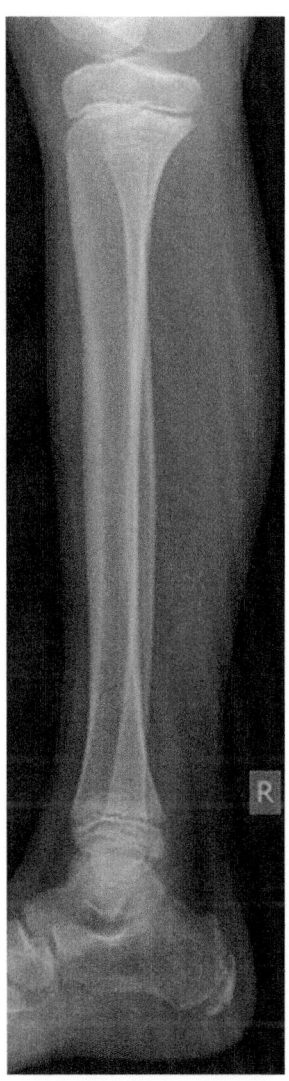

Normal	Abnormal	Diagnosis/Abnormality (only if abnormal)

Image 24

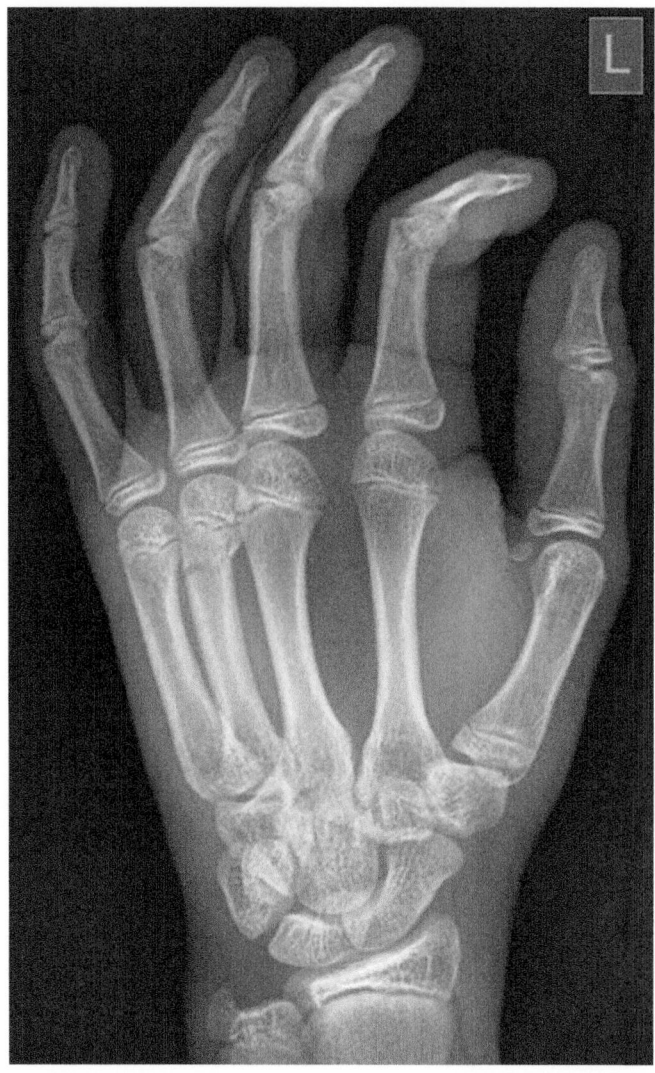

Normal	Abnormal	Diagnosis/Abnormality (only if abnormal)

Image 25

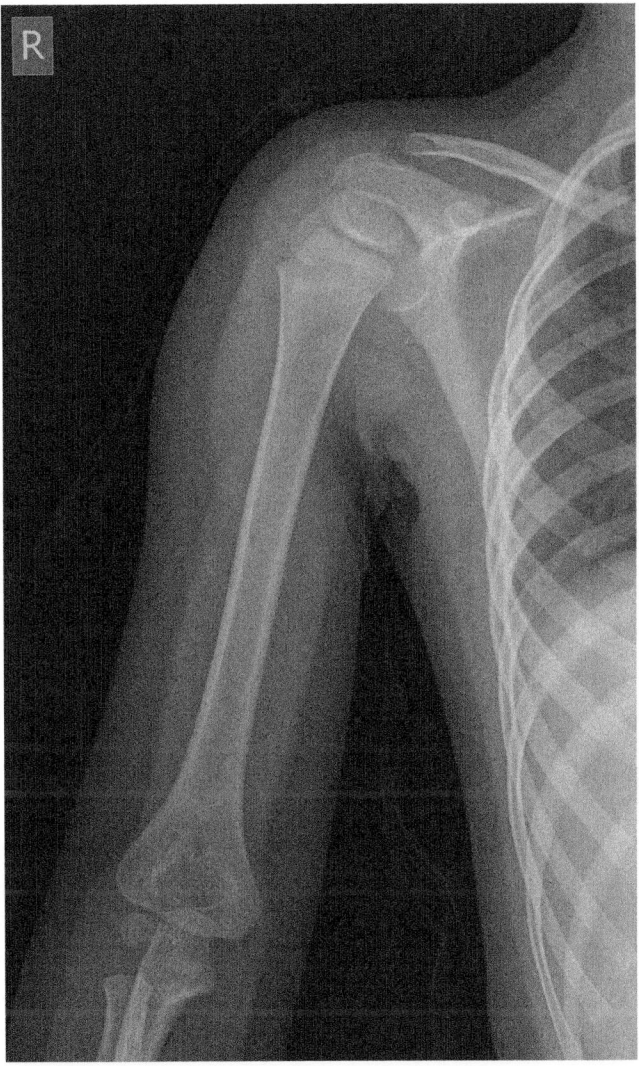

Normal	Abnormal	Diagnosis/Abnormality (only if abnormal)

Image 26

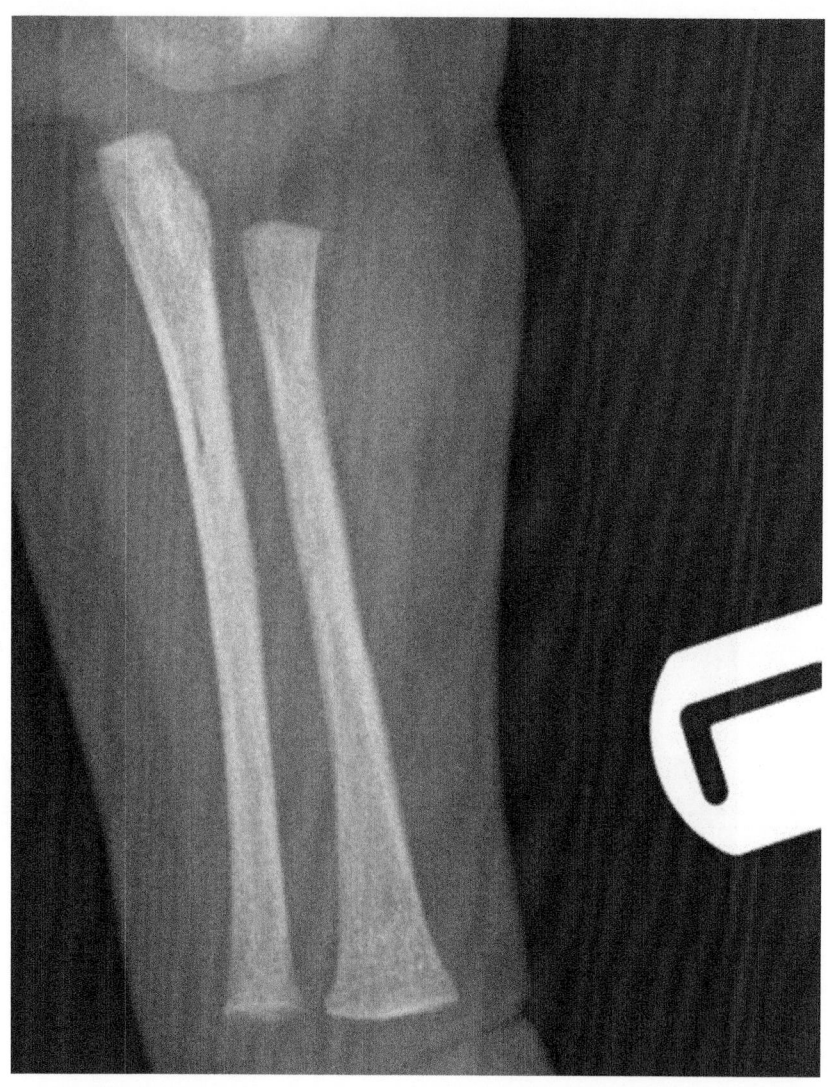

Normal	Abnormal	Diagnosis/Abnormality (only if abnormal)

Image 27

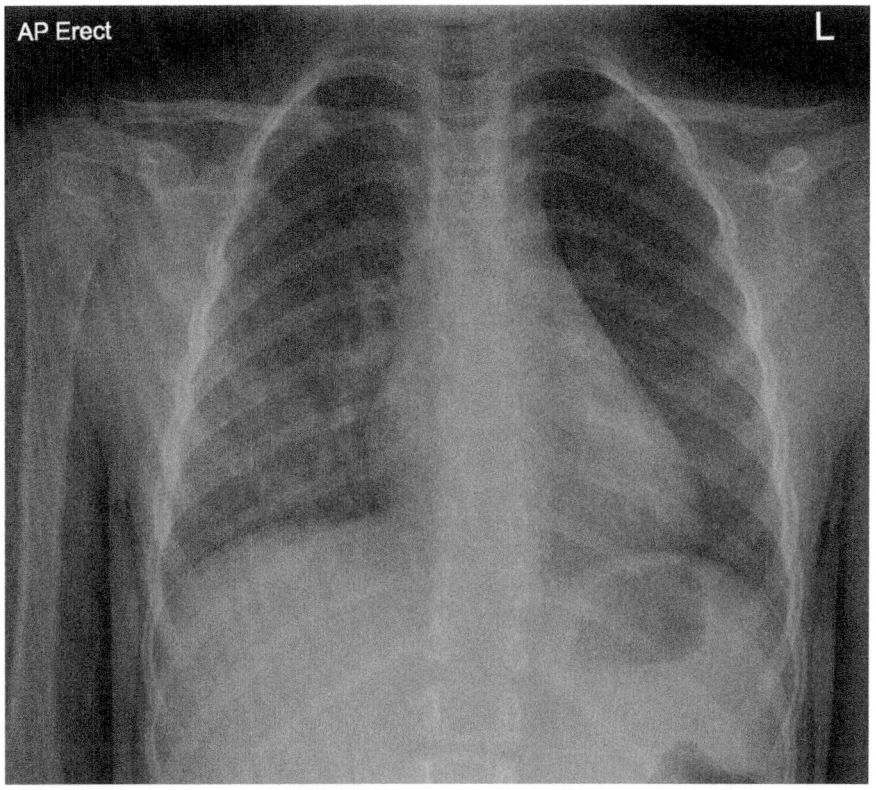

Normal	Abnormal	Diagnosis/Abnormality (only if abnormal)

Image 28

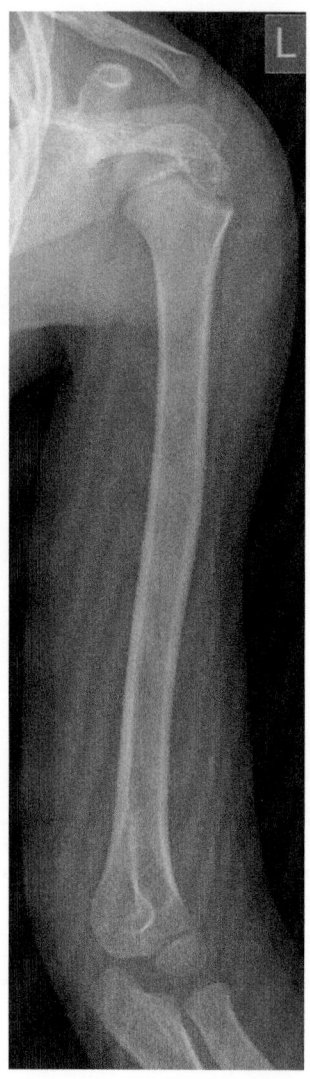

Normal	Abnormal	Diagnosis/Abnormality (only if abnormal)

Image 29

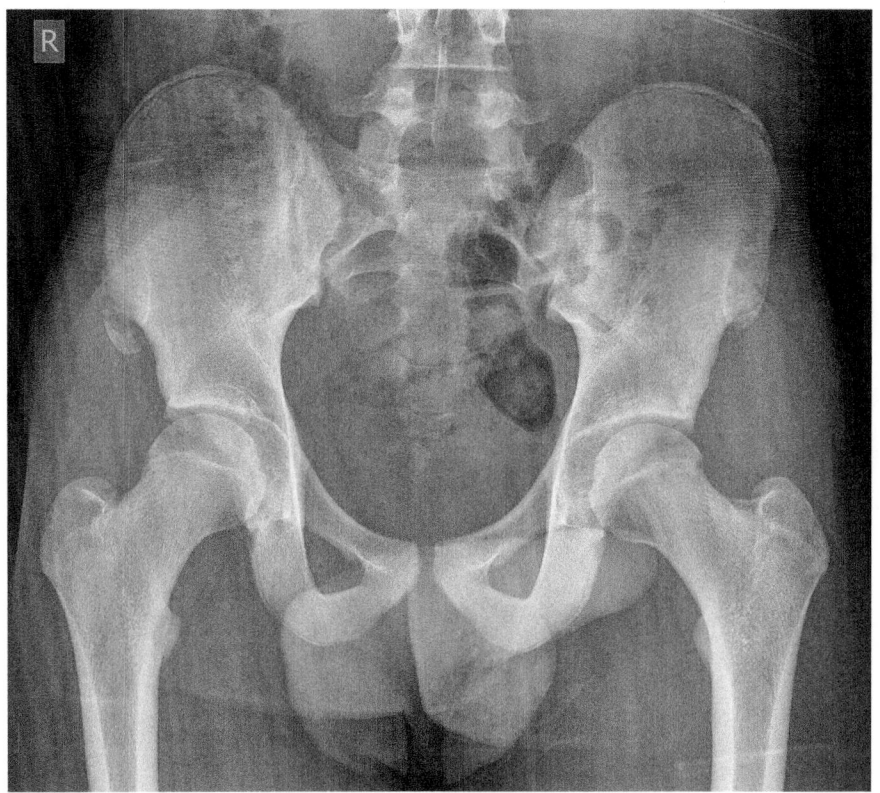

Normal	Abnormal	Diagnosis/Abnormality (only if abnormal)

Image 30

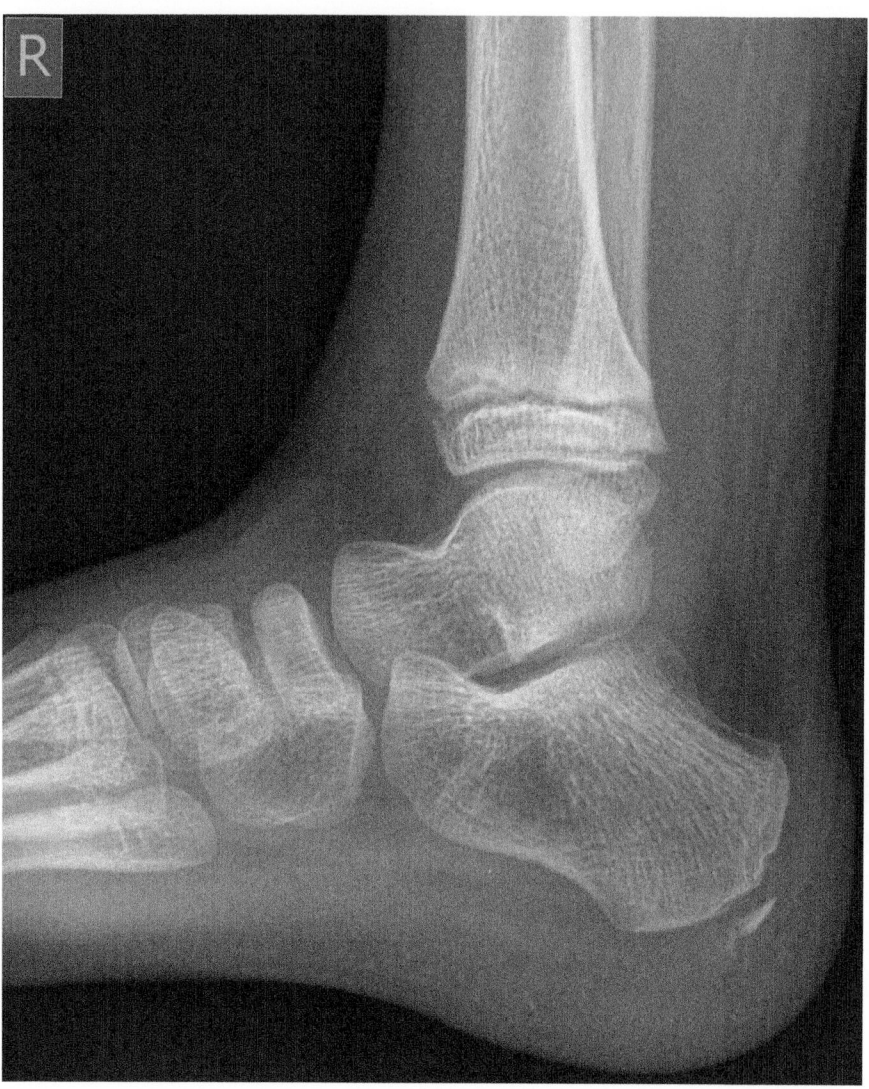

Normal	Abnormal	Diagnosis/Abnormality (only if abnormal)

6.2   Answers

Image	Normal	Abnormal	Diagnosis/abnormality (only if abnormal)
1		✓	Left Tillaux #
2		✓	Right supracondylar #
3	✓		
4		✓	# left fourth toe proximal phalanx
5		✓	Vertebra plana T9
6		✓	# base left first metatarsal
7	✓		
8		✓	# base left fifth metatarsal
9		✓	Avulsion # right medial epicondyle
10		✓	Buckle # base left little finger proximal phalanx
11	✓		
12	✓		
13		✓	Diffuse bony sclerosis
14		✓	Lucent lesion left parietal bone
15	✓		
16		✓	Left lower lobe collapse
17		✓	Buckle # left distal radius
18		✓	Increased soft tissue density pelvis/paucity pelvic bowel gas/ pelvic mass
19		✓	Healing avulsion # left anterior inferior iliac spine (AIIS)
20		✓	Buckle # left proximal tibia
21	✓		
22		✓	Buckle #s left distal radius and ulna
23	✓		
24		✓	Transverse # left ring finger metacarpal neck
25	✓		
26	✓		
27	✓		
28	✓		
29		✓	Avulsion # right anterior superior iliac spine (ASIS)
30	✓		

6.3   Explanations

1. **Left Tillaux #**
   The distal tibial physis fuses from medial to lateral with the lateral aspect fusing at around the age of 12–15 years.

   A Salter-Harris 3 fracture through the *lateral* aspect of the distal tibial epiphysis is known as a Tillaux fracture (after the French surgeon and anatomist). In these injuries which occur in older children and adolescents, the medial aspect of the distal tibial epiphysis has fused and is not involved. This fracture is associated with an avulsion of the anterior tibiofibular ligament following an abduction-external rotation mechanism of injury.

   A triplanar fracture is seen in a younger age group than the Tillaux fracture before distal tibial physeal fusion has begun. It is a complex Salter-Harris 4 fracture, and as the name suggests, involves three planes centred around the distal tibial physis:
   - A vertical fracture through the lateral aspect of the epiphysis
   - A horizontal fracture through the physis
   - An oblique (posteriorly orientated) fracture though the metaphysis

   As such, any contemporaneous lateral/orthogonal projection must be carefully evaluated for extension through the posterior aspect of the distal tibial metaphysis. If there is *any* uncertainty regarding the type of fracture sustained, evaluation with CT is indicated, particularly as small vertically orientated fractures can be overlooked. The degree of fracture fragment displacement determines management: open reduction and internal fixation (ORIF) is indicated where there is lateral talar displacement of greater than 1 mm.

   See the explanation for Test 1, Image 30 for the Salter-Harris classification.

2. **Right supracondylar fracture**

4. **# left fourth toe proximal phalanx**
   The fracture is magnified below:

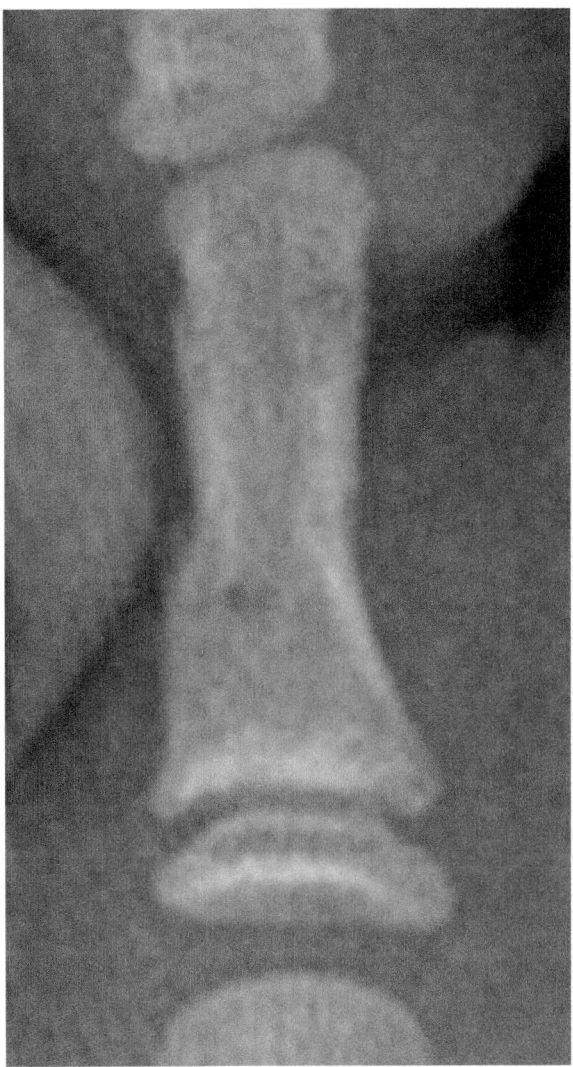

5. **Vertebra plana T9**

   Vertebra plana describes the advanced collapse of a vertebral body having lost almost all its anterior, middle and posterior height. See the advanced collapse of the T9 vertebral body in the magnified image below and compare it with the adjacent vertebral bodies:

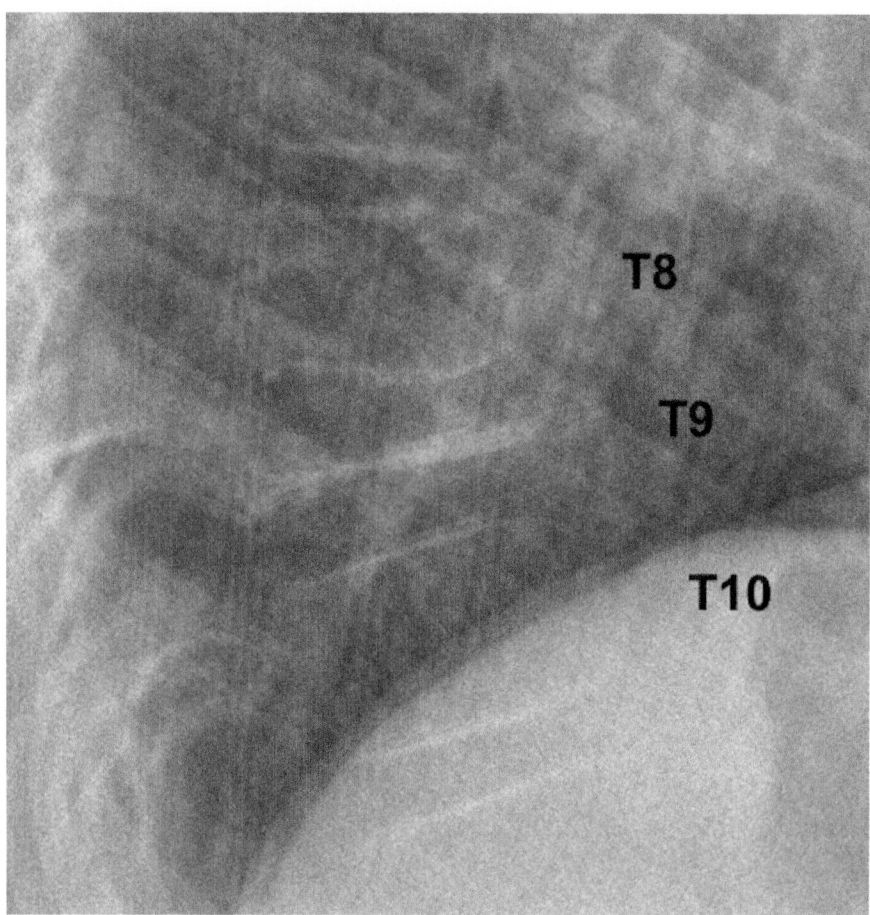

The T9 vertebral body can be identified by either counting up from lumbosacral junction (the lowest wholly imaged vertebral body in this case is L5) or identifying where the lowest most rib articulates with the T12 vertebral body and counting up. These methods are not perfect because they assume that the spinal segmentation is normal and that there are 12 pairs of ribs, which may not be the case in every child. Nevertheless, where the entire thoracolumbar spine is not available for review, it is safest to assume that the lowermost pair of ribs articulate with T12. You can add this as a note in your report and mention it should it come up in your viva. For the purposes of the Rapid Reporting examination, you are unlikely to be penalised if you report this as 'vertebra plana of a lower thoracic vertebral body'.

The most common cause of vertebra plana in *children*, as in this case, is Langerhans' cell histiocytosis (LCH). The differential diagnosis of a *single* level vertebra plana in children also includes:

- Ewing's sarcoma
- Aneurysmal bone cyst (ABC)
- Osteomyelitis (look for the associated loss of disc height)

The differential diagnosis of *multiple* vertebra plana in *children* includes:

- Gaucher's disease (see the explanation for Test 1, Image 1)
- Lymphoma
- Metastatic disease
- Fractures

6. **# base left first metatarsal**

Note the step in the medial cortex of the base of the left first metatarsal. The fracture is magnified below:

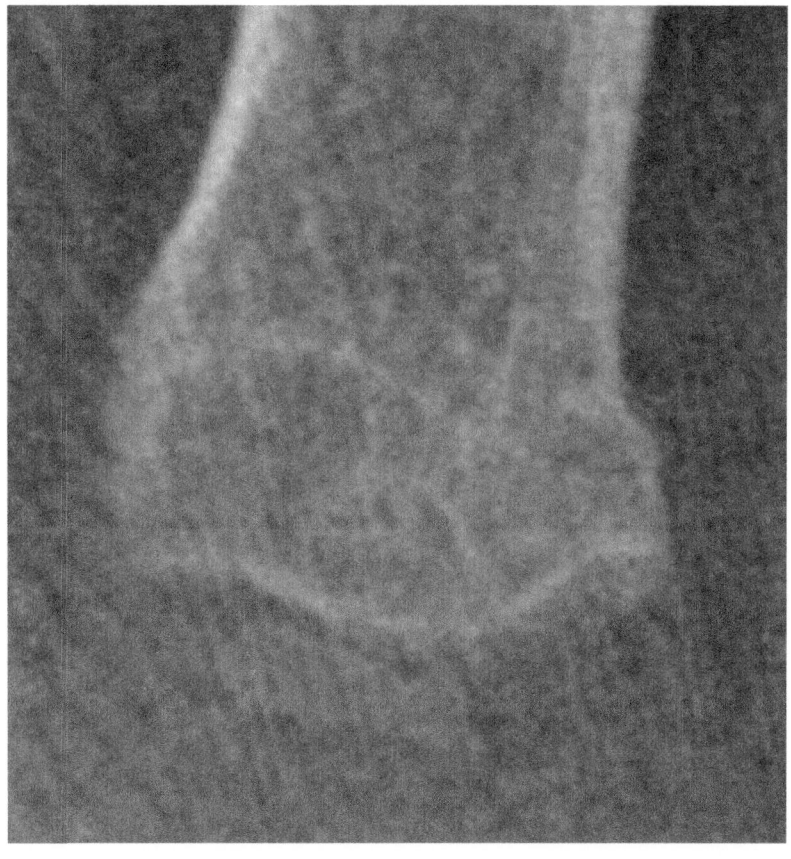

8. **# base left fifth metatarsal**
   See the explanation for Test 1, Image 7.

9. **Avulsion # right medial epicondyle**
   These are the most common avulsion injuries of the elbow in children and adolescents. This radiograph demonstrates the displaced medial epicondyle avulsion fracture with significant overlying soft tissue swelling. Whilst fairly obvious on this radiograph, sometimes the soft tissue swelling may be the only sign of an injury, particularly in those children aged less than 7 years when the medial apophysis has not yet begun to ossify. In such cases, there may be subtle widening of the physis, displacement, and/or angulation of the apophysis.

   The medial epicondyle ossification centre is classed as an *apophysis* as it does not contribute to the longitudinal growth of the humerus or the formation of the elbow joint. Apophyses are sites of ligament or tendon attachment. Knowledge of the normal ossification centres of the elbow and the sequence and timing of ossification, best remembered using the mnemonic **CRITOE**, is essential because an avulsed ossification centre may mimic another (normal) apophysis if significantly displaced:
   - **C**apitellum: 3–12 months (up to 1 year)
   - **R**adial head: 5 years
   - **I**nternal (medial) epicondyle: 5–7 years
   - **T**rochlear: 9–10 years
   - **O**lecranon: 9–11 years
   - **E**xternal (lateral) epicondyle: 10–12 years

   All centres are usually ossified by the age of 12 years; the ossification centres generally appear earlier in females than in males. Any apparently missing ossification centre(s) appearing in the wrong sequence should be viewed suspiciously and the elbow scrutinised for injury.

   Avulsion of the medial epicondyle ossification centre results from extreme valgus when a child falls on to an outstretched arm (FOOSH). This can temporarily open the joint space in which the avulsed medical epicondyle ossification centre can be displaced, simulating the trochlear ossification centre. This is a significant injury that should *not* be missed—retention of the avulsion fragment in the joint space can lead to severe articular damage and early secondary osteoarthritis.

10. **Buckle # base left little finger proximal phalanx**
    This fracture may be missed if you do not look through the overlying bones, thus reinforcing the need for careful inspection of every bone. The acute step in the dorsal cortex of the base of the proximal phalanx is consistent with an acute fracture, seen in the magnified image below:

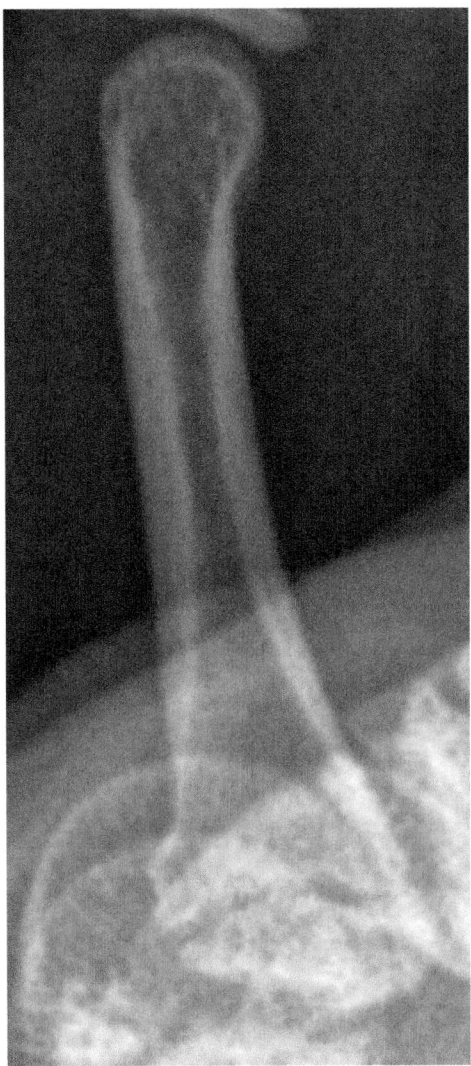

Note also the associated soft tissue swelling on the original image.

11. **Normal left elbow radiograph**

This radiograph is normal. As with any rule, there are always exceptions. In most children, the anterior humeral line (as discussed in Test 1, Image 28) will pass through the middle third of the capitellum (i.e. the line will bisect the capitellum). In some normal children however, this line will pass through the anterior third. Furthermore, there are no secondary signs of acute injury: there is no fracture or effusion and the radiocapitellar alignment is normal.

13. **Diffuse bony sclerosis**

The differential for diffuse bony sclerosis in children can be divided into the broad categories of **PIMS:**

- Poisoning:
  - Lead
  - Fluorosis
  - Hypervitaminosis D
  - Chronic hypervitaminosis A
- Idiopathic:
  - Caffey disease: see the explanation for Test 5, Image 2
  - Idiopathic hypercalcaemia of infancy
- Metabolic:
  - Renal osteodystrophy
- Skeletal dysplasia:
  - Osteopetrosis
  - Pyknodysostosis

The sclerosis in this case was secondary to pyknodysostosis, a rare autosomal recessive skeletal dysplasia characterised by osteosclerosis and short stature.

14. **Lucent lesion left parietal bone**

The lucent lesion, which was secondary to LCH in this case, is magnified below:

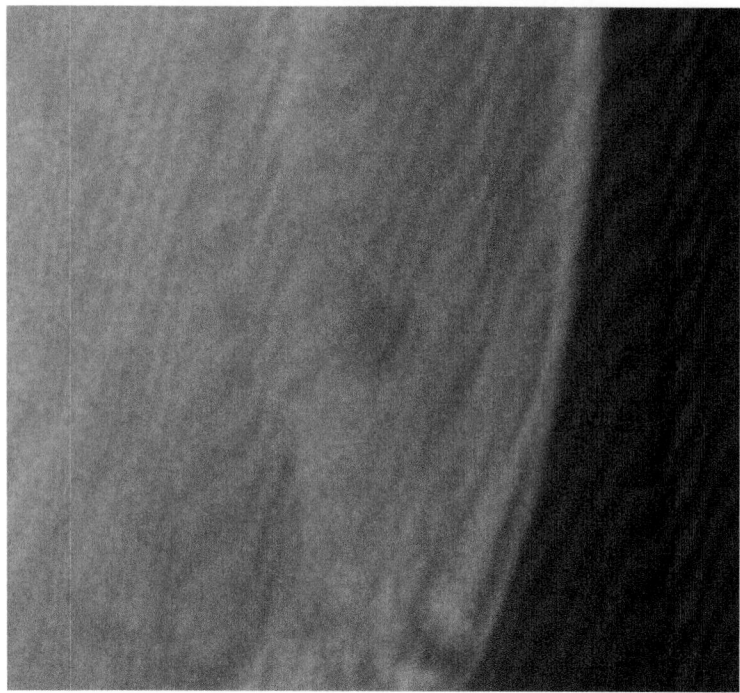

The differential diagnosis for a lucent skull lesion in a *child* is wide and includes:
- Eosinophilic granuloma/LCH
- Metastases:
  - Neuroblastoma
  - Medulloblastoma
  - Leukaemia
- Osteomyelitis
- Dermoid/epidermoid
- Fibrous dysplasia
- Haemangioma
- Leptomeningeal cyst: these can present as enlarging scalp masses, result from an extension of post-traumatic encephalomalacia and are typically seen a few months post-trauma. They complicate approximately 1% of skull fractures and are known by the misnomer, 'growing skull fractures'
- Surgical defect, e.g. previous burr hole

16. **Left lower lobe collapse**

This radiograph demonstrates the distinctive features of a left lower lobe collapse, including:
- Volume loss in the left hemithorax
- Elevation of the left hemidiaphragm (in this example there is gastric distention and an air-fluid level; in the absence of the gastric distension, the border of the left hemidiaphragm would usually be obscured/obliterated)
- Mediastinal deviation to the left
- Increased retrocardiac/posteromedial left lung opacity
- Edge of the collapsed left lower lobe creates a 'double cardiac contour'

A common cause of lobar collapse in children is mucous plugging in the setting of asthma or airways inflammation/infection. Foreign body inhalation/ aspiration is also an important cause which should *always* be considered.

17. **Buckle # left distal radius**

The subtle buckling of the distal radial cortex, magnified below, may be overlooked but it is a genuine finding:

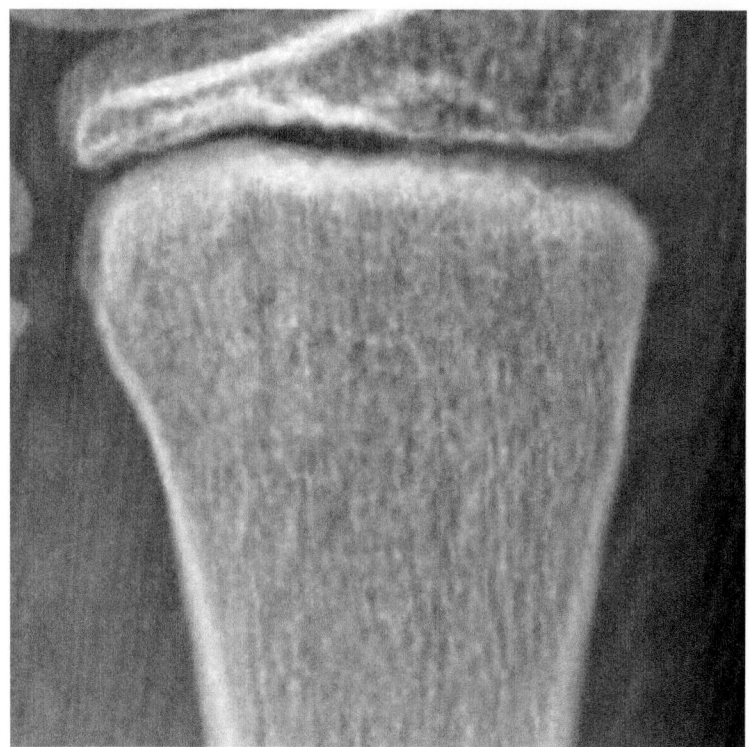

18. **Increased soft tissue density pelvis/paucity pelvic bowel gas/pelvic mass**
    The paucity of bowel gas in the pelvis is noticeable once you know to look for
    it. 'Standing back' to evaluate the radiograph, one's eye is drawn to this area
    where there is an increased opacification alongside a paucity of bowel gas.
    Compare this radiograph with the one from Image 19 in this test. Furthermore,
    the gas-filled bowel loop in the central abdomen is displaced superiorly imply-
    ing that there is something displacing it.

    This 14-year-old female presented with abdominal pain. Following this
    radiograph, a transabdominal ultrasound was performed which revealed a
    large, distended fluid-filled structure with internal echoes. The anatomy was
    difficult to delineate on ultrasound given its size. An MRI revealed a haemato-
    metrocolpos—a blood-filled distended uterus and vagina. The most common
    cause for this is an imperforate hymen which prevents the evacuation of men-
    strual blood. Occasionally, the distension can be so great as to cause ureteric
    obstruction and dilation of the proximal renal tracts (hydronephrosis). There
    may also be an associated Mullerian duct anomaly/malformation:
    • Mullerian agenesis
    • Obstructing vaginal septum
    • Unicornuate uterus
    • Bicornuate uterus
    • Uterus didelphys
    • Septated uterus

The kidneys should always be assessed for urinary tract malformations which are associated with Mullerian duct anomalies.

The differential for this radiographic appearance could also include: bladder outflow obstruction/urinary retention; megaureter; or other pelvic mass such as a rhabdomyosarcoma, large adnexal mass/cyst, or hydrosalpinx. A gravid uterus should also be considered in any young female of child-bearing age.

19. **Healing avulsion # left anterior inferior iliac spine (AIIS)**
There is irregularity of the left AIIS consistent with a healing injury. See the explanation for Test 4, Image 13. The AIIS is the insertion for the rectus femoris tendon.

20. **Buckle # left proximal tibia**
Buckle or transverse fractures of the proximal tibial metaphysis are more commonly known as 'trampoline fractures'. These typically occur in children aged 2–5 years of age and are thought to result when a second, usually heavier child causes the trampoline surface to recoil upwards to meet the 'descending' child who is usually younger/lighter. The 'excessive load' is thought to result in this characteristic fracture pattern seen in the magnified image below (the subtle bulge in the medial cortex of the proximal tibia):

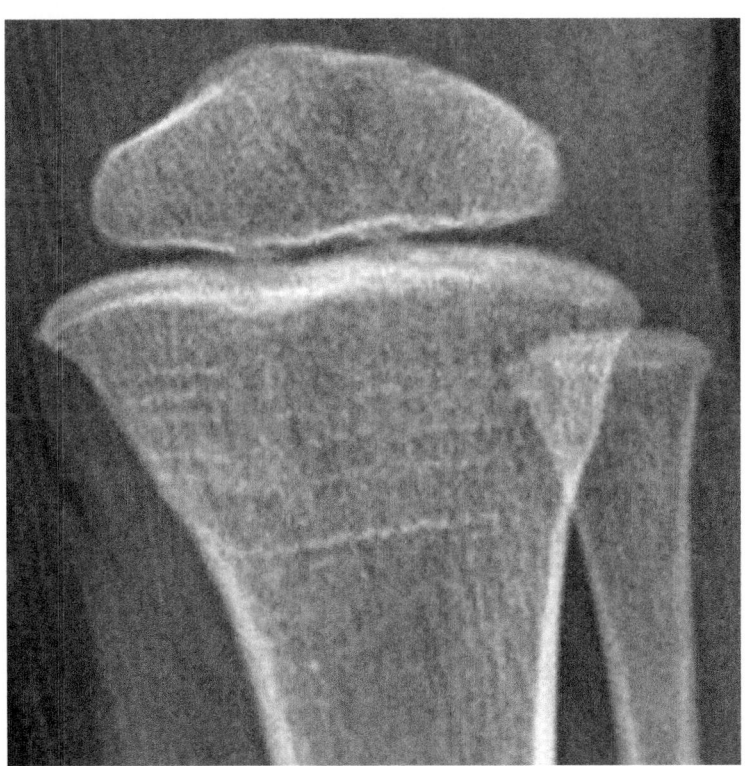

There is a documented propensity for these fractures to develop a late valgus angulation deformity, known as Cozen's phenomenon (named for the orthopaedic surgeon who first described this deformity). This is usually self-limiting and resolves in 1–2 years following the acute injury. Whilst better remodelling potential may be expected in younger children, corrective hemi-epiphysiodesis may sometimes be required. Early recognition of this complication is important so that early orthopaedic assessment and appropriate management can be instigated, if required.

22. **Buckle #s left distal radius and ulna**
    See explanation for Test 1, Image 18 and the Introduction section.

24. **Transverse # left ring finger metacarpal neck**

26. **Normal left forearm radiograph**
    This radiograph is normal. The subperiosteal bone collars visualised at the left distal radius and ulna metaphyses are normal. See the explanation for Test 5, Image 6.

29. **Avulsion # right anterior superior iliac spine (ASIS)**
    See the explanation for Test 4, Image 13. The anterior superior iliac spine is the insertion for the sartorius and tensor fascia latae tendons.

Further Reading

Image 1

Lukies M, Gaillard F et al (2018) Tillaux fracture. https://radiopaedia.org/articles/tillaux-fracture. Accessed May 2018

Smithius R (2018) Ankle – special fracture cases. Detection of 'not so obvious' fractures. http://www.radiologyassistant.nl/en/p50335f3cb7dc9/ankle-special-fracture-cases.html. Accessed July 2018

Weerakkody Y, Gaillard F et al (2018) Triplane fracture. https://radiopaedia.org/articles/triplane-fracture. Accessed May 2018

Image 5

Bell DJ, Skorupka K et al (2018) Vertebra plana. https://radiopaedia.org/articles/vertebra-plana. Accessed May 2018

Wheeless CR (2012) Eosinophilic Granuloma of the Spine. http://www.wheelessonline.com/ortho/eosinophilic_granuloma_of_the_spine. Accessed May 2018

Image 9

Jones J, Bronson R et al (2018) Medial epicondyle fracture. https://radiopaedia.org/articles/medial-epicondyle-fracture-1. Accessed May 2018

Jones J et al (2018) Ossification centres of the elbow. https://radiopaedia.org/articles/ossification-centres-of-the-elbow. Accessed May 2018

Smithuis R (2018) Elbow – fractures in children. http://www.radiologyassistant.nl/en/p58c4d-d5b9219a/elbow-fractures-in-children.html. Accessed June 2018

St-Amant M, Gaillard F et al (2018) Elbow ossification mnemonic. https://radiopaedia.org/articles/elbow-ossification-mnemonic. Accessed May 2018

Image 11

Jones J et al (2018) Anterior humeral line. https://radiopaedia.org/articles/anterior-humeral-line. Accessed July 2018

Image 13

Hacking C, Salam H et al (2018) Generalised increased bone density in children. https://radiopaedia.org/articles/generalised-increased-bone-density-in-children. Accessed May 2018

Ihde LL, Forrester DM, Gottsegen CJ et al (2011) Sclerosing bone dysplasias: review and differentiation from other causes of osteosclerosis. Radiographics 31(7):1865–1882

Sharma R, Dixon A et al (2018) Pyknodysostosis. https://radiopaedia.org/articles/pyknodysostosis. Accessed May 2018

Image 14

Kang O, Gaillard F et al (2018) Solitary lucent skull lesion. https://radiopaedia.org/articles/solitary-lucent-skull-lesion. Accessed May 2018

Sharma R, St-Amant M et al (2018) Leptomeningeal cyst. https://radiopaedia.org/articles/leptomeningeal-cyst. Accessed May 2018

Image 16

Gaillard F et al (2018) Left lower lobe collapse. https://radiopaedia.org/articles/left-lower-lobe-collapse. Accessed May 2018

Image 18

Bickle I et al (2018) Haematometrocolpos. https://radiopaedia.org/articles/haematometrocolpos. Accessed May 2018

Images 19 and 29

See the references for Test 4, Image 13

Image 20

Batta NS, Dixon A et al (2018) Trampoline fracture. https://radiopaedia.org/articles/trampoline-fracture. Accessed June 2018

Bruyeer E, Geusens E, Catry F et al (2012) 'Trampoline fracture' of the proximal tibia in children: report of 3 cases and review of literature. JBR-BTR 95(1):10–12

Dorman S, Jariwala A, Campbell D (2013) Cozen's phenomenon: a reminder. Scott Med J 58(3):e10–e13

Knipe H, Teng J et al (2018) Cozen fracture. https://radiopaedia.org/articles/cozen-fracture-1. Accessed June 2018

Test 7

7.1   Images

Image 1

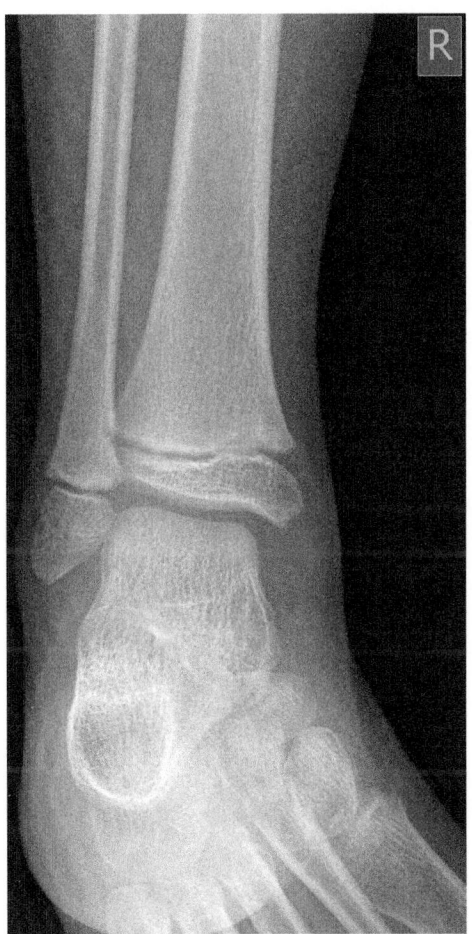

Normal	Abnormal	Diagnosis/Abnormality (only if abnormal)

M. Paddock, A. C. Offiah, *Paediatric Radiology Rapid Reporting for FRCR Part 2B*,
https://doi.org/10.1007/978-3-030-01965-5_7

Image 2

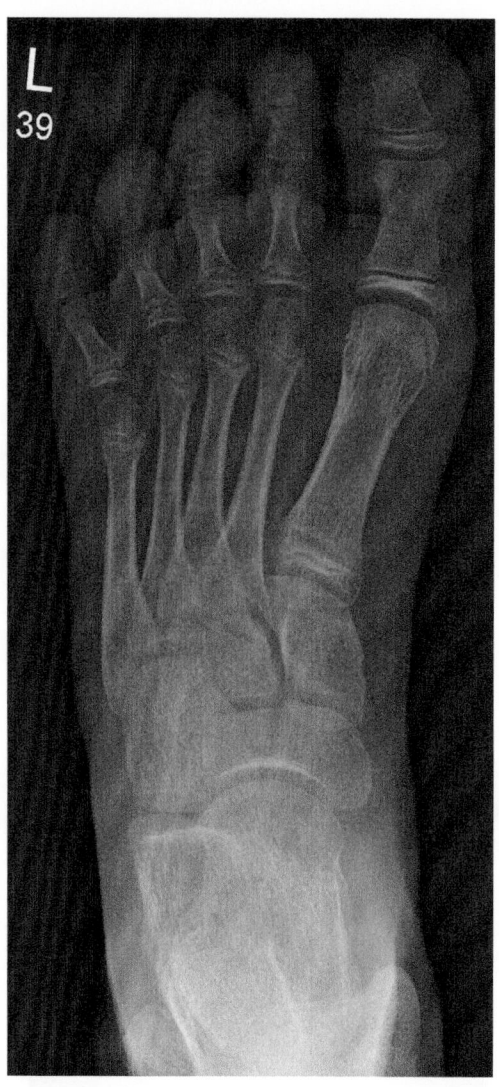

Normal	Abnormal	Diagnosis/Abnormality (only if abnormal)

Image 3

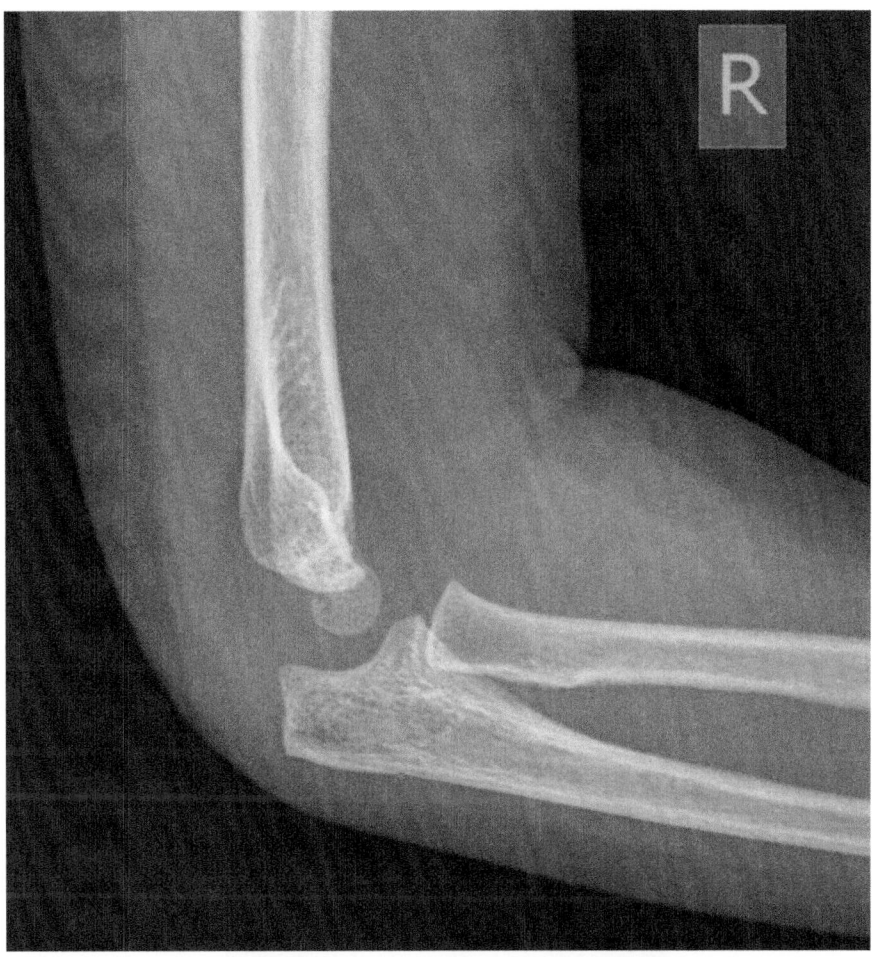

Normal	Abnormal	Diagnosis/Abnormality (only if abnormal)

Image 4

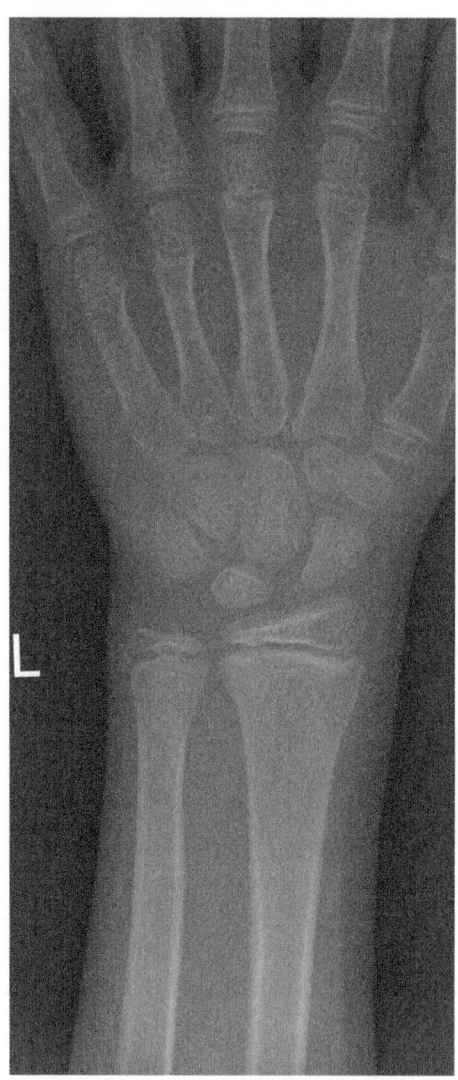

Normal	Abnormal	Diagnosis/Abnormality (only if abnormal)

Image 5

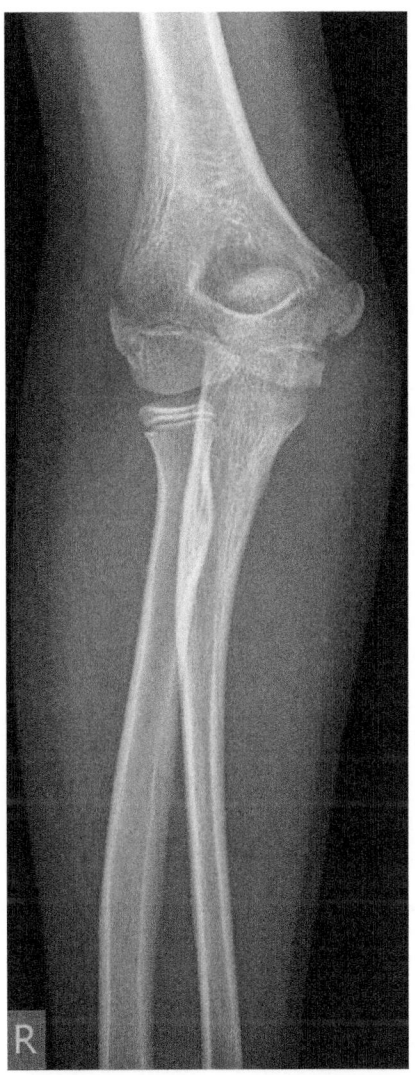

Normal	Abnormal	Diagnosis/Abnormality (only if abnormal)

Image 6

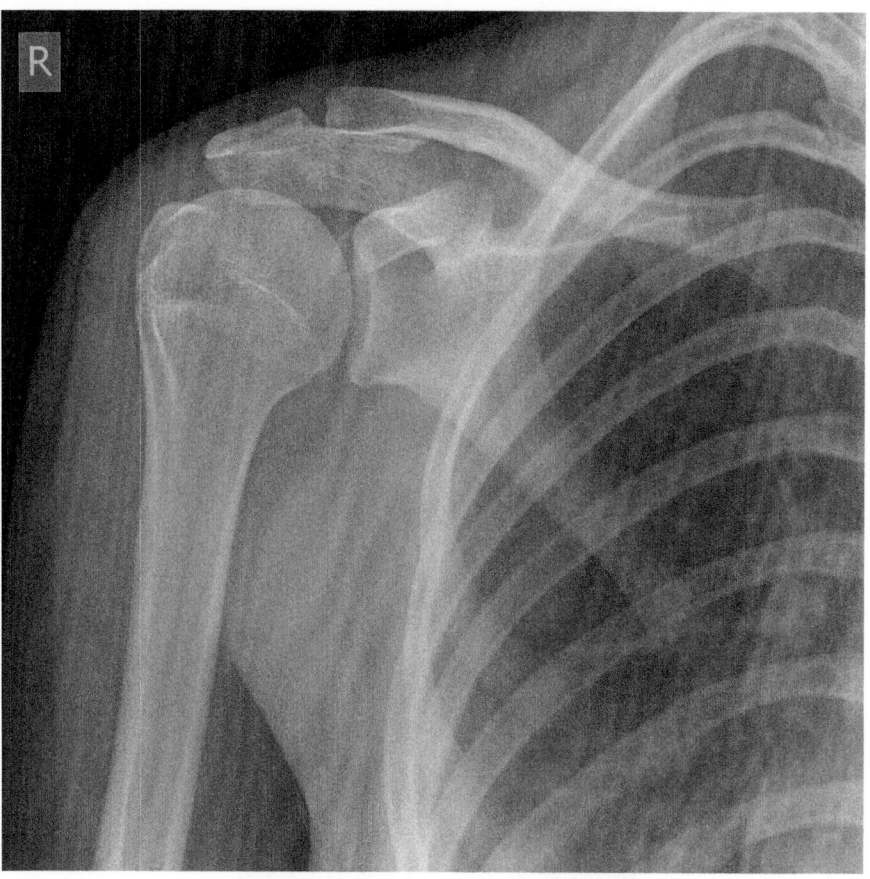

Normal	Abnormal	Diagnosis/Abnormality (only if abnormal)

Image 7

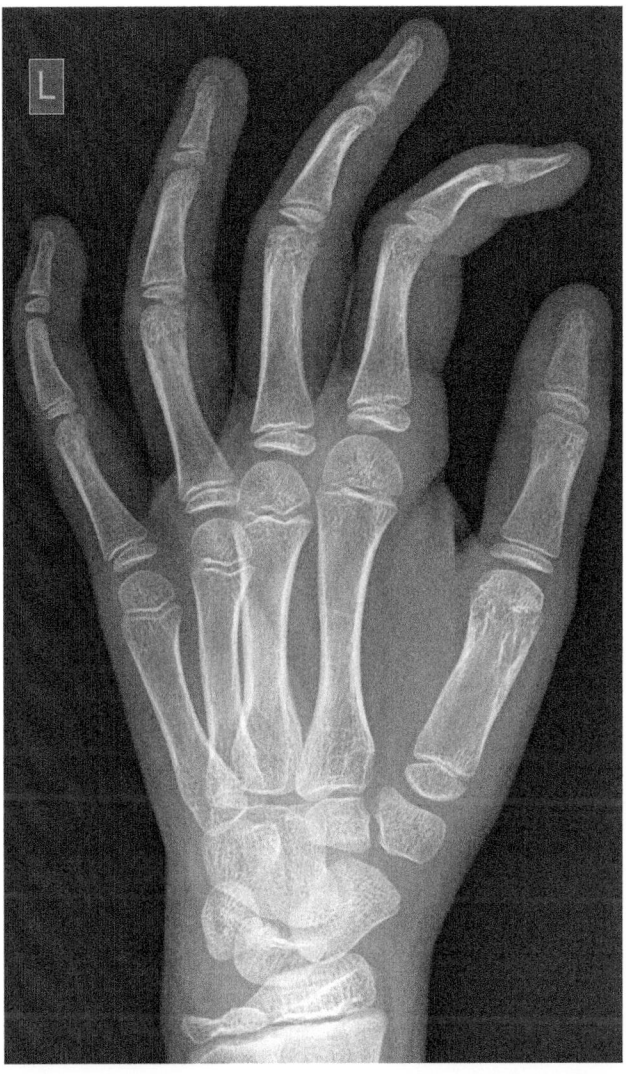

Normal	Abnormal	Diagnosis/Abnormality (only if abnormal)

Image 8

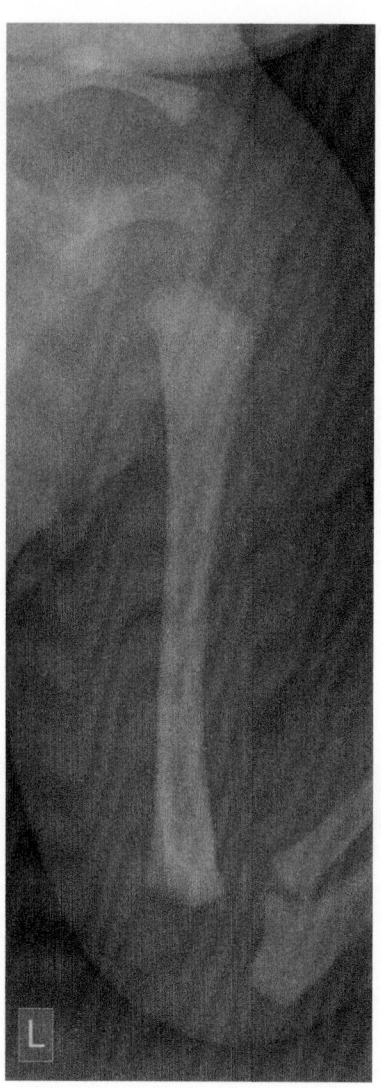

Normal	Abnormal	Diagnosis/Abnormality (only if abnormal)

Image 9

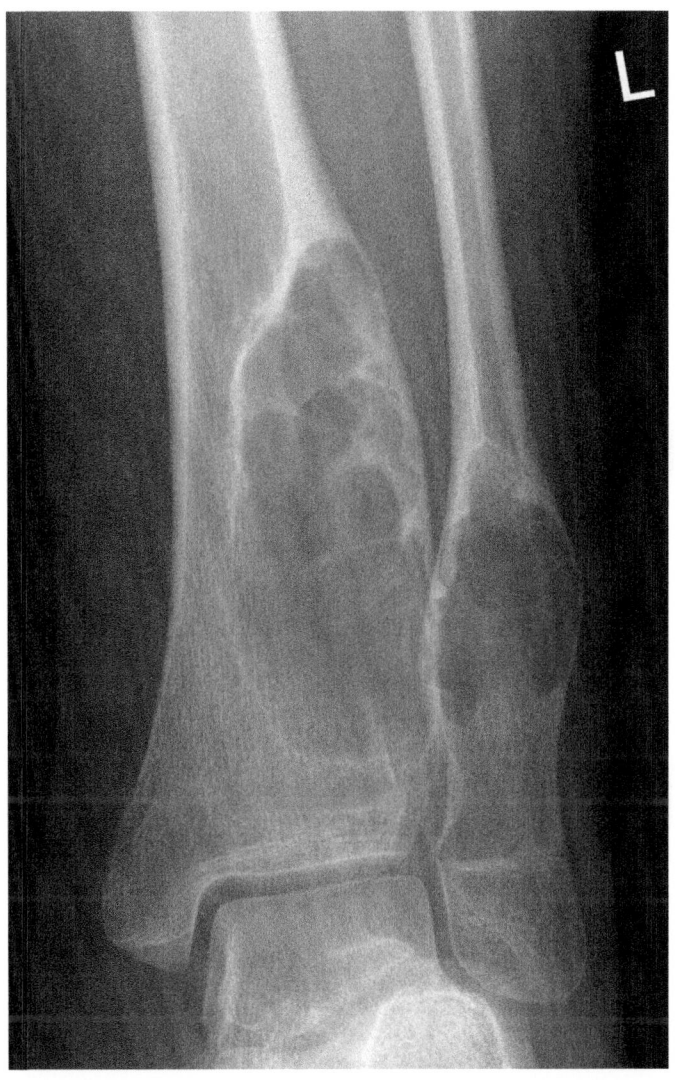

Normal	Abnormal	Diagnosis/Abnormality (only if abnormal)

Image 10

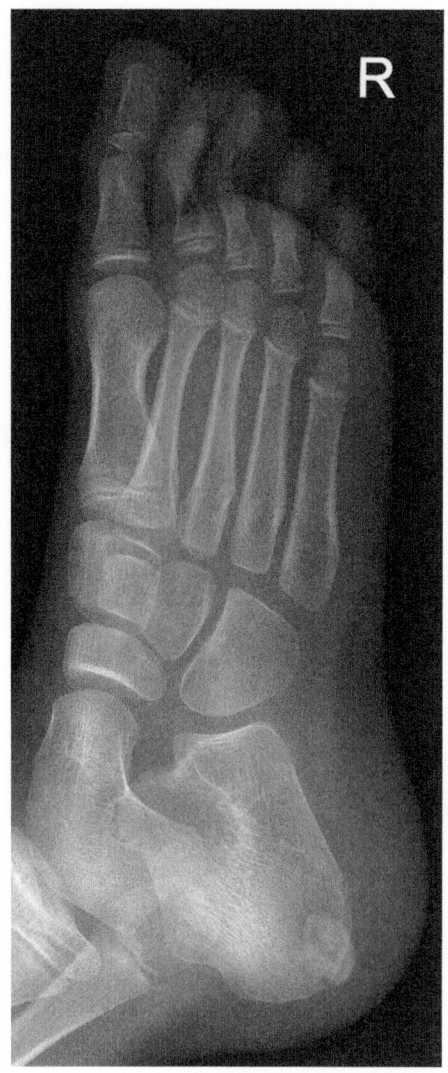

Normal	Abnormal	Diagnosis/Abnormality (only if abnormal)

Image 11

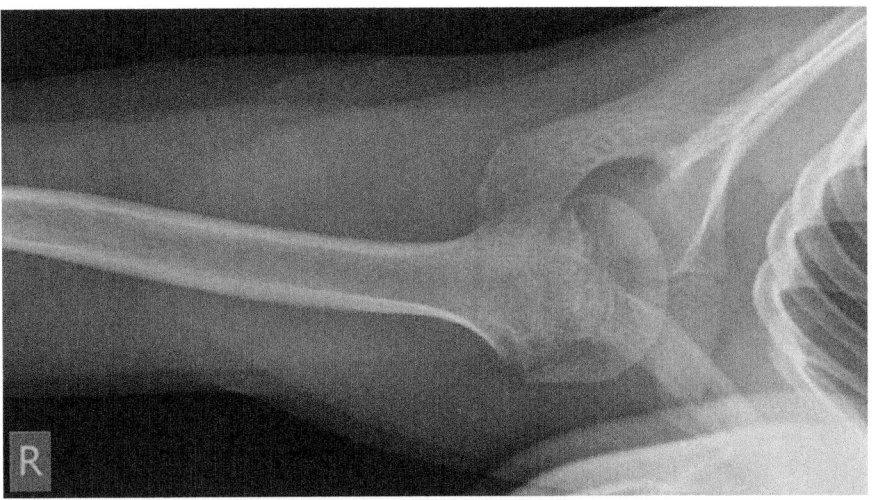

Normal	Abnormal	Diagnosis/Abnormality (only if abnormal)

Image 12

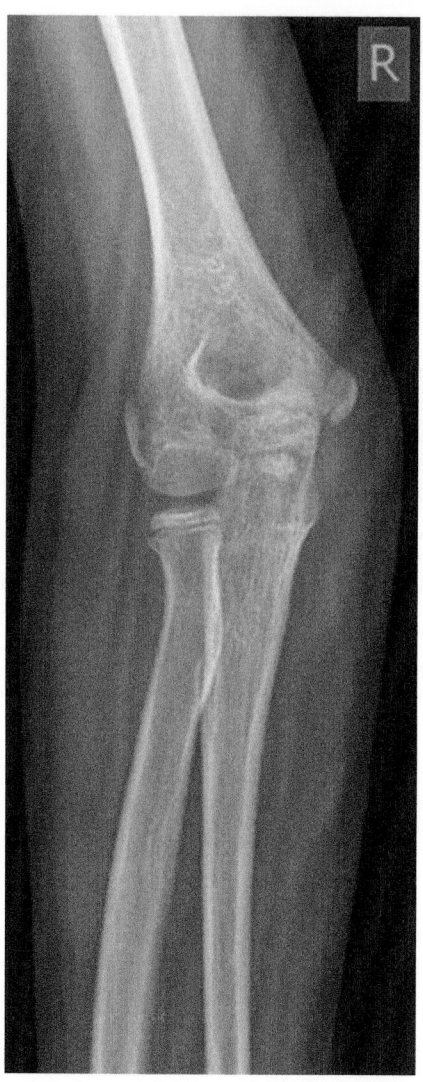

Normal	Abnormal	Diagnosis/Abnormality (only if abnormal)

Image 13

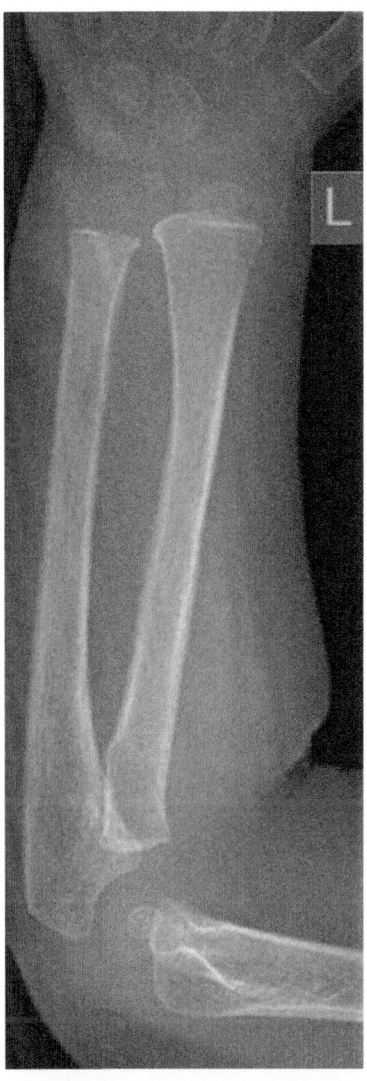

Normal	Abnormal	Diagnosis/Abnormality (only if abnormal)

Image 14

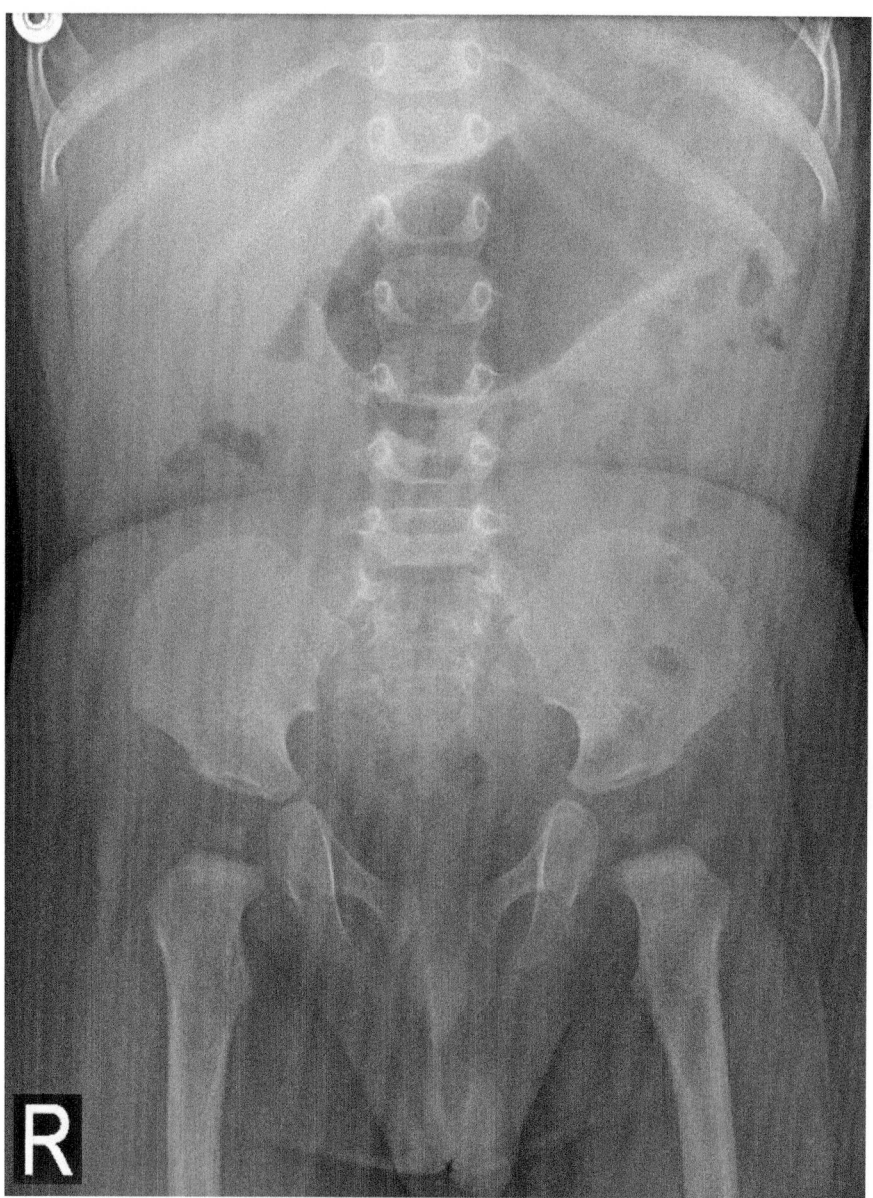

Normal	Abnormal	Diagnosis/Abnormality (only if abnormal)

Image 15

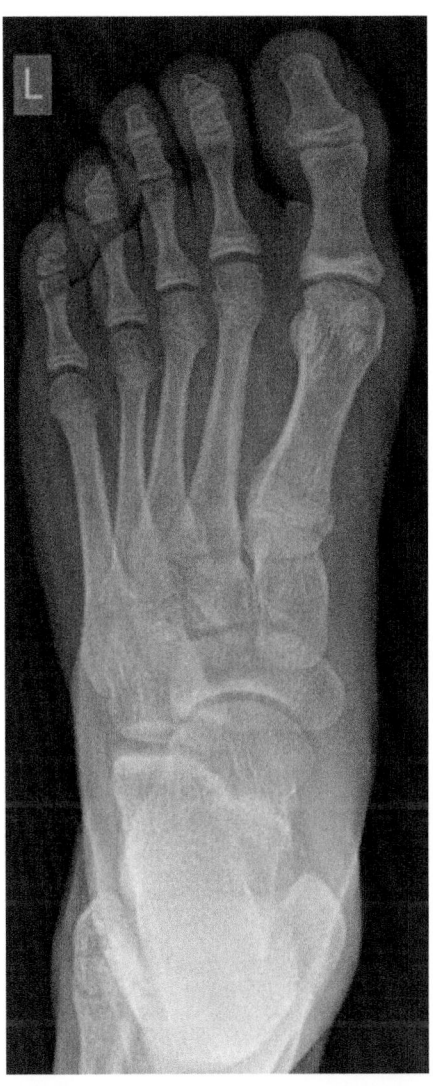

Normal	Abnormal	Diagnosis/Abnormality (only if abnormal)

Image 16

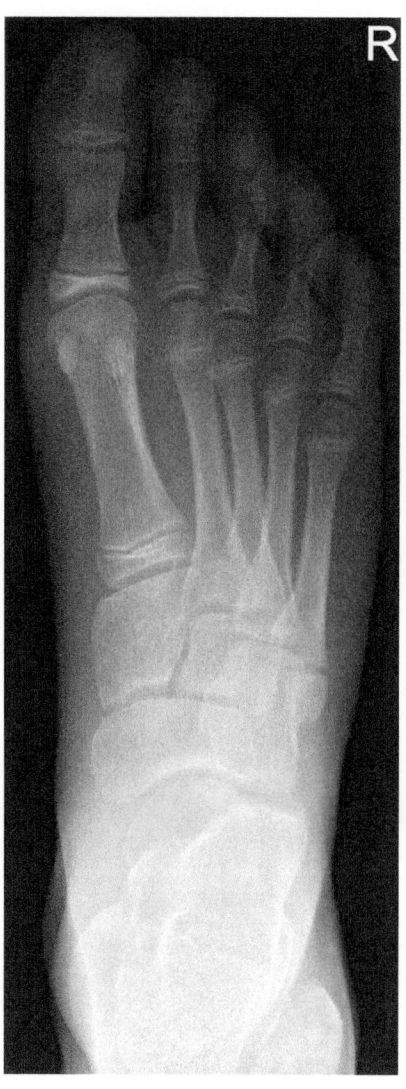

Normal	Abnormal	Diagnosis/Abnormality (only if abnormal)

Image 17

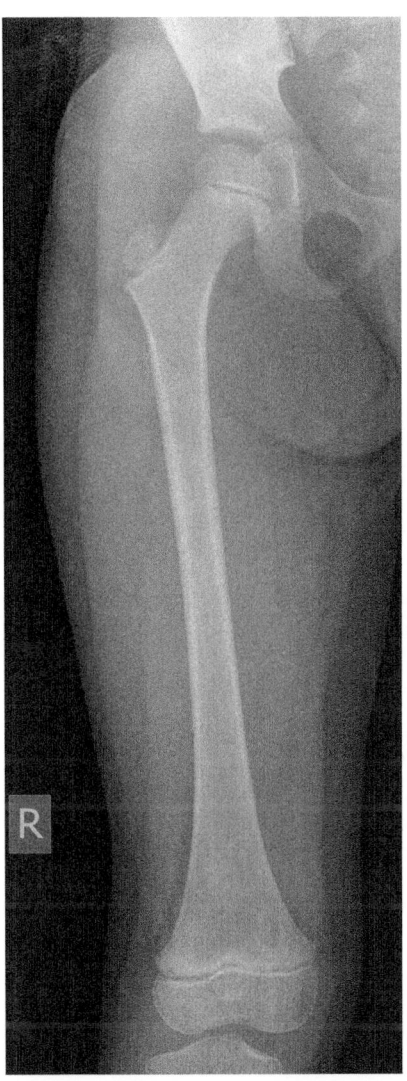

Normal	Abnormal	Diagnosis/Abnormality (only if abnormal)

Image 18

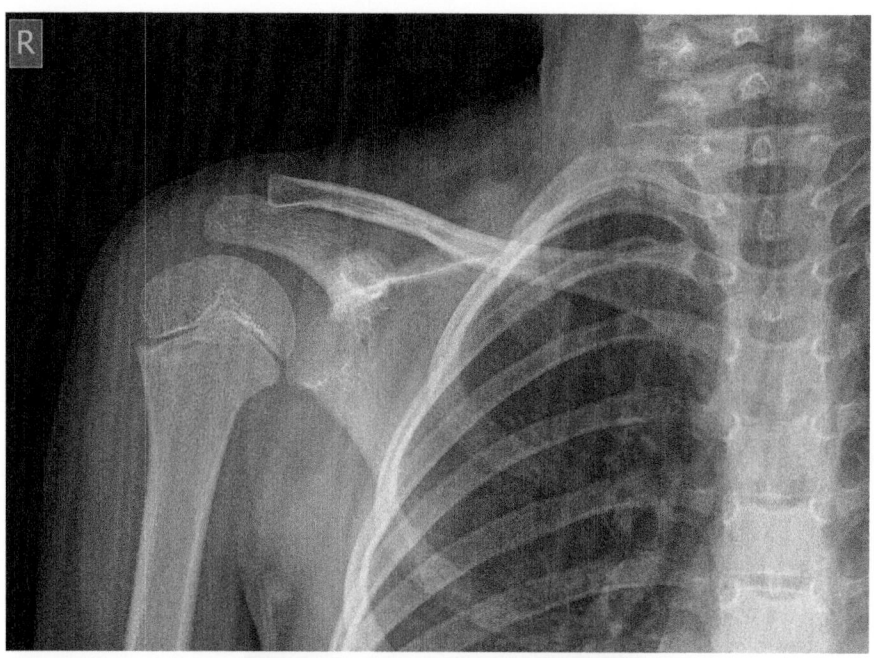

Normal	Abnormal	Diagnosis/Abnormality (only if abnormal)

Image 19

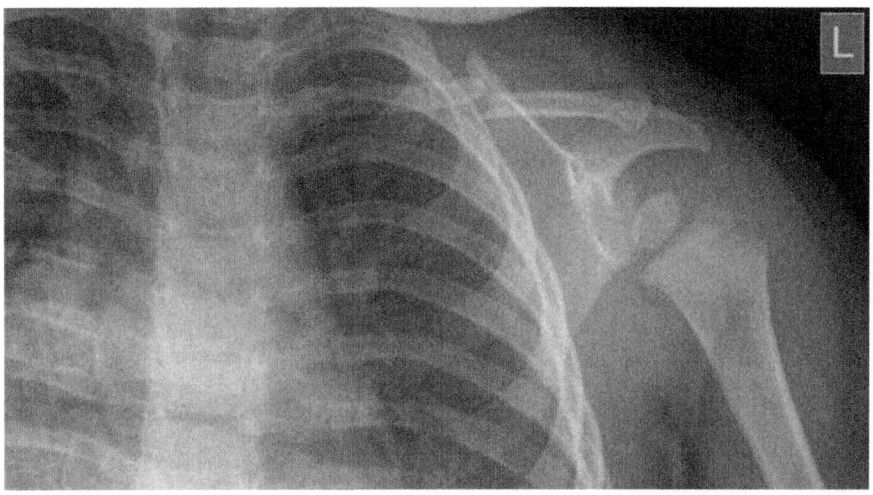

Normal	Abnormal	Diagnosis/Abnormality (only if abnormal)

Image 20

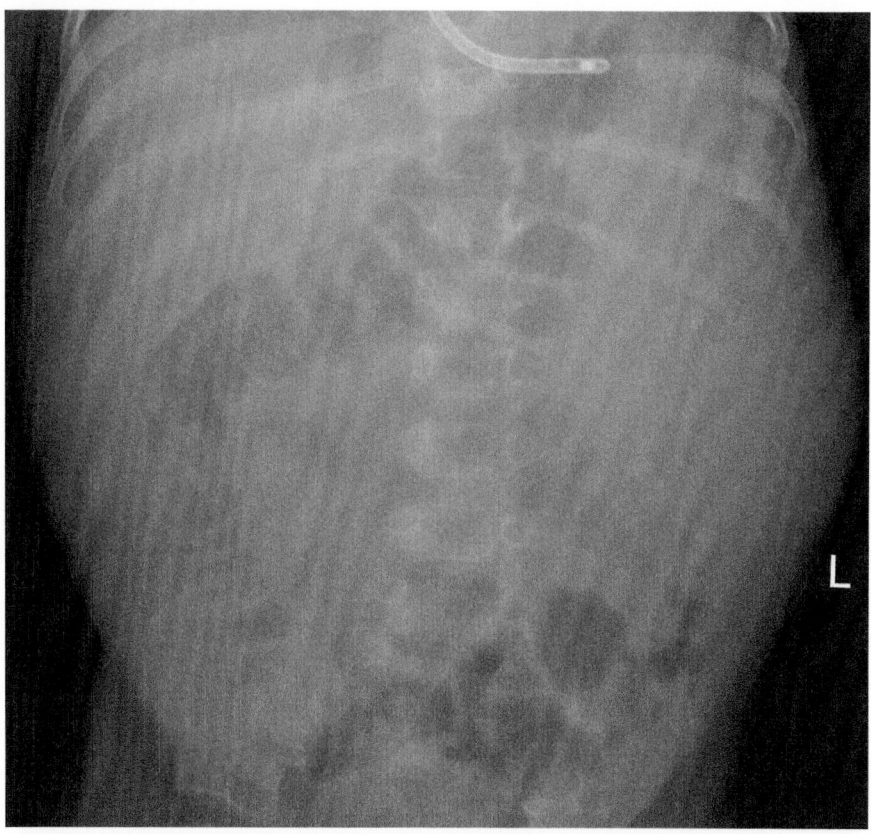

Normal	Abnormal	Diagnosis/Abnormality (only if abnormal)

Image 21

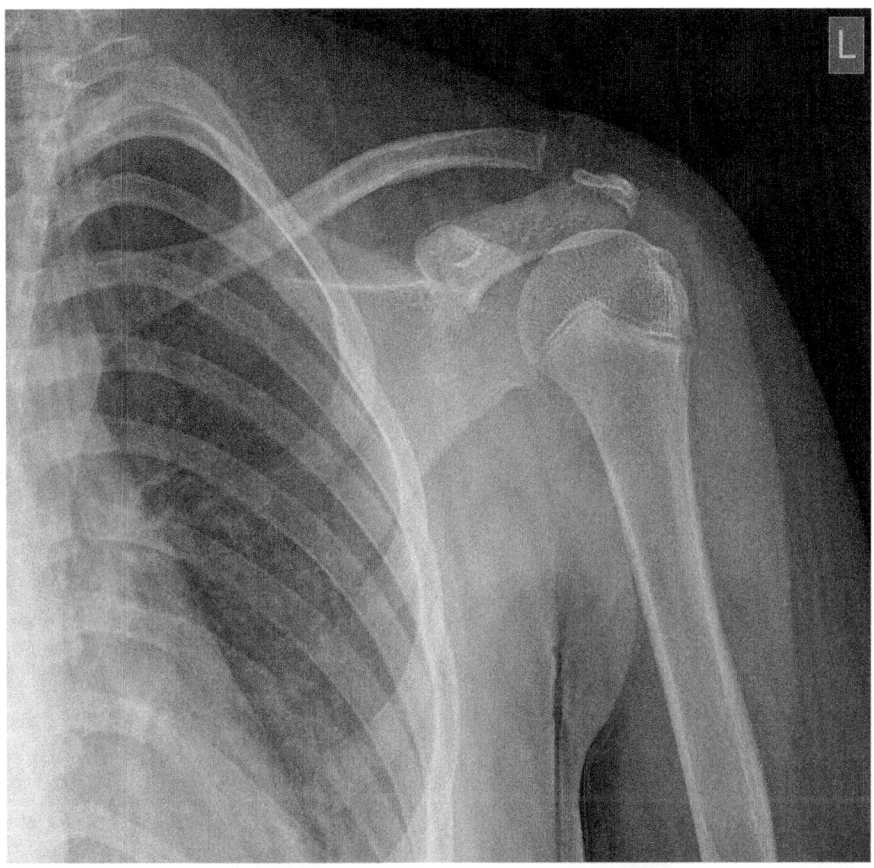

Normal	Abnormal	Diagnosis/Abnormality (only if abnormal)

Image 22

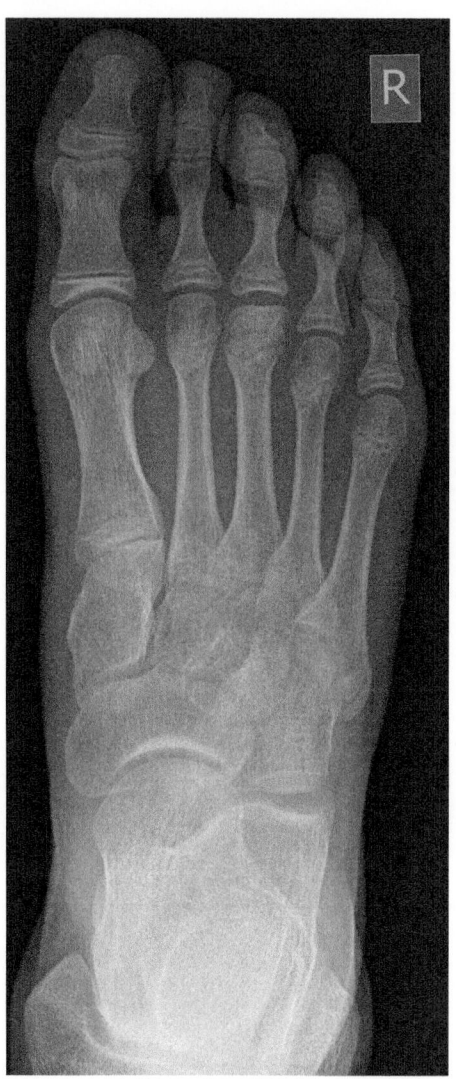

Normal	Abnormal	Diagnosis/Abnormality (only if abnormal)

Image 23

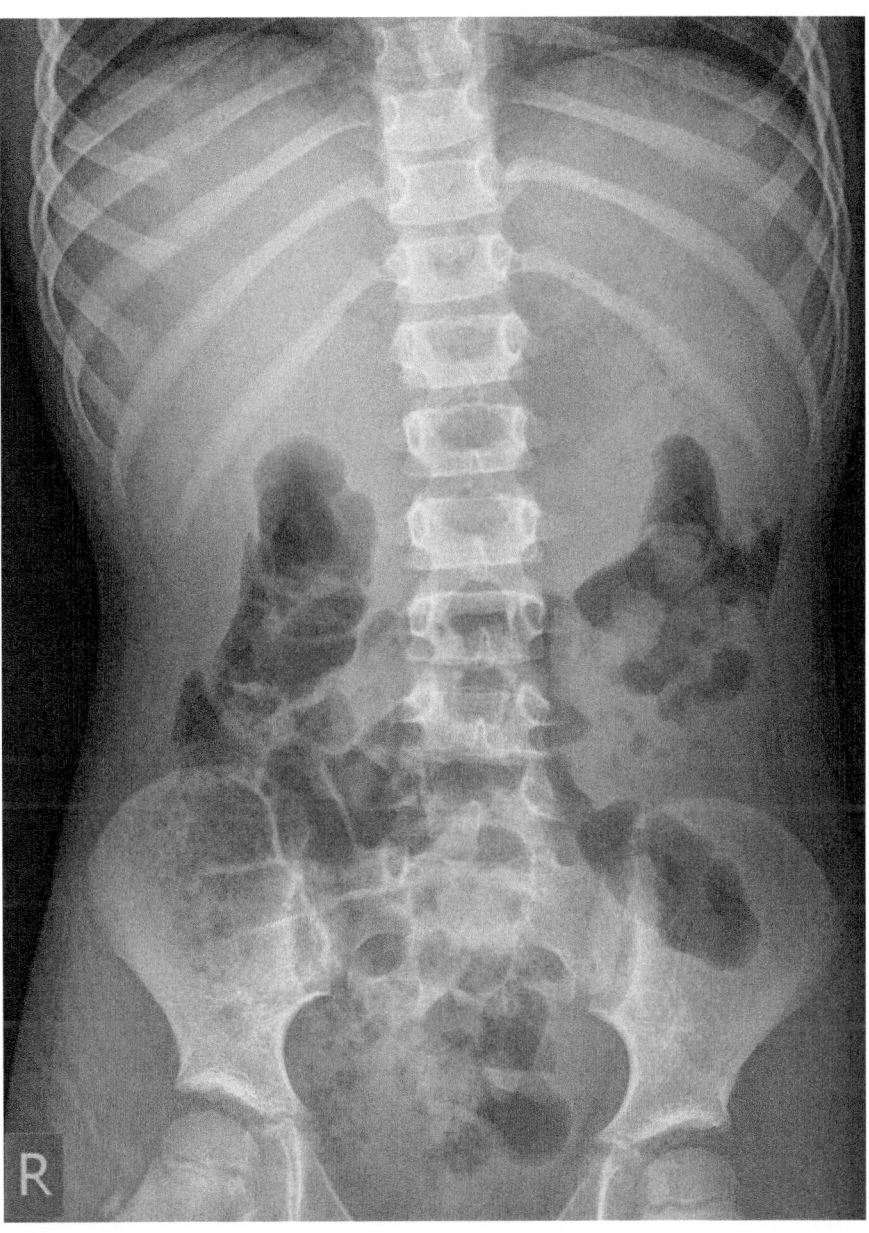

Normal	Abnormal	Diagnosis/Abnormality (only if abnormal)

Image 24

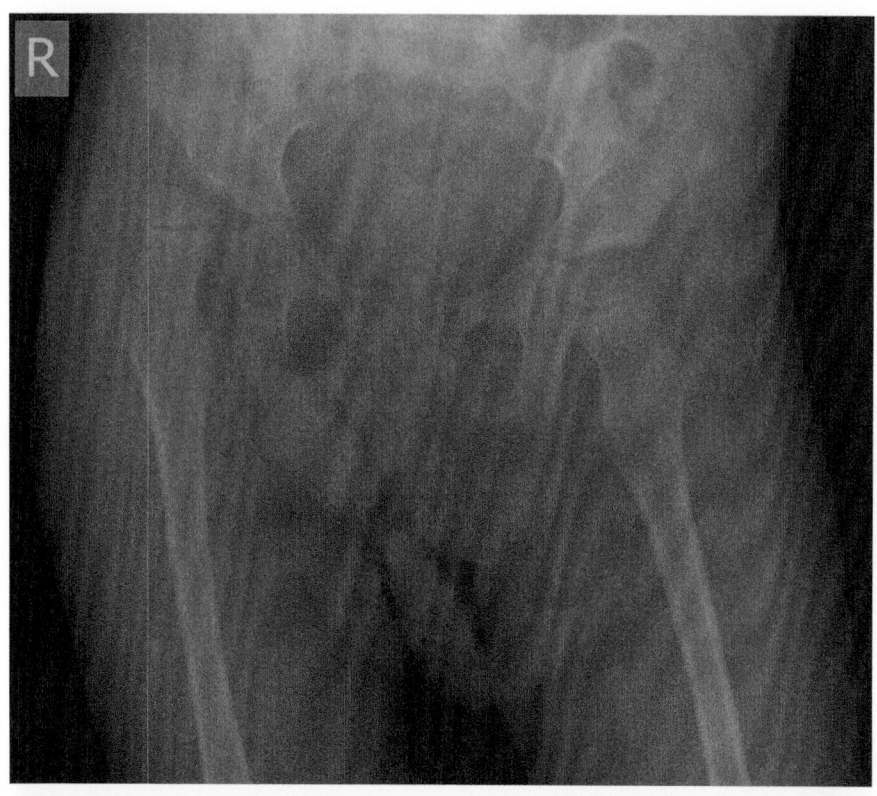

Normal	Abnormal	Diagnosis/Abnormality (only if abnormal)

Image 25

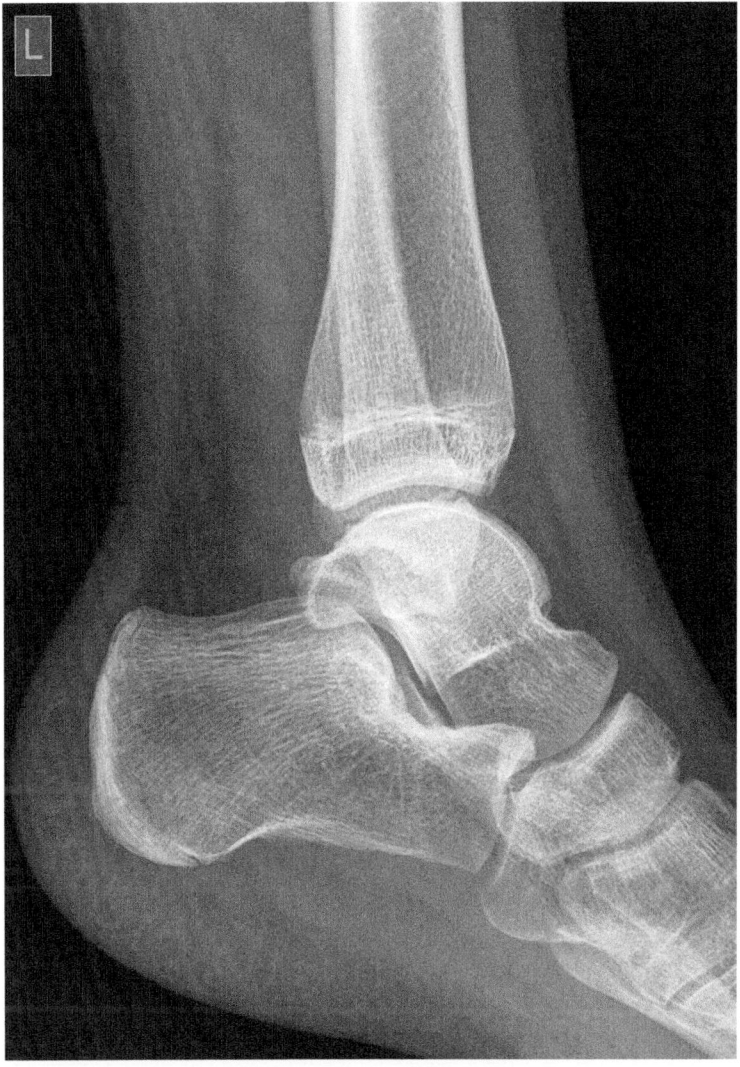

Normal	Abnormal	Diagnosis/Abnormality (only if abnormal)

Image 26

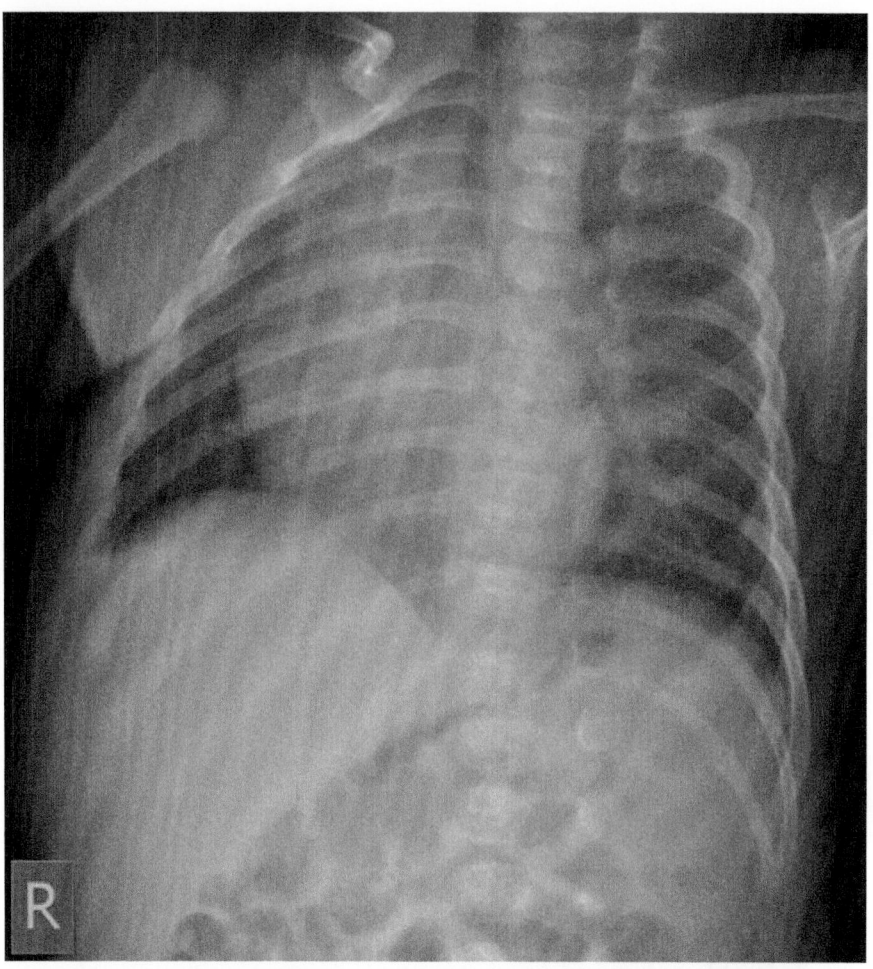

Normal	Abnormal	Diagnosis/Abnormality (only if abnormal)

Image 27

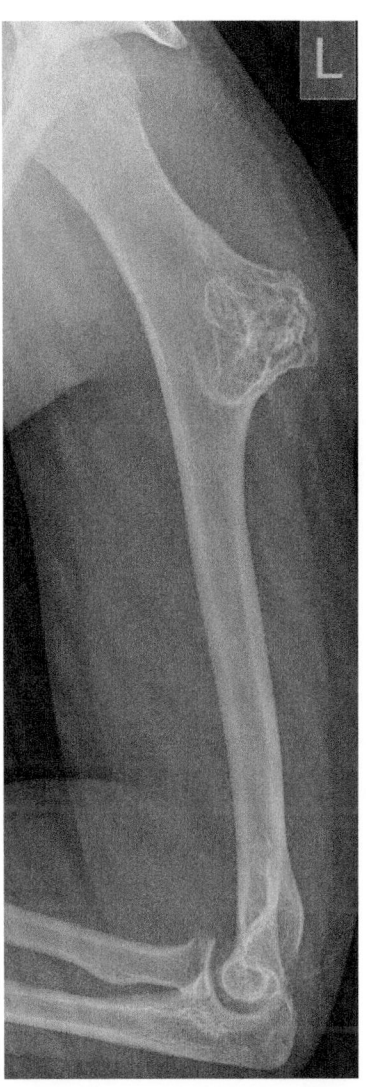

Normal	Abnormal	Diagnosis/Abnormality (only if abnormal)

Image 28

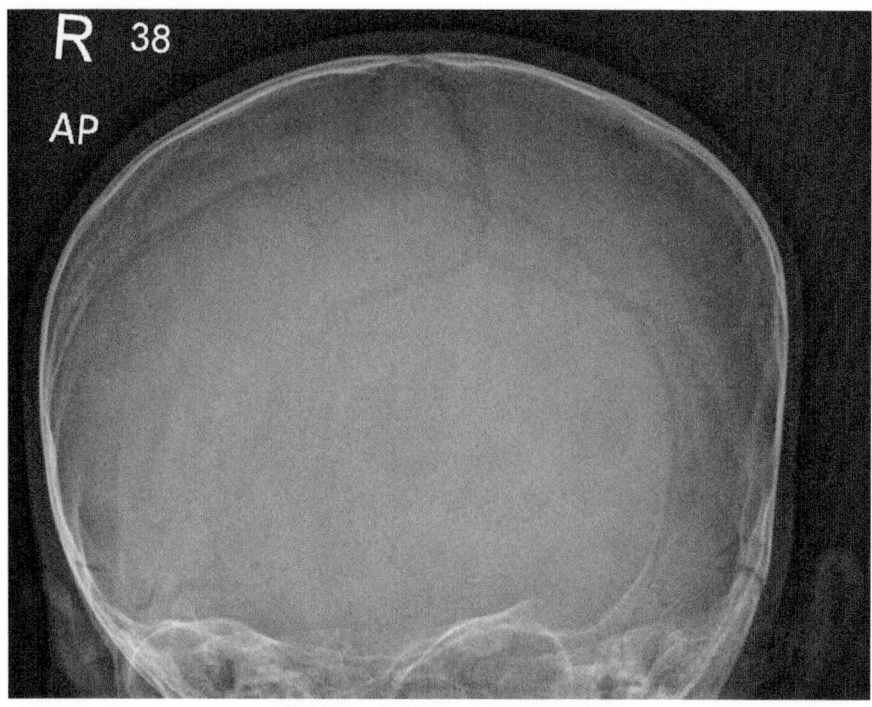

Normal	Abnormal	Diagnosis/Abnormality (only if abnormal)

Image 29

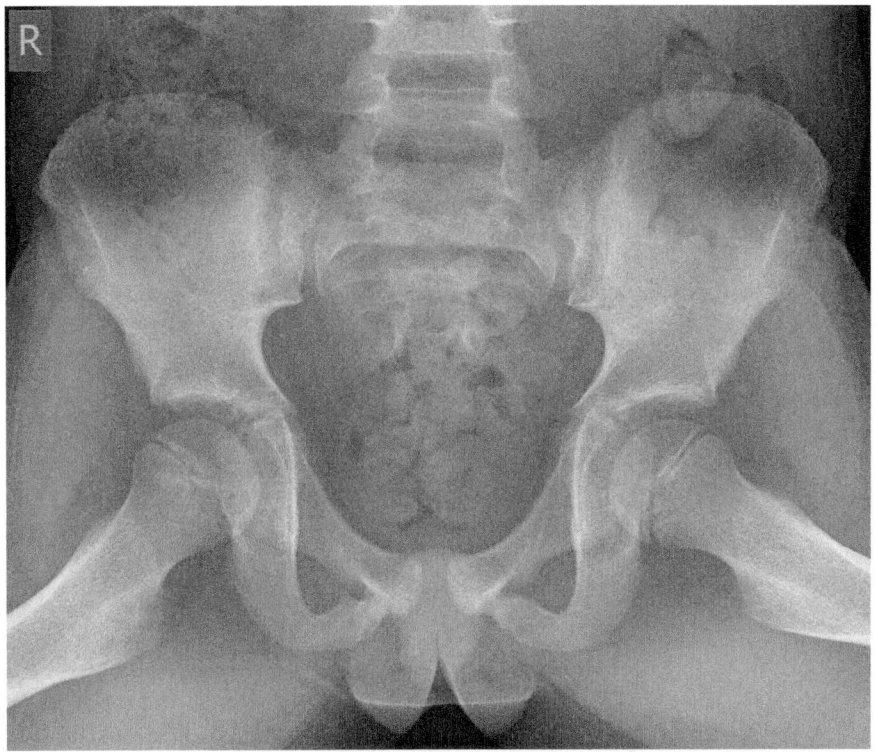

Normal	Abnormal	Diagnosis/Abnormality (only if abnormal)

Image 30

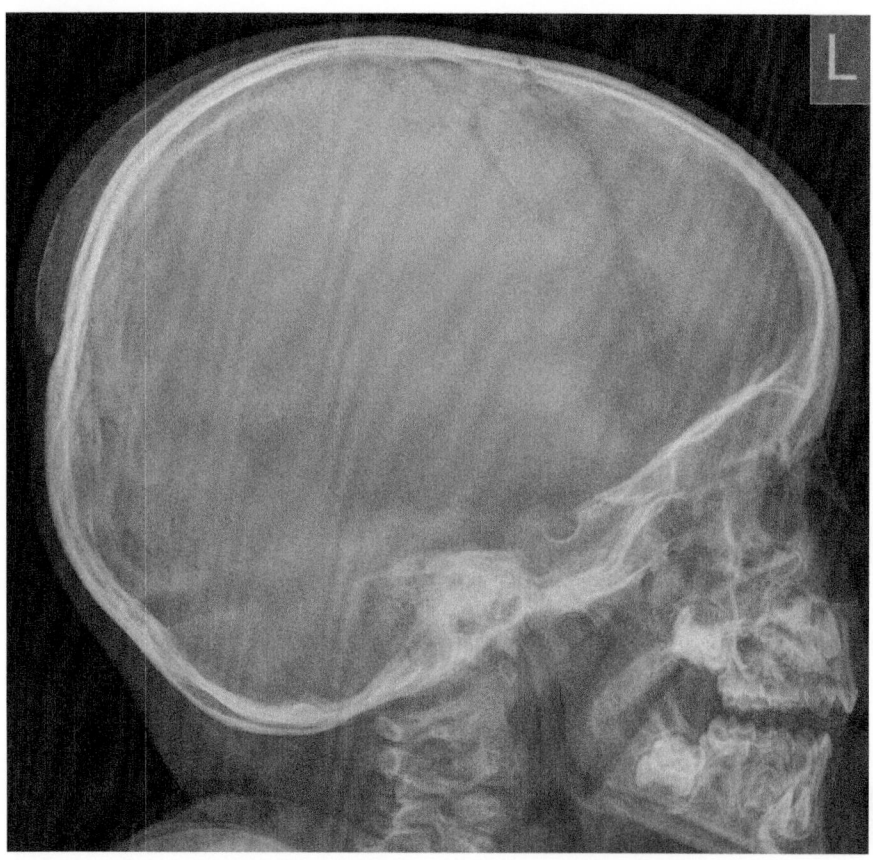

Normal	Abnormal	Diagnosis/Abnormality (only if abnormal)

7.2   Answers

Image	Normal	Abnormal	Diagnosis/abnormality (only if abnormal)
1	✓		
2		✓	Buckle # base left little toe proximal phalanx
3		✓	Minimally displaced right olecranon #
4		✓	Buckle # left distal radius
5	✓		
6	✓		
7	✓		
8		✓	# left clavicle
9		✓	Fibrous dysplasia left distal tibia and fibula
10	✓		
11	✓		
12		✓	Right radial neck #
13		✓	Periosteal reaction left distal ulna
14	✓		
15	✓		
16		✓	# base right fifth metatarsal
17	✓		
18	✓		
19		✓	# left clavicle
20		✓	Left upper quadrant mass
21	✓		
22		✓	Freiberg infraction third metatarsal epiphysis
23	✓		
24		✓	Developmental dysplasia right hip
25	✓		
26		✓	Acute #s left seventh and eighth posterior ribs
27		✓	Exostosis metadiaphysis left humerus
28	✓		
29	✓		
30		✓	Calcified occipital scalp collection

7.3   Explanations

2. **Buckle # base left little toe proximal phalanx**

3. **Minimally displaced right olecranon fracture**
   Careful evaluation of each bone reveals a cortical step of the olecranon consistent with an acute minimally displaced fracture. This fracture is intra-articular resulting in an associated joint effusion (elevation of both the anterior and posterior fat pads)—remember that elbow effusions do not only result from supracondylar and radial neck fractures. As discussed in prior elbow radiograph explanations, the alignment must always be assessed: in this radiograph, the anterior humeral and radiocapitellar alignment is normal. The fracture is magnified below:

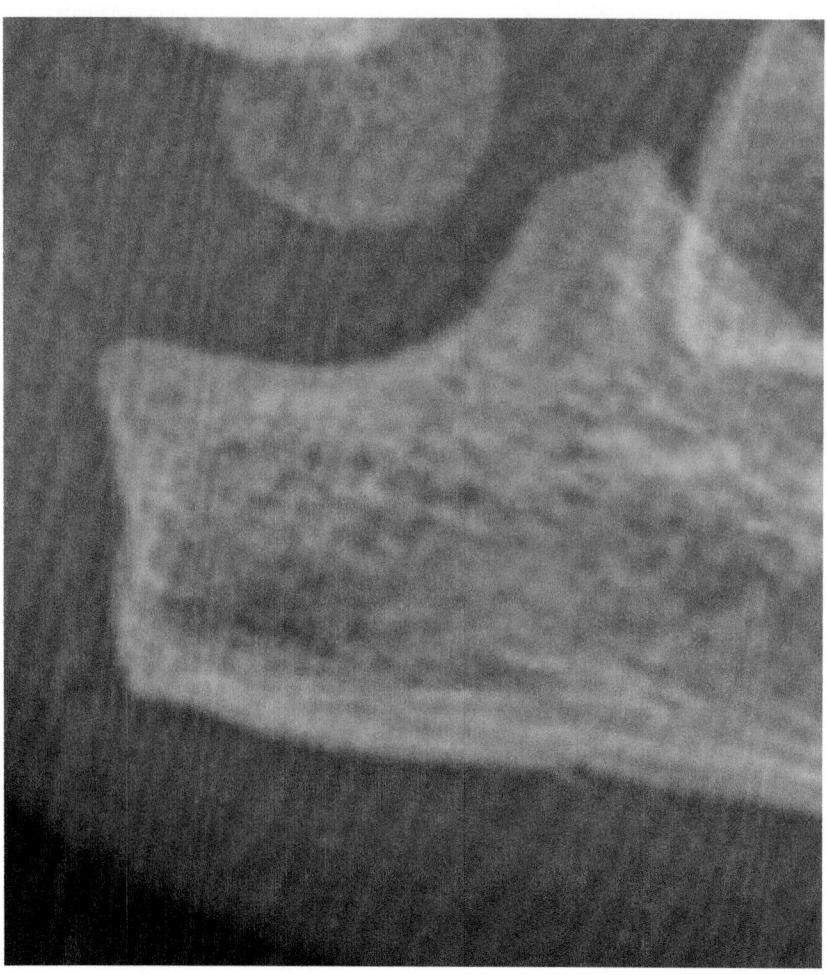

4. **Buckle # left distal radius**

8. **# left clavicle**

This term male neonate was born by normal vaginal delivery. The midwife reported feeling a click on delivery of the left anterior shoulder. Whilst normal movements of the left arm were initially reported, crepitus and deformity of the left clavicle were noted on palpation. This solitary humeral radiograph was performed. In some centres, only one projection may be performed (as in this case) which is why you must be methodical when evaluating the bony structures. If there is radiological suspicion of fracture, a further/dedicated view of the area of concern would be justified.

Careful assessment of the left clavicle reveals a minimally displaced midshaft fracture with overlapping fragments resulting in the increased density. The fracture is magnified in the image below:

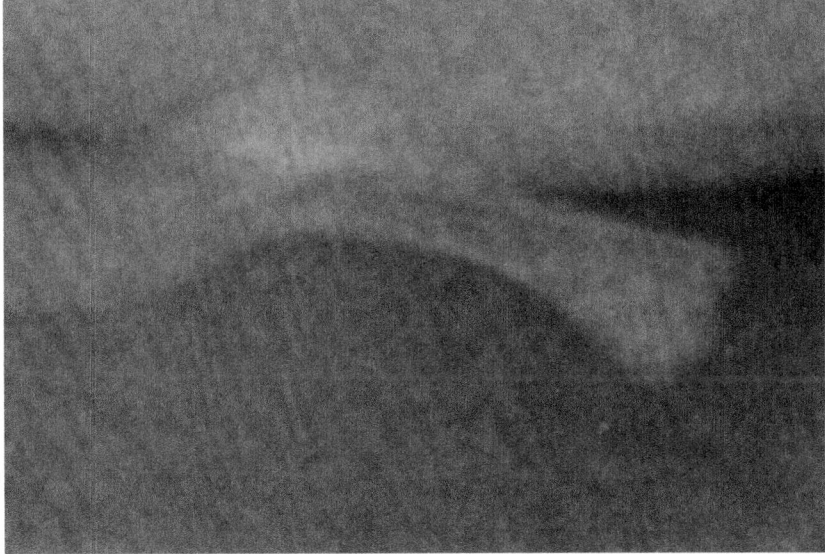

Often, these injuries are missed on clinical examination. It is important to consider the clinical and birth history in any infant younger than 3 months old that is presented with an unexplained injury or one that is identified on radiography performed for another indication.

The follow-up radiograph 6 weeks later demonstrated abundant callus formation consistent with a healing fracture. A further follow-up radiograph performed 6 months following the initial injury showed that the left clavicle had completely healed and remodelled. A clavicular fracture is the commonest bony birth injury and may result from shoulder dystocia or traumatic delivery, as in this case. Beyond 3 months of age, any birth-related fracture should have healed completely which is important to remember in the context of an unexplained injury when inflicted injury (physical abuse) is a possibility.

9. **Fibrous dysplasia left distal tibia and fibula**
   See the explanation for Test 3, Image 10.

10. **Normal right calcaneal apophysis**
    This radiograph is normal. The morphology of the calcaneal apophysis can be variable across all ages. Secondary ossification usually occurs in the plantar third of the apophysis by 7 years of age with fusion of the physis beginning from around the age of 12 years and completing from around 15 years (but this may be later in males). In this oblique radiograph, the calcaneal apophysis is projected over the body of the calcaneus and its appearance is entirely normal.

11. **Normal right shoulder radiograph**
    This radiograph is normal. Contemporaneous AP and dedicated clavicle projections confirm that there is no fracture. The lucent line medial to the right humeral head is the physis for the coracoid ossification centre which has not yet fused.

12. **Right radial neck #**
    Compare the radial neck in this image with that from Image 5 from this test— the acute cortical step in the right proximal radial metaphysis (neck) in this image is apparent.

13. **Periosteal reaction left distal ulna**

This finding is subtle, but real, and is appreciated even when comparing the original image with the magnified one below:

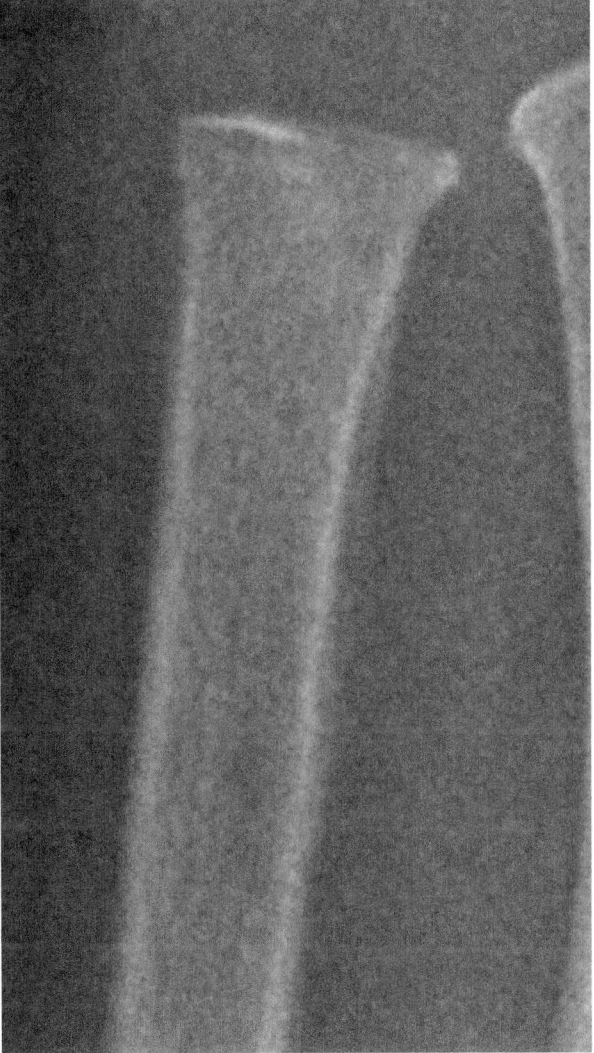

This radiograph was performed to assess for any underlying evidence of osteo-myelitis post drainage of a left wrist abscess. The periosteal reaction on both sides of the distal ulna meta/diaphysis appears multilamellated, i.e. not benign (see the explanation for Test 5, Image 2). Furthermore, in the clinical context of local abscess the changes must be considered secondary to osteomyelitis. Radiographic changes of osteomyelitis may include: focal osteopenia, lysis, and/or cortical loss; endosteal scalloping; and loss of bony trabecular architecture.

The metaphysis is the primary site of infection in osteomyelitis but due to the transphyseal vessels (those which extend from the metaphysis across the physis and into the epiphysis) in those aged less than 18 months, direct extension of the infection into the epiphysis can result in destruction of the epiphyseal cartilage, disrupting growth. This epiphyseal extension contributes to the higher incidence of septic arthritis in this age group.

The most common organism resulting in haematogenous osteomyelitis in infants and children is *Staphylococcus aureus*. However, there has been an increase in cases of *Kingella kingae* over recent years in Europe and the Middle East, becoming the most common pathogen causing osteomyelitis or septic arthritis in young children from these areas. Notably, in patients with sickle cell disease, *Salmonella* infection is more common. Importantly, one-third of children with osteomyelitis have a history of recent trauma.

Tip for the viva:
- Normal radiographic appearances do not exclude osteomyelitis: periosteal reaction may not be apparent on radiographs for up to 14 days. If there is ongoing clinical concern in children, follow-up radiography should be performed 5–7 days following the initial radiographs (and 10–14 days in adults).

14. **Normal abdominal radiograph**
    When infants and children cry (a common occurrence when radiography is being performed), they can swallow a lot of air distending their stomach, as seen in this radiograph. There is no air-fluid level to indicate gastric outflow obstruction. The remainder of the bowel gas pattern and the bony structures are normal. Both hips are in joint.

Tip for the viva:
- On every abdominal radiograph, you must always assess the hip joints, particularly when performed for other indications, as you may be the first person to detect the subluxation in a dysplastic hip or the early changes of Perthes disease.

16. **# base right fifth metatarsal**

19. **# left clavicle**
    This 11-month-old female was presented to ED after rolling off the bed and not using her left arm. The radiograph reveals a midshaft left clavicular fracture. It was felt that the fracture was likely to have resulted from the mechanism of injury offered by the parents. There were no other concerns and no further imaging or investigations were performed.

As clinical radiologists, it is imperative that we, as well as our ED and paediatric colleagues, are satisfied that any fracture in a pre-ambulant infant has a satisfactory explanation/appropriate mechanism of injury.

20. **Left upper quadrant mass**
    There is an appreciable paucity of bowel gas in the left upper quadrant with medial displacement of the splenic flexure colon. Note the focus of calcification within the mass just inferior to the anterior end of the left 12th rib. Following this radiograph, an ultrasound and MRI were performed which demonstrated a large mass and MIBG scintigraphy confirmed a diagnosis of neuroblastoma.

    Tip for the viva:
    • Be sure to assess the bones for any aggressive features to suggest metastases in the context of an abdominal mass.

22. **Freiberg infraction third metatarsal epiphysis**
    This is osteochondrosis of the metatarsal heads, typically the second metatarsal head but the third, as in this case, and fourth metatarsal heads may be affected, also. It is thought to result from either an acute or repetitive trauma (as in this 11-year-old gymnast presenting with foot pain) and presents with swelling and pain on weight-bearing. The radiographic features include metatarsal head flattening, sclerosis and cortical thickening, and widening of the affected metatarsal joint. The changes may be bilateral in up to 10% of cases.

    Tip for the viva:
    • Flattening of the metatarsal head in the absence of other associated radiographic findings of osteochondrosis may be seen in up to 10% of the asymptomatic population.

24. **Developmental dysplasia right hip**
    See the explanation for Test 2, Image 17. There is a small medial portion of the right proximal femoral epiphysis which is in joint (covered by the acetabulum). As such, the right hip is laterally subluxed and not yet dislocated.

25. **Normal left ankle radiograph**
    See the explanation for Test 4, Image 5 regarding the os trigonum.

26. **Acute #s left seventh and eighth posterior ribs**

    See the explanation for Test 2, Image 14. The fractures are better visualised in the magnified image below:

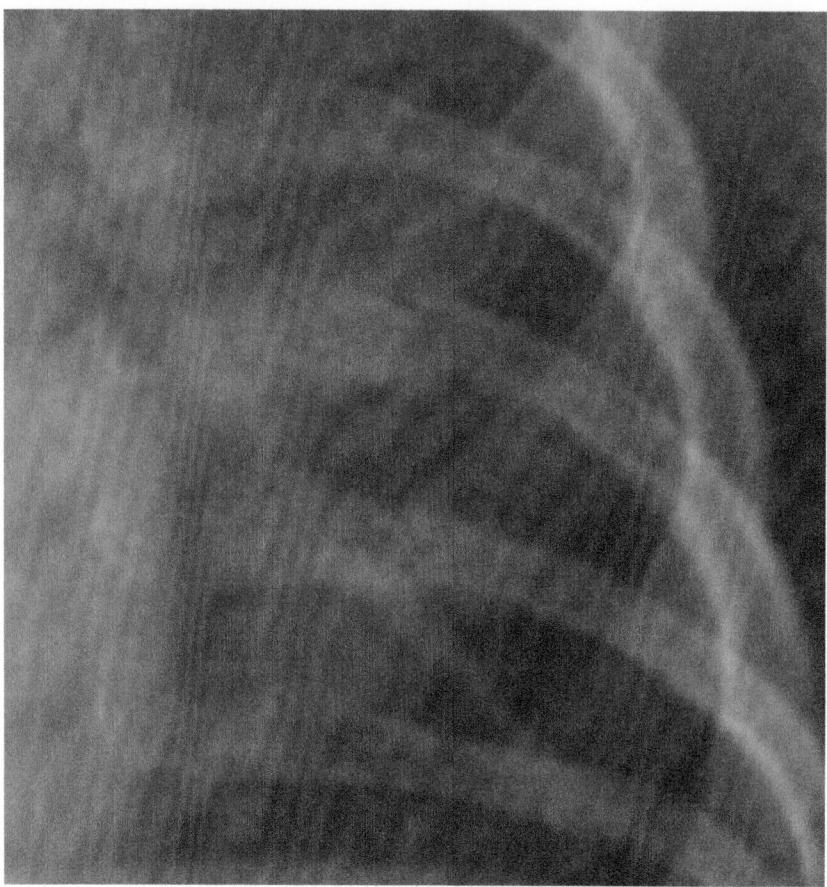

27. **Exostosis metadiaphysis left humerus**

    Exostoses are benign bony outgrowths that arise from the surface of the bone, typically in the appendicular skeleton. The medullary cavity of the exostosis is usually continuous with the parent bone. These develop during childhood, can present at any age, and are most frequently encountered incidentally. When exostoses are capped with cartilage, they are known as osteochondromas and can be considered a chondroid neoplasm. Osteochondromas may be congenital or result from previous trauma to the physis. They typically grow *away* from the adjacent joint. Given that they represent growth of the physis in an abnormal direction, they often stop growing once skeletal maturity has been reached, i.e. when the physes have fused. If they are sporadic and solitary, they have a low malignant potential (approximately 1%) but this is much higher in the context of hereditary multiple exostoses (HME), ranging from 5 to 25%—they may degenerate into low-grade malignancies, chondrosarcomas, in up to 85% of cases.

Ultrasound is accurate in assessing the presence of a cartilage cap. CT will demonstrate the cartilage cap also; however, MRI is the best modality to assess for cartilage thickness, surrounding soft tissue and marrow oedema, and in particular malignant degeneration—a cartilage cap measuring over *1.5 cm* is suspicious for malignant change. The mnemonic **GLADPAST** can be used to remember the features of sarcomatous degeneration of an osteochondroma:

- **G**rowth after skeletal maturity
- **L**ucency (new)
- **A**dditional scintigraphic activity
- **D**estruction (cortical)
- **P**ain after puberty
- **A**nd
- **S**oft tissue mass
- **T**hickened cartilage cap greater than 1.5 cm

This 14-year-old female originally presented at the age of 10 years with shoulder pain and the exostosis was demonstrated on radiography. Presentation is usually with pain from local pressure effects of the osteochondroma, pathological fracture, or malignant degeneration.

Tip for the viva:
- When an exostosis/osteochondroma has been identified, look for features of an aggressive bone lesion suggesting malignant degeneration on radiography (i.e. cortical irregularity/bone destruction, wide zone of transition, associated soft tissue mass) and look for other exostoses suggesting a diagnosis of HME (which, in case you are asked, is autosomal dominant).

28. **Normal skull radiograph**
This radiograph is normal. The obliquity of this AP projection allows the cranial sutures to be well visualised. Correlate with the reference from Test 2, Image 24.

30. **Calcified occipital scalp collection**

This child was referred by her GP for an ultrasound of the scalp because of a large, non-tender, fluctuant cystic swelling at the vertex. The ultrasound revealed a compressible subcutaneous fluid collection. She disclosed that she had hit her head on a door handle. Subsequent radiography, as shown, demonstrated a calcified occipital scalp collection seen in the magnified image below:

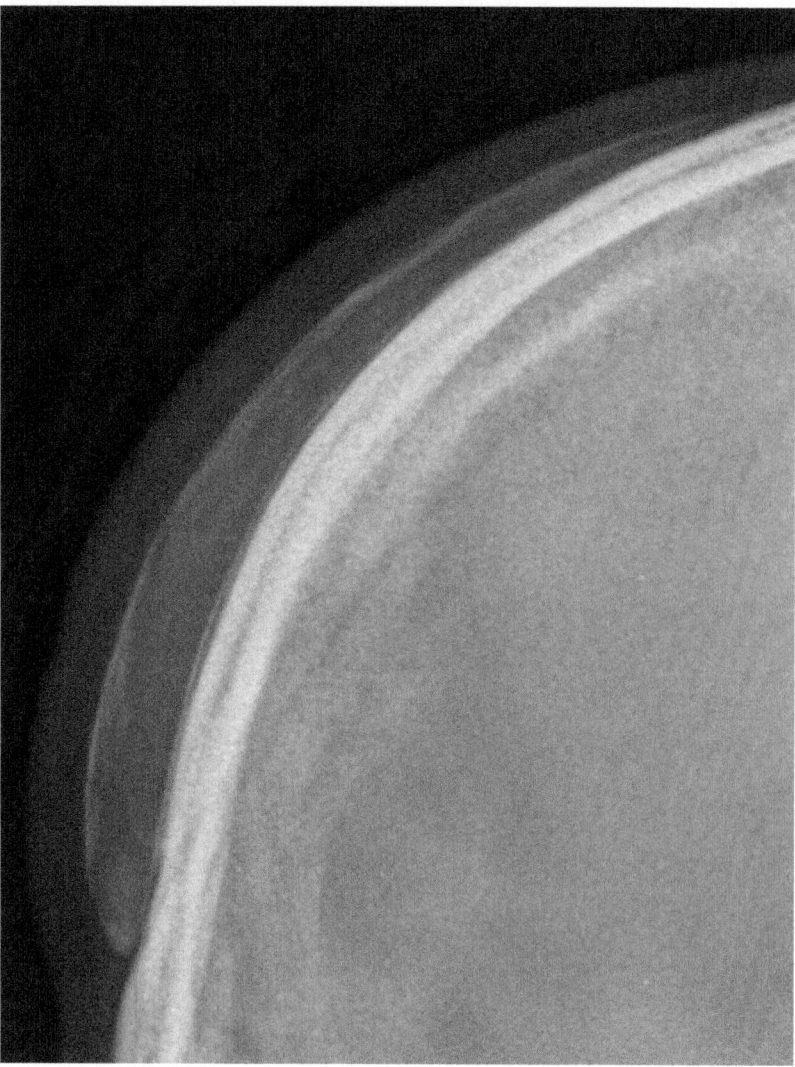

This collection was confirmed on CT to be subgaleal in location, crossing over the sagittal suture. This location cannot be reliably ascertained from this lateral radiograph so identifying it as a calcified occipital scalp collection is sufficient for the examination.

When considering the three main types of scalp haematoma (caput succedaneum, subgaleal haematoma, and cephalohaematoma), it is helpful to remember the layers of the scalp which can be best remembered using the mnemonic, **SCALP**:

- **S**kin—a subcutaneous (below the skin) collection of serosanguinous fluid/haematoma is known as *caput succedaneum* (from the Latin, literally *head + substitute*, presumably referring to how the normal head shape is temporarily 'substituted' for another). These collections usually result from pressure on the presenting part of the skull from the dilating cervix and/or bony pelvis during a prolonged second stage of labour. Although they can be ill-defined and may cross the midline if extensive, these are usually simple and self-limiting.
- **C**onnective tissue
- **A**poneurosis—this tough sheet of fibrous connective tissue, is also known as the epicranial aponeurosis or *galea* (from the Latin, meaning 'helmet'). Its anterior attachment, the frontalis muscle inserts on the frontal bone, and its posterior attachment, the occipitalis muscle, inserts on the external occipital protuberance of the occipital bone. Subgaleal haematomas are found beneath the galea but above the loose connective tissue and commonly occur following a ventouse/vacuum delivery. Not being bound by sutures, they may extend from the orbits to the nape of the neck (anterior to posterior aponeurotic insertions, as above) and feel ill-defined on clinical examination. They are potentially lethal and there have been reported neonatal deaths secondary to extensive subgaleal haemorrhage because neonates can lose a significant amount of their circulating blood volume following a traumatic/difficult delivery (the average circulating volume of a neonate is approximately 300 mL and the aponeurotic space may hold up to 260 mL): thus, prompt recognition is vital.
- **L**oose connective tissue
- **P**eriosteum—the periosteum is the outer most layer that covers bones. Haematomas found in the potential subperiosteal space (the space between the periosteum and the bone) are known as cephalohaematomas and result from rupture of subperiosteal vessels usually from birth trauma/assisted delivery (forceps, ventouse/vacuum delivery). Given their location, cephalohaematomas are bound by the periosteum and therefore *cannot* cross suture lines, thus distinguishing them from subgaleal haematomas which *can* cross suture lines. Cephalohaematomas can be thought of as extradural haematomas but on the external side of the skull. Cephalohaematomas may be unilateral or bilateral and when long-standing, will usually calcify and gradually resolve by incorporation into the underlying skull (which may result in deformity).

Representative figures of all the described collections are available in the references.

Further Reading

Image 8

Please see the Test 2, Image 14 references regarding the imaging of suspected physical abuse in infants and young children.

Image 10

Rossi I, Rosenburg Z, Zember J (2016) Normal skeletal development and imaging pitfalls of the calcaneal apophysis: MRI features. Skeletal Radiol 45(4):483–493

Image 13

Jaramillo D, Dormans JP, Delgado J et al (2017) Haematogenous osteomyelitis in infants and children: imaging of a changing disease. Radiology 283(3):629–643
Skandhan AKP, Gaillard F et al (2018) Osteomyelitis. https://radiopaedia.org/articles/osteomyelitis. Accessed May 2018

Image 22

Talusan PG, Diaz-Collado PJ, Reach JS Jr (2014) Freiberg's infraction: diagnosis and treatment. Foot Ankle Spec 7(1):52–56
Thurston M, Jones J et al (2018) Freiberg disease. https://radiopaedia.org/articles/freiberg-disease. Accessed May 2018

Image 27

Bell DJ, Gaillard F et al (2018) Osteochondroma. https://radiopaedia.org/articles/osteochondroma. Accessed May 2018
Murphy A, Jones J et al (2018) Exostosis. https://radiopaedia.org/articles/exostosis. Accessed May 2018
Murphey MD, Choi JJ, Kransdorf MJ et al (2000) Imaging of osteochondroma: variants and complications with radiologic-pathologic correlation. Radiographics 20(5):1407–1434

Image 30

Chaturvedi A, Chaturvedi A, Stanescu AL et al (2018) Mechanical birth-related trauma to the neonate: an imaging perspective. Insights Imaging 9(1):103–118
Davis DJ (2001) Neonatal subgaleal haemorrhage: diagnosis and management. CMAJ 164(10):1452–1453
Jones J et al (2018) Layers of the scalp mnemonic. https://radiopaedia.org/articles/layers-of-the-scalp-mnemonic. Accessed June 2018
Hacking C et al (2018) Caput succedaneum. https://radiopaedia.org/articles/caput-succedaneum. Accessed June 2018

Hacking C, Jones J (2018a) Galea aponeurotica. https://radiopaedia.org/articles/galea-aponeuro-tica. Accessed June 2018

Hacking C, Jones J (2018b) Subgaleal haematoma. https://radiopaedia.org/articles/subgaleal-hae-matoma-2. Accessed June 2018

Hacking C, Gaillard F et al (2018). Cephalohaematoma. https://radiopaedia.org/articles/cephalo-haematoma. Accessed June 2018

Test 8

8

8.1 Images

Image 1

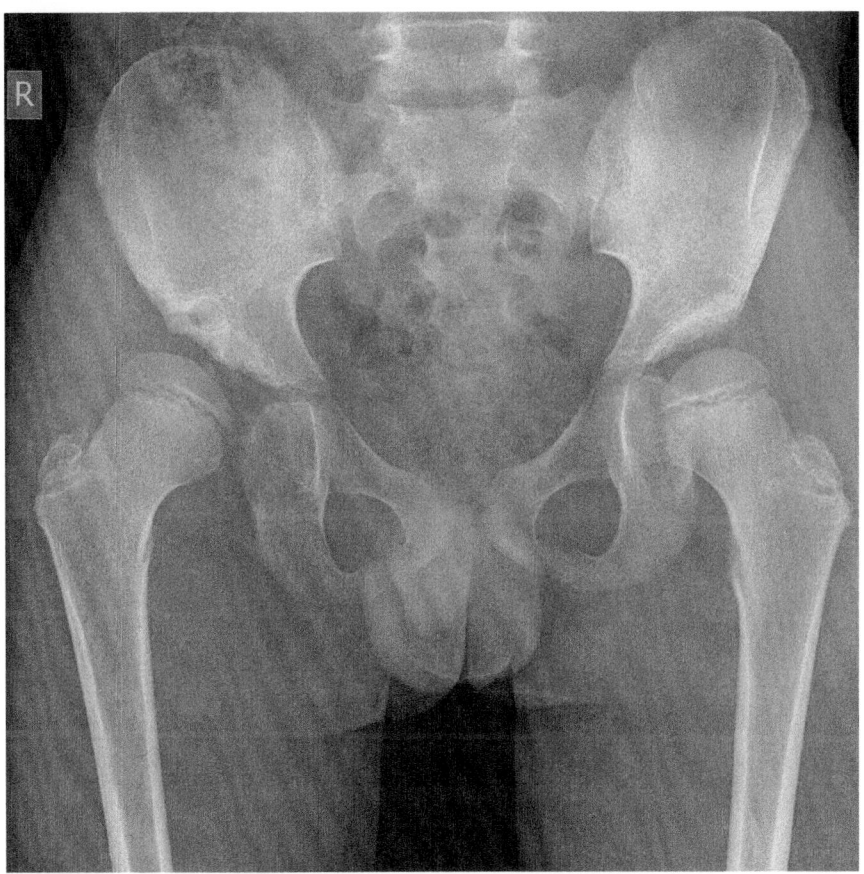

Normal	Abnormal	Diagnosis/Abnormality (only if abnormal)

© Springer Nature Switzerland AG 2019
M. Paddock, A. C. Offiah, *Paediatric Radiology Rapid Reporting for FRCR Part 2B*,
https://doi.org/10.1007/978-3-030-01965-5_8

Image 2

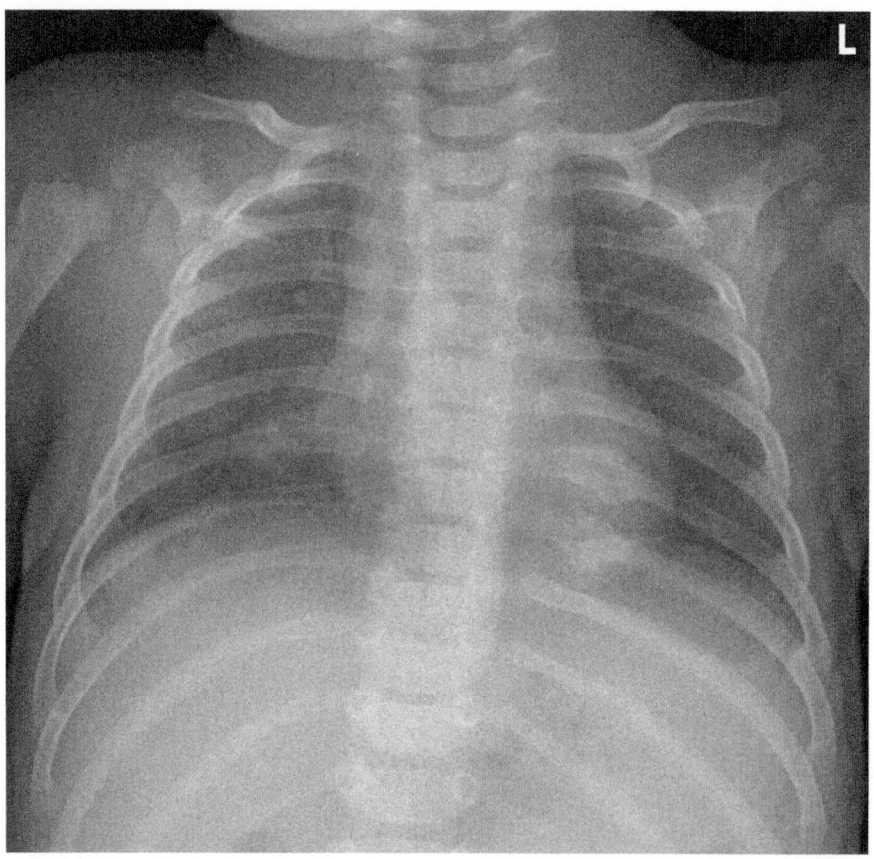

Normal	Abnormal	Diagnosis/Abnormality (only if abnormal)

Image 3

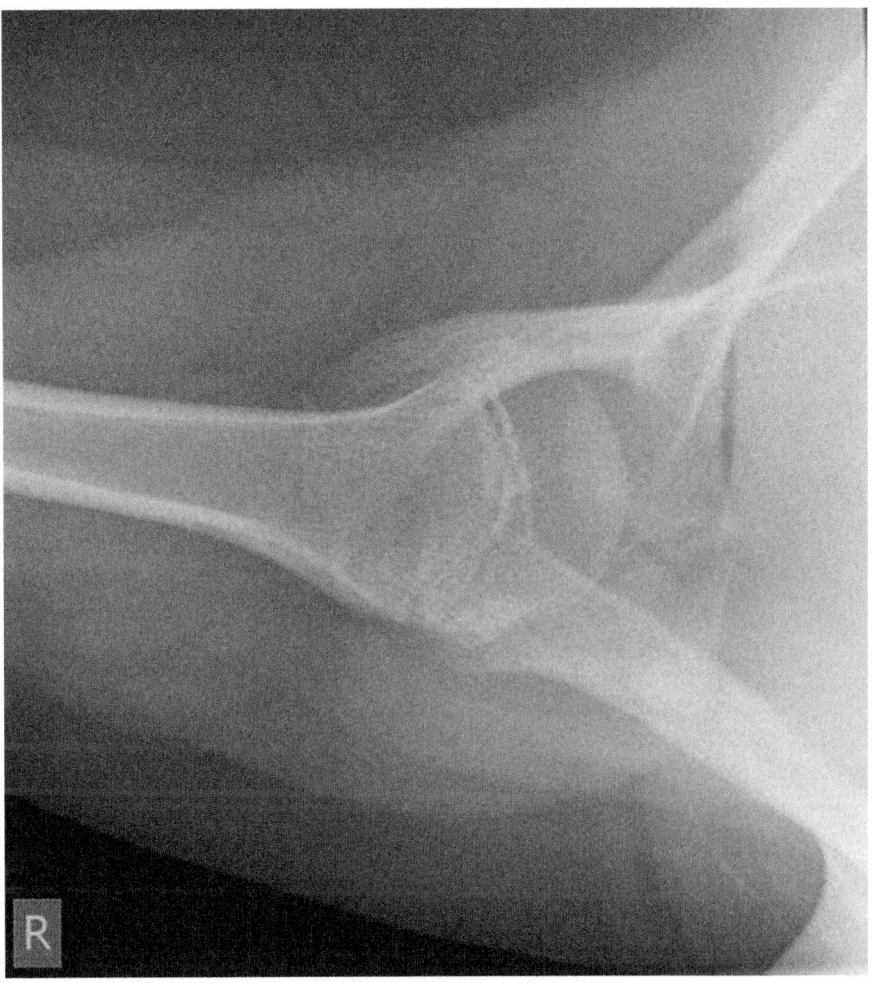

Normal	Abnormal	Diagnosis/Abnormality (only if abnormal)

Image 4

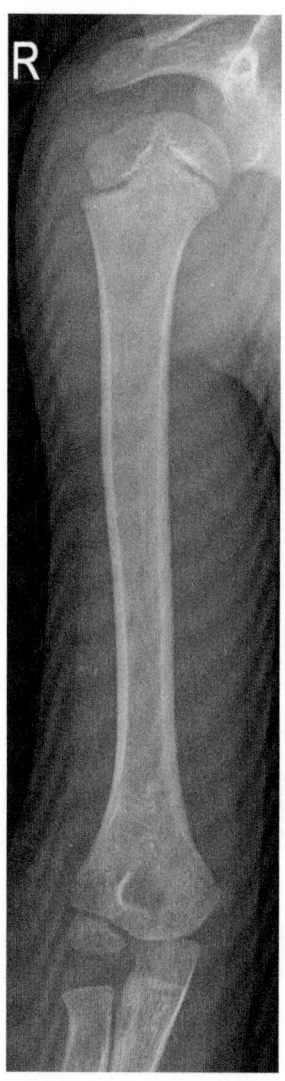

Normal	Abnormal	Diagnosis/Abnormality (only if abnormal)

Image 5

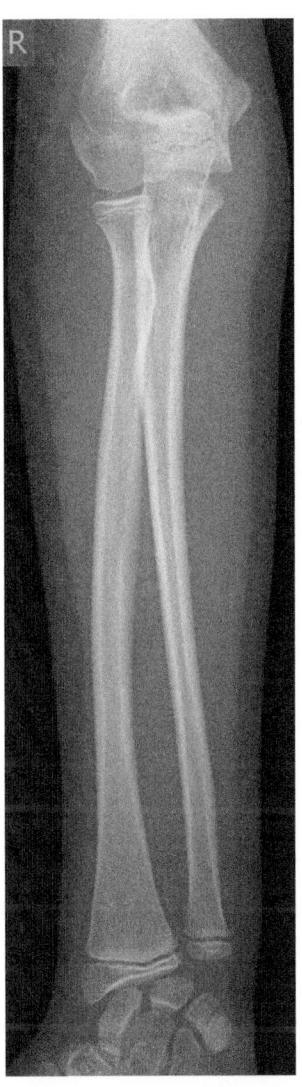

Normal	Abnormal	Diagnosis/Abnormality (only if abnormal)

Image 6

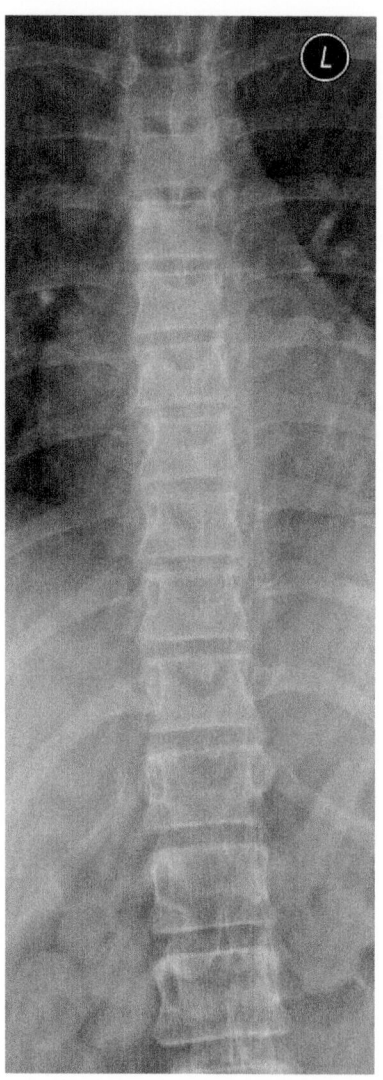

Normal	Abnormal	Diagnosis/Abnormality (only if abnormal)

Image 7

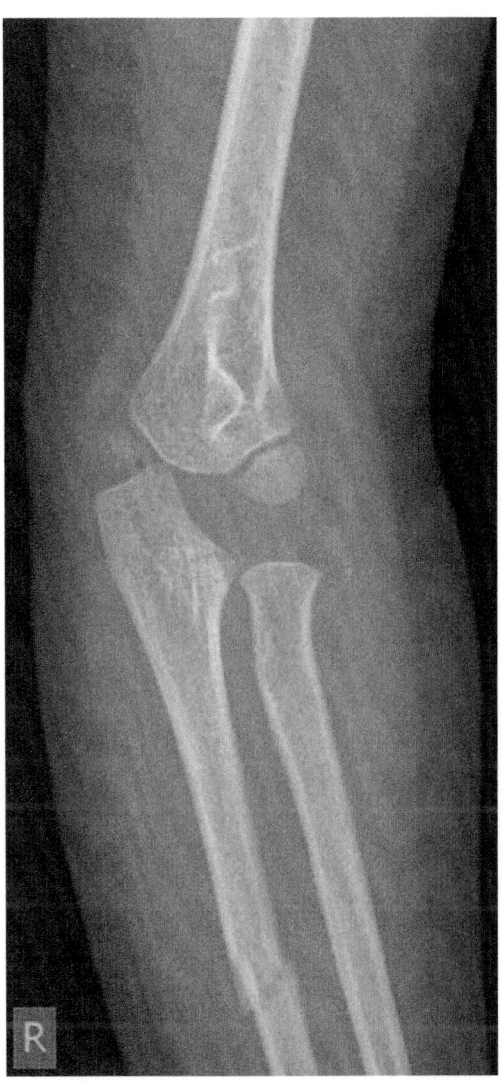

Normal	Abnormal	Diagnosis/Abnormality (only if abnormal)

Image 8

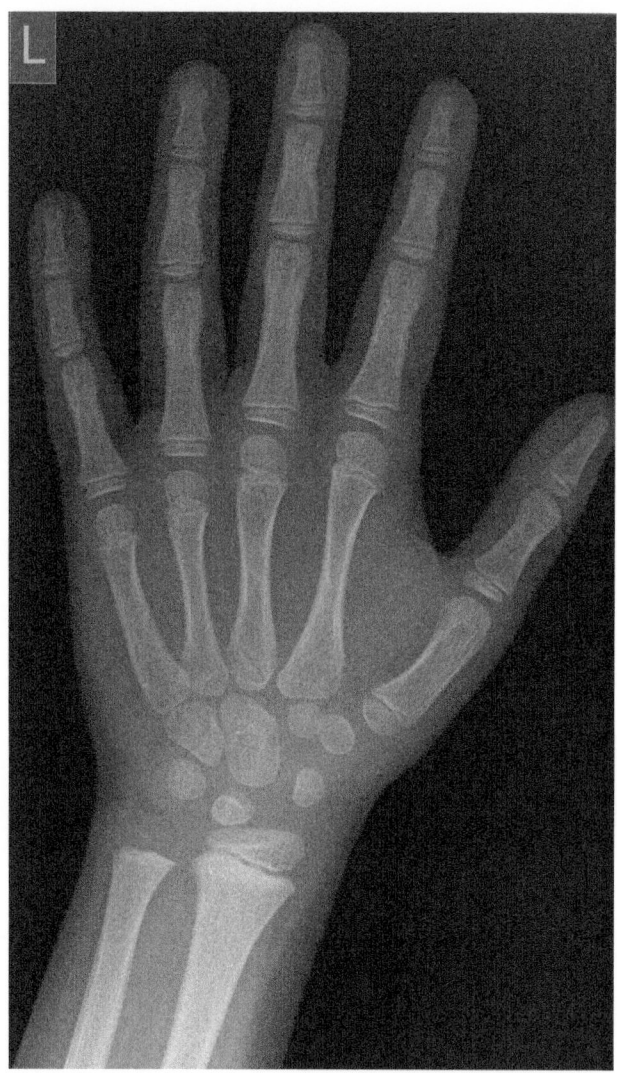

Normal	Abnormal	Diagnosis/Abnormality (only if abnormal)

Image 9

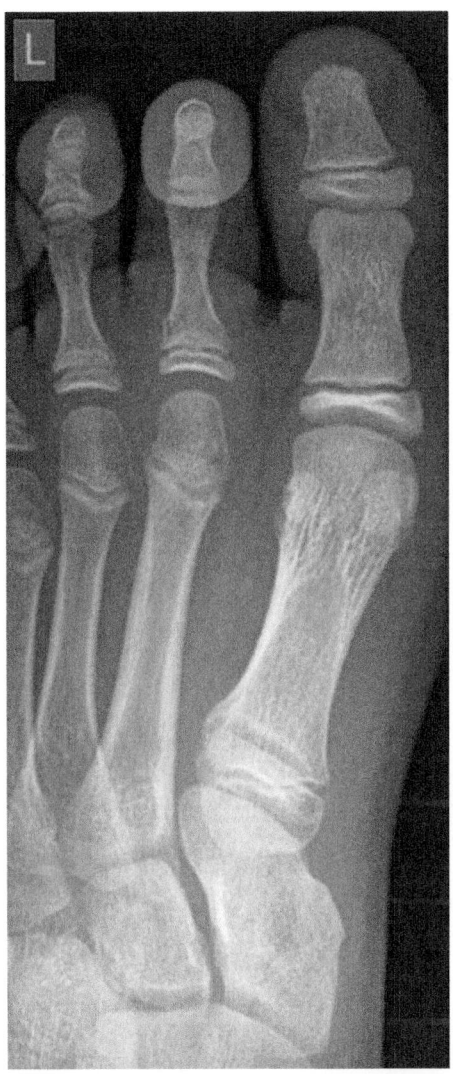

Normal	Abnormal	Diagnosis/Abnormality (only if abnormal)

Image 10

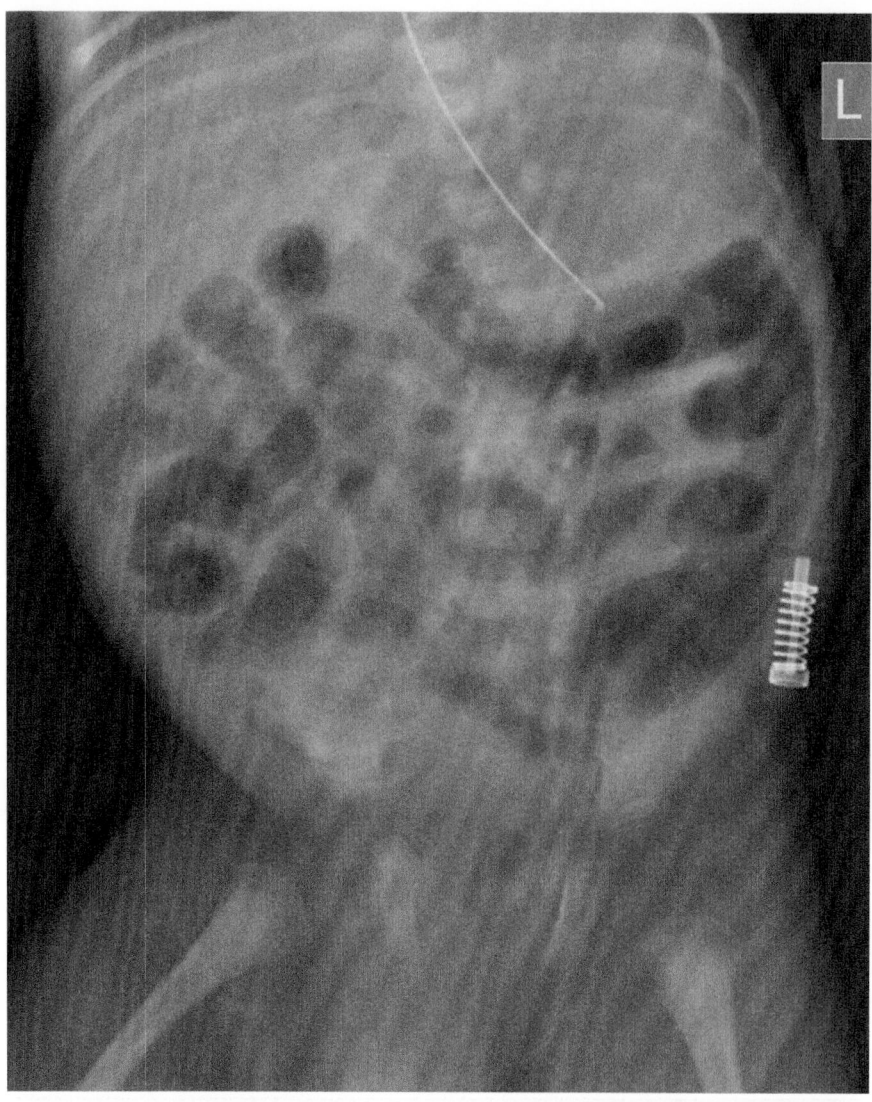

Normal	Abnormal	Diagnosis/Abnormality (only if abnormal)

Image 11

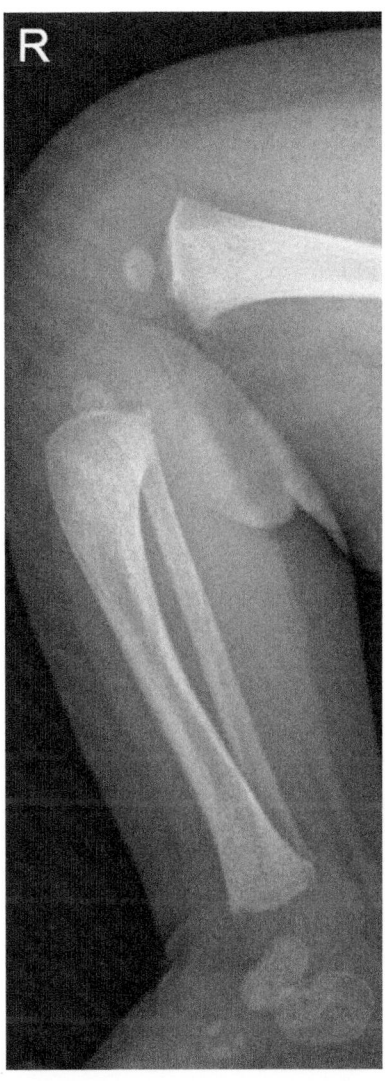

Normal	Abnormal	Diagnosis/Abnormality (only if abnormal)

Image 12

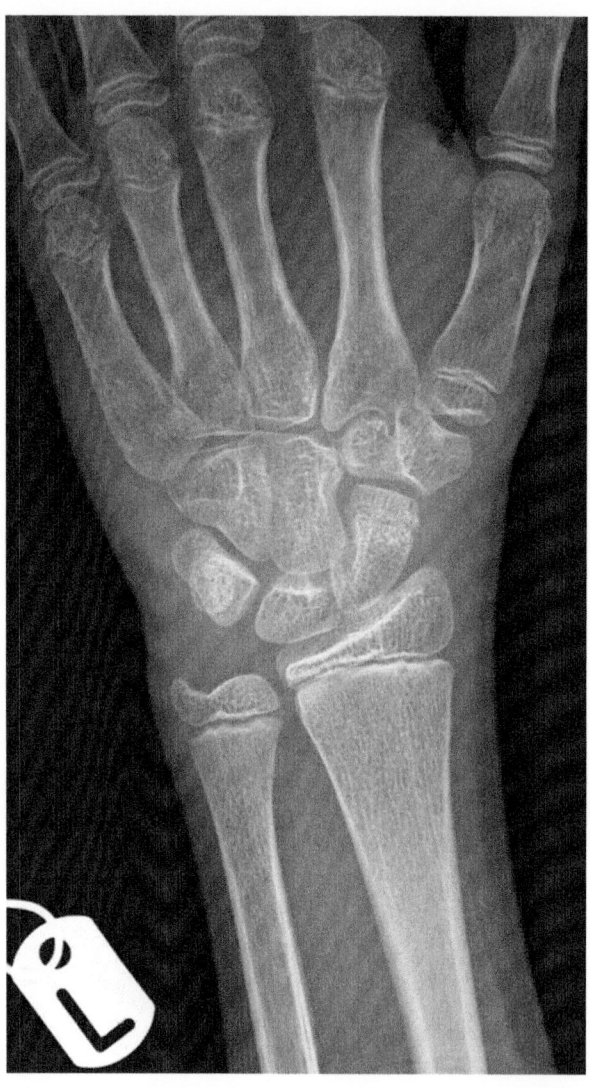

Normal	Abnormal	Diagnosis/Abnormality (only if abnormal)

Image 13

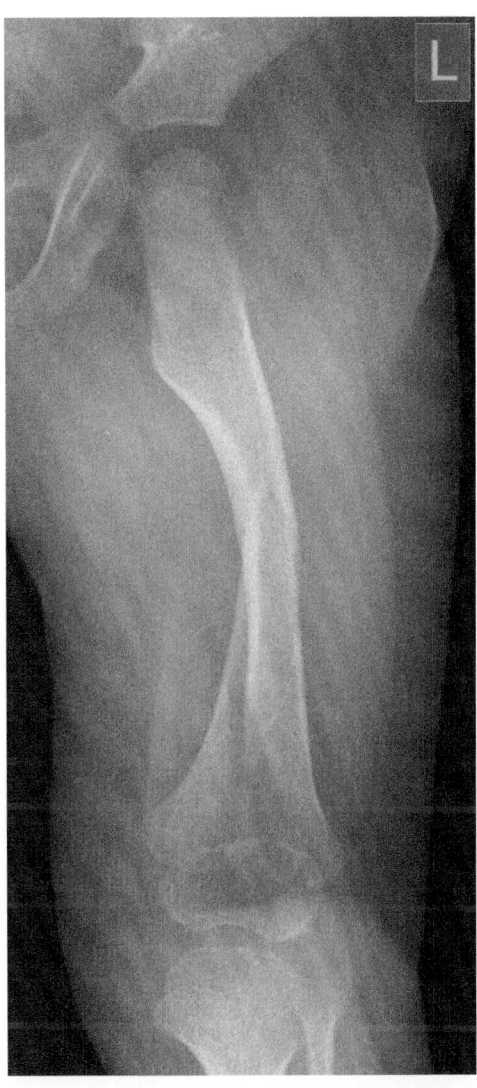

Normal	Abnormal	Diagnosis/Abnormality (only if abnormal)

Image 14

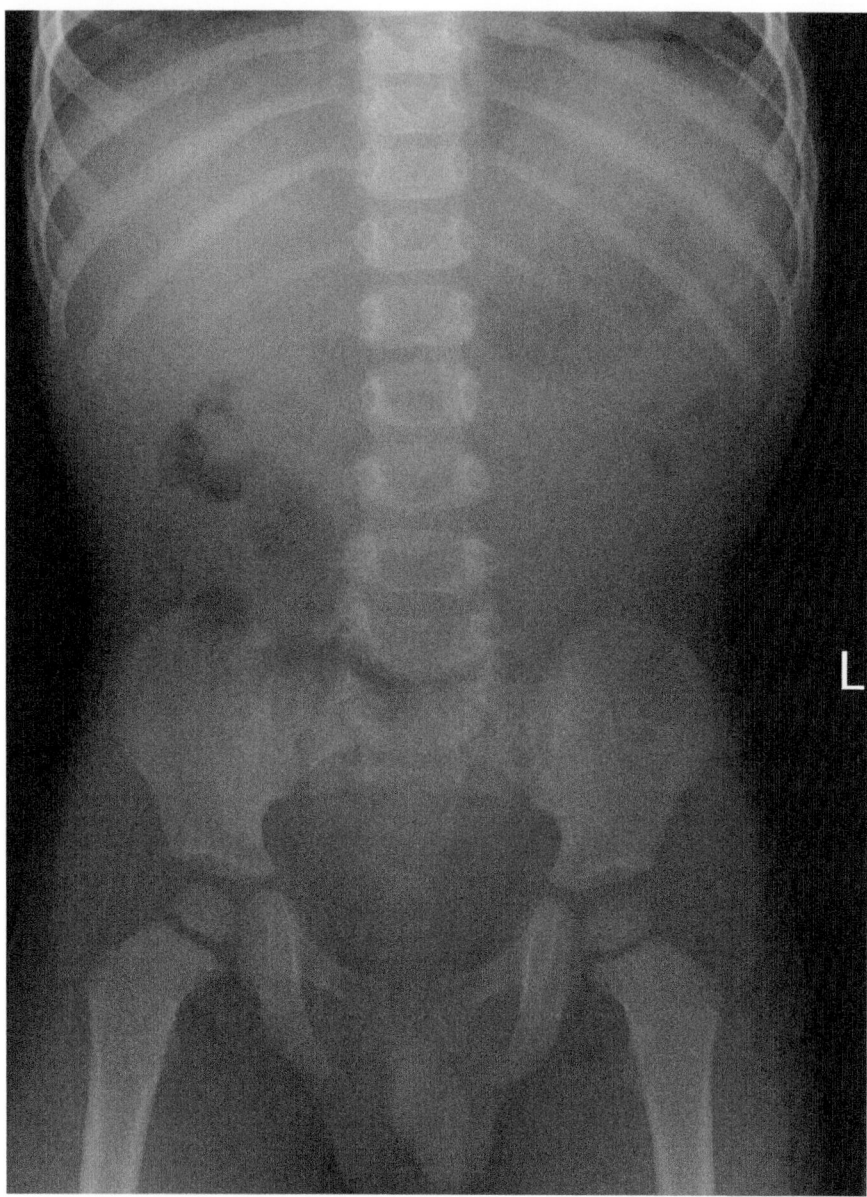

Normal	Abnormal	Diagnosis/Abnormality (only if abnormal)

Image 15

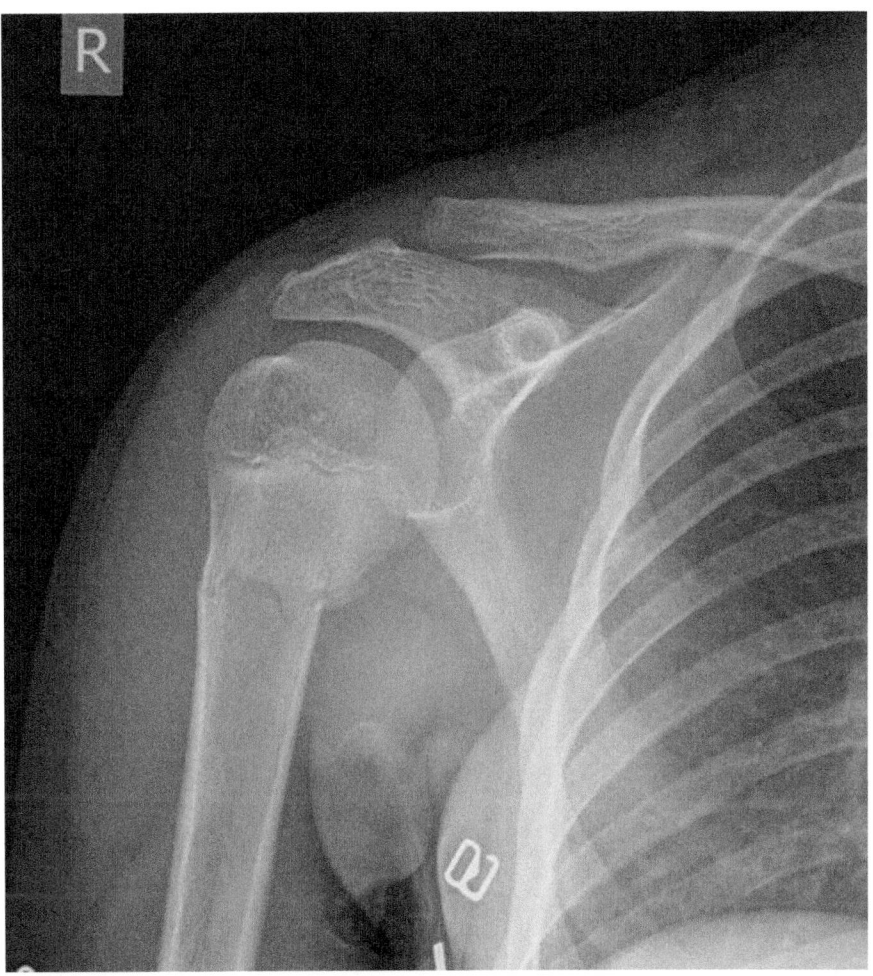

Normal	Abnormal	Diagnosis/Abnormality (only if abnormal)

Image 16

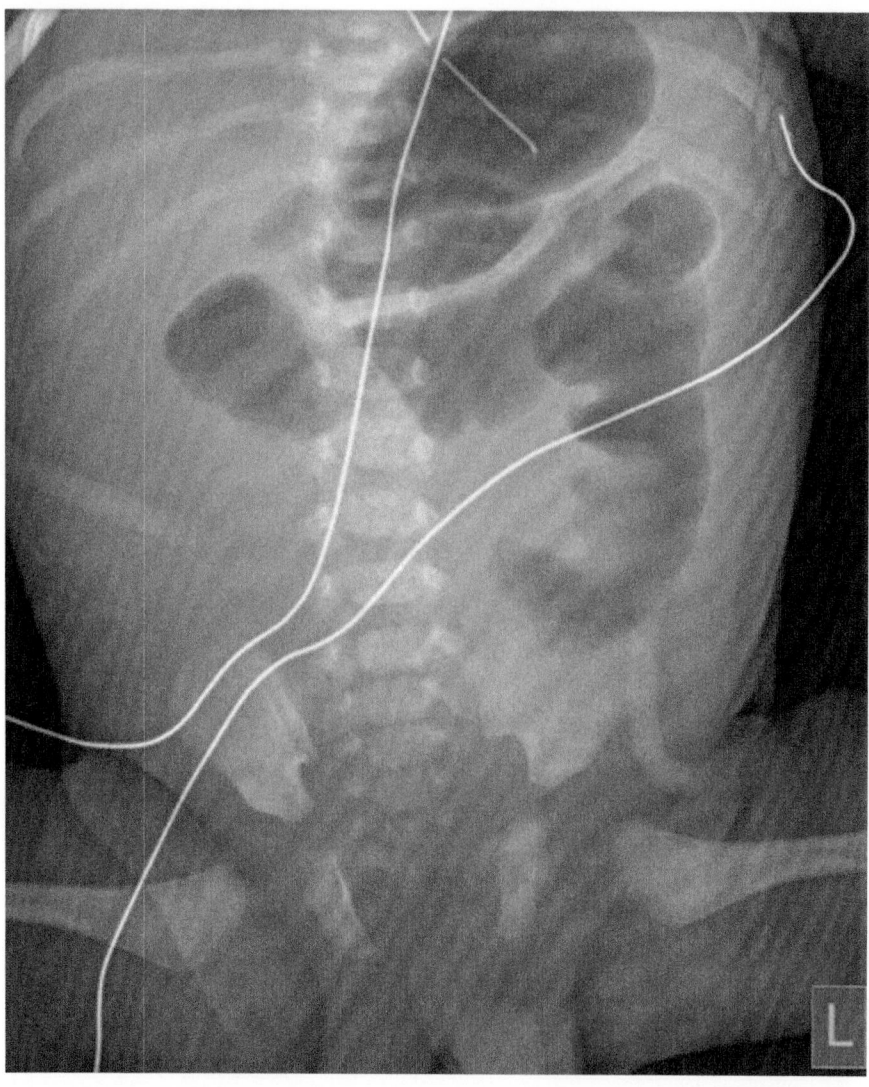

Normal	Abnormal	Diagnosis/Abnormality (only if abnormal)

Image 17

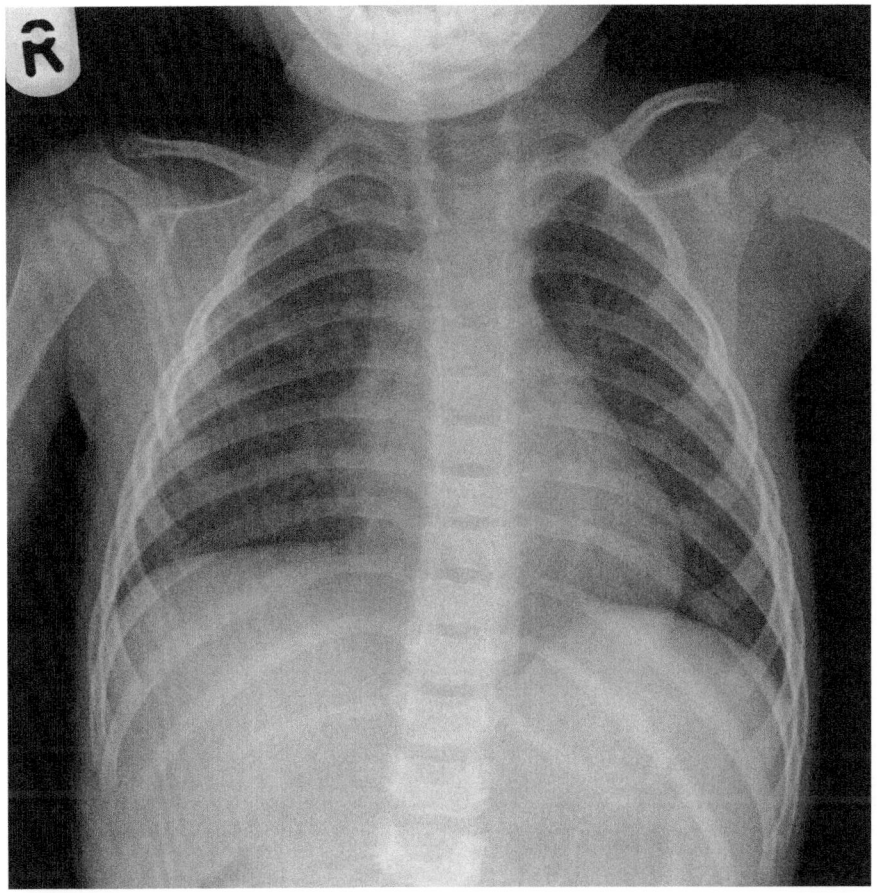

Normal	Abnormal	Diagnosis/Abnormality (only if abnormal)

Image 18

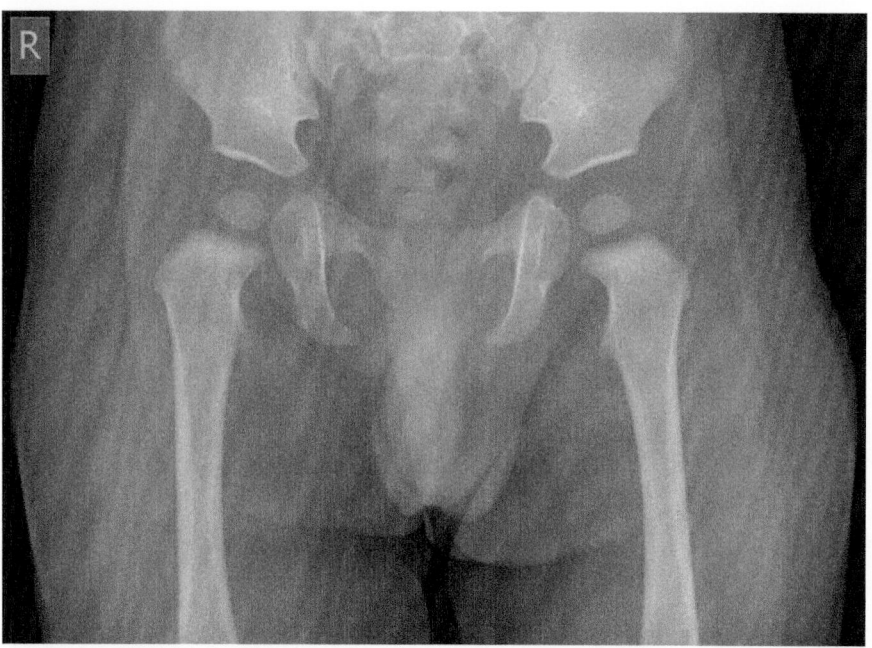

Normal	Abnormal	Diagnosis/Abnormality (only if abnormal)

Image 19

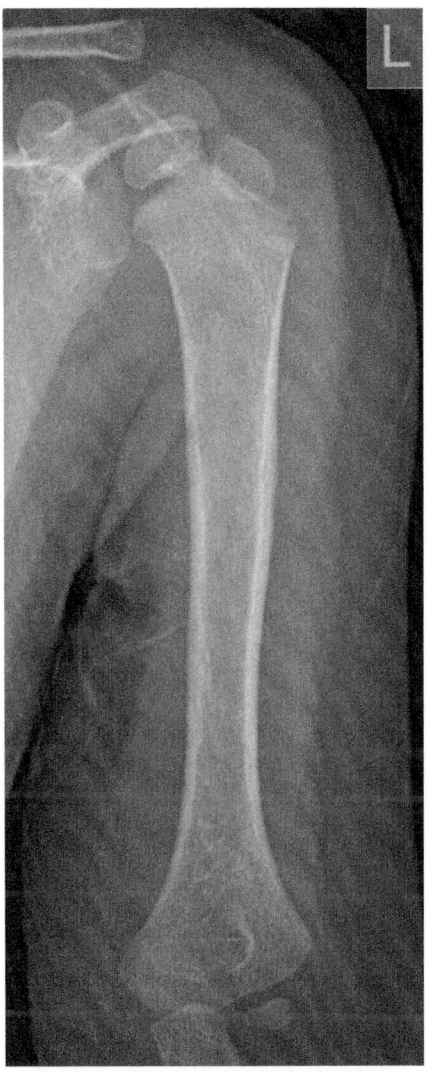

Normal	Abnormal	Diagnosis/Abnormality (only if abnormal)

Image 20

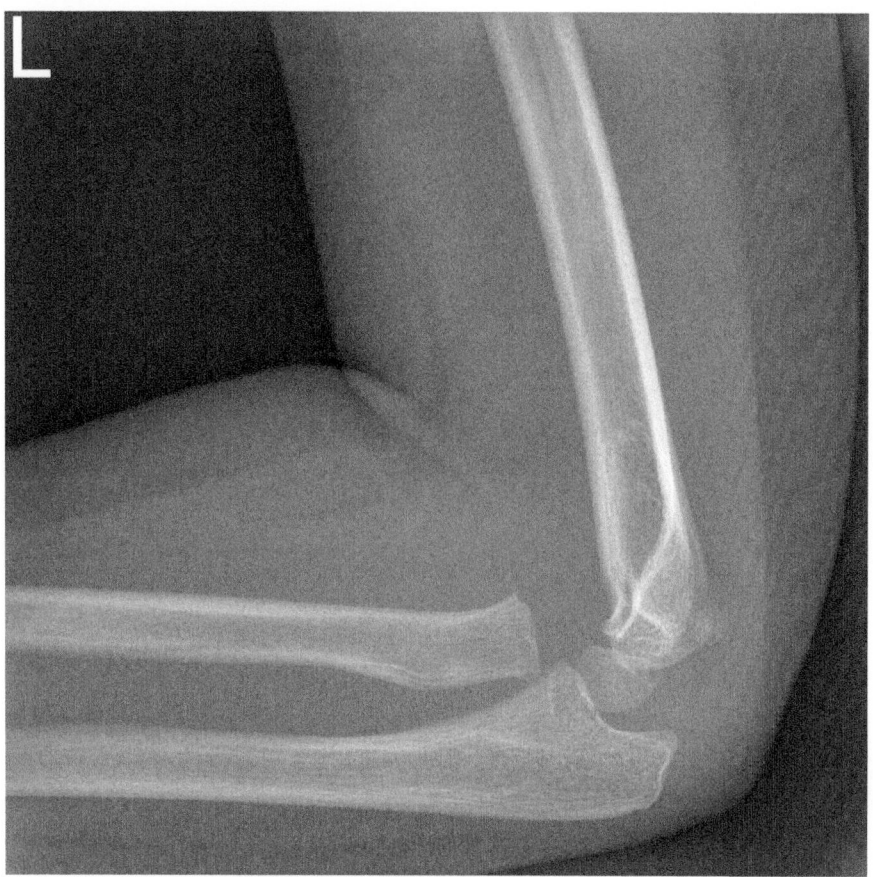

Normal	Abnormal	Diagnosis/Abnormality (only if abnormal)

Image 21

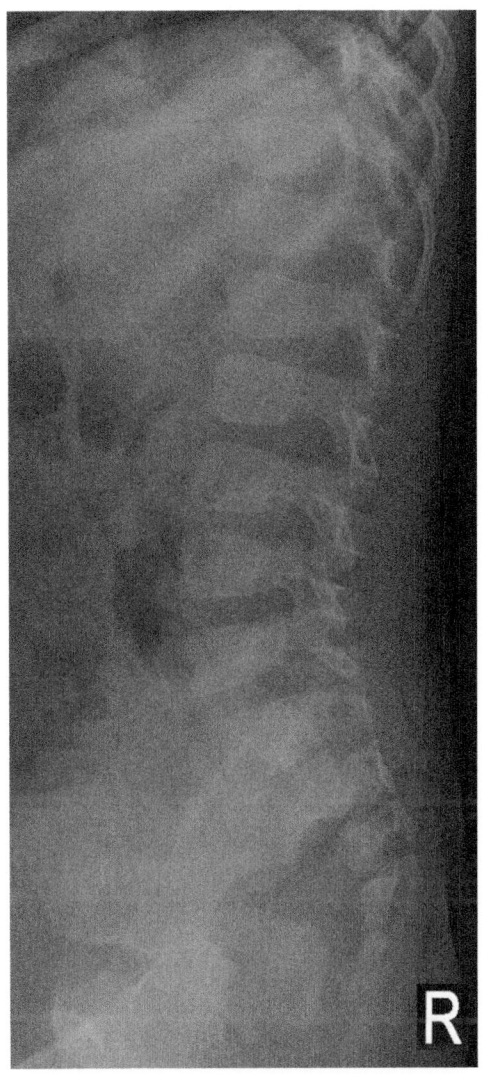

Normal	Abnormal	Diagnosis/Abnormality (only if abnormal)

Image 22

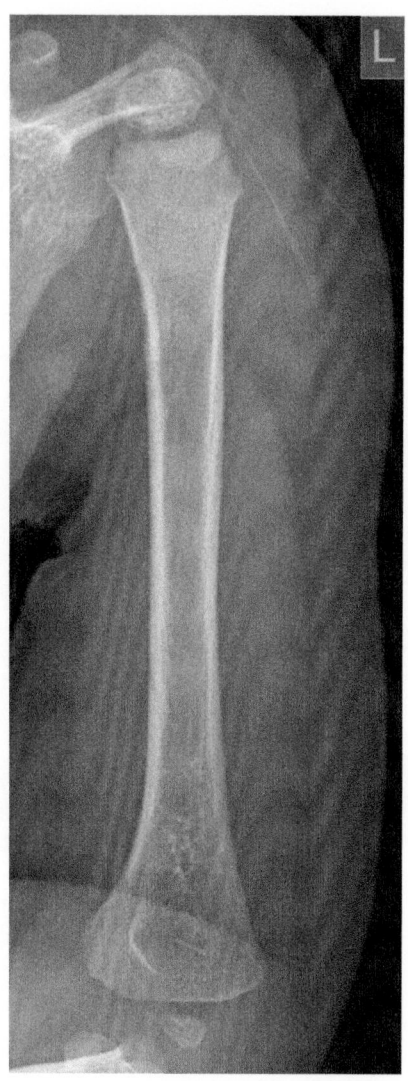

Normal	Abnormal	Diagnosis/Abnormality (only if abnormal)

Image 23

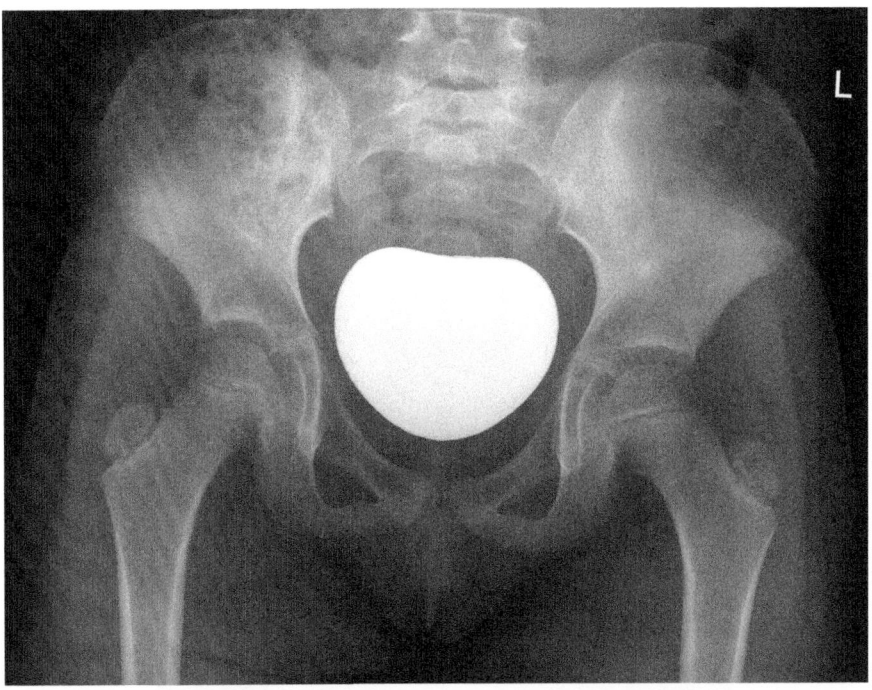

Normal	Abnormal	Diagnosis/Abnormality (only if abnormal)

Image 24

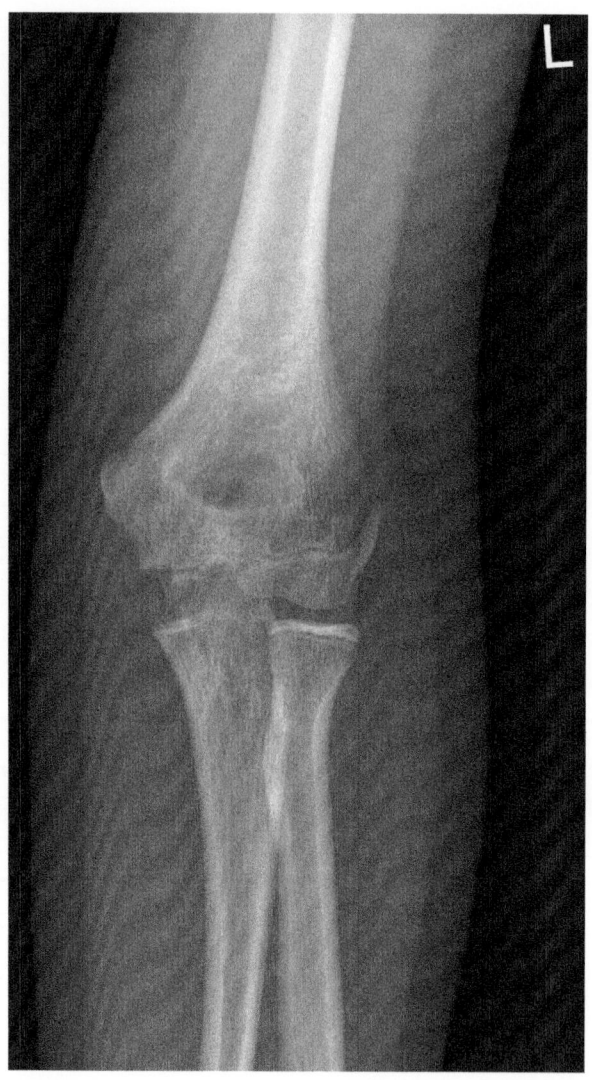

Normal	Abnormal	Diagnosis/Abnormality (only if abnormal)

Image 25

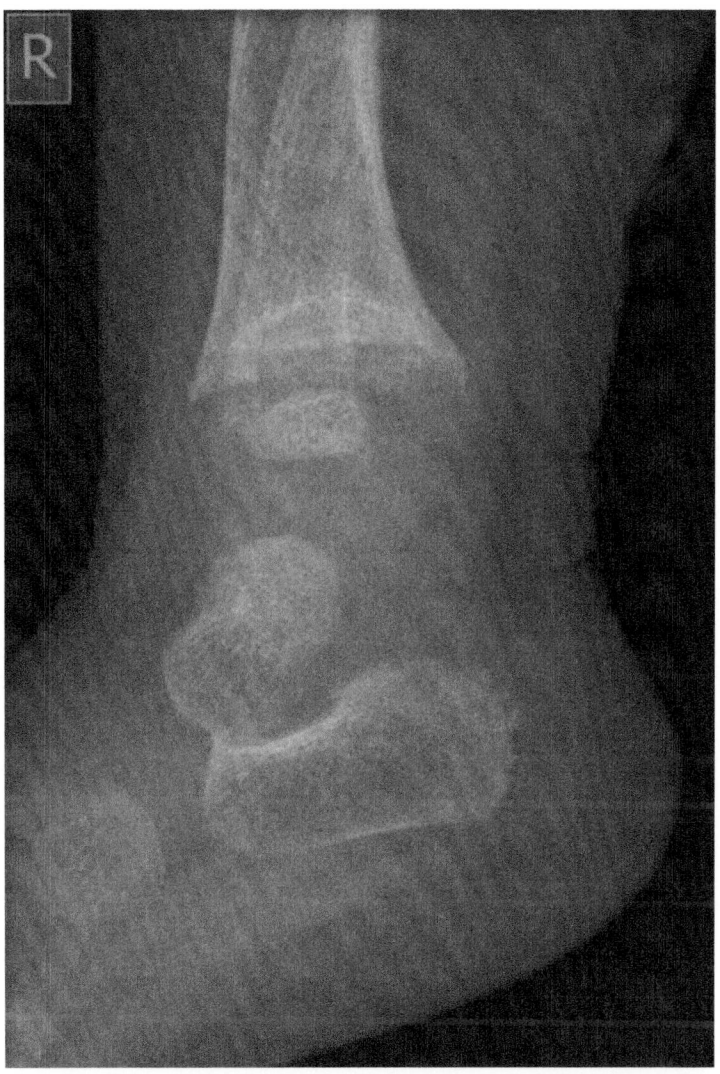

Normal	Abnormal	Diagnosis/Abnormality (only if abnormal)

Image 26

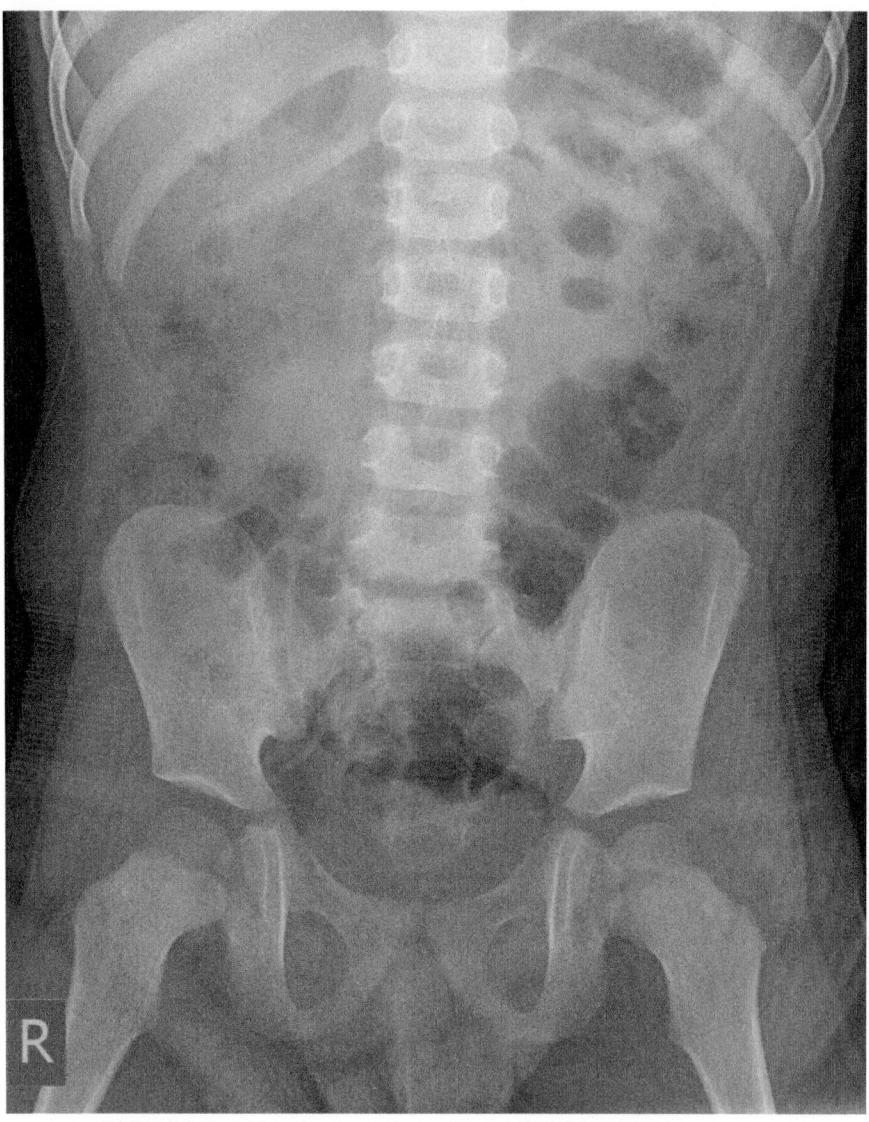

Normal	Abnormal	Diagnosis/Abnormality (only if abnormal)

Image 27

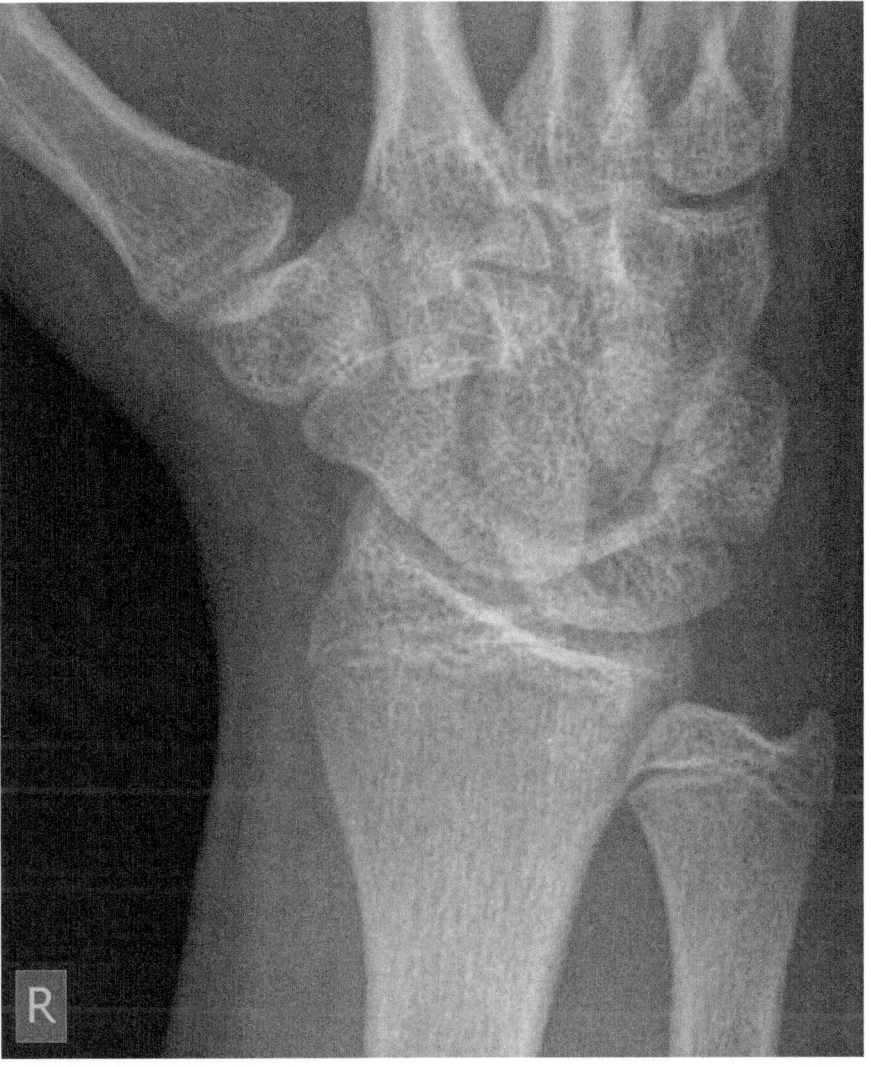

Normal	Abnormal	Diagnosis/Abnormality (only if abnormal)

Image 28

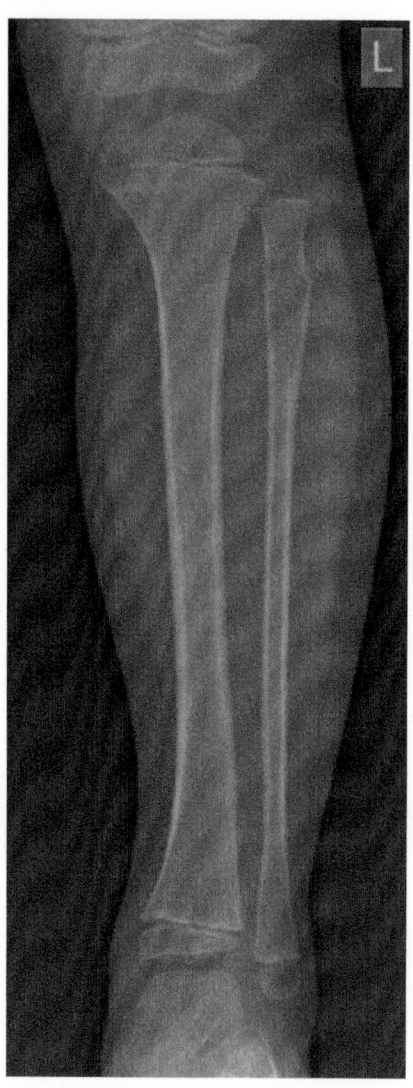

Normal	Abnormal	Diagnosis/Abnormality (only if abnormal)

Image 29

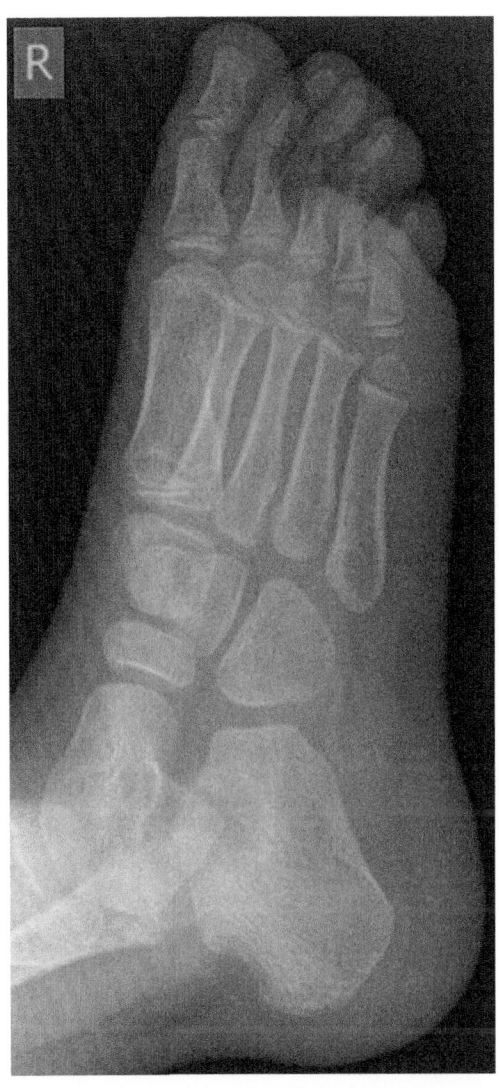

Normal	Abnormal	Diagnosis/Abnormality (only if abnormal)

Image 30

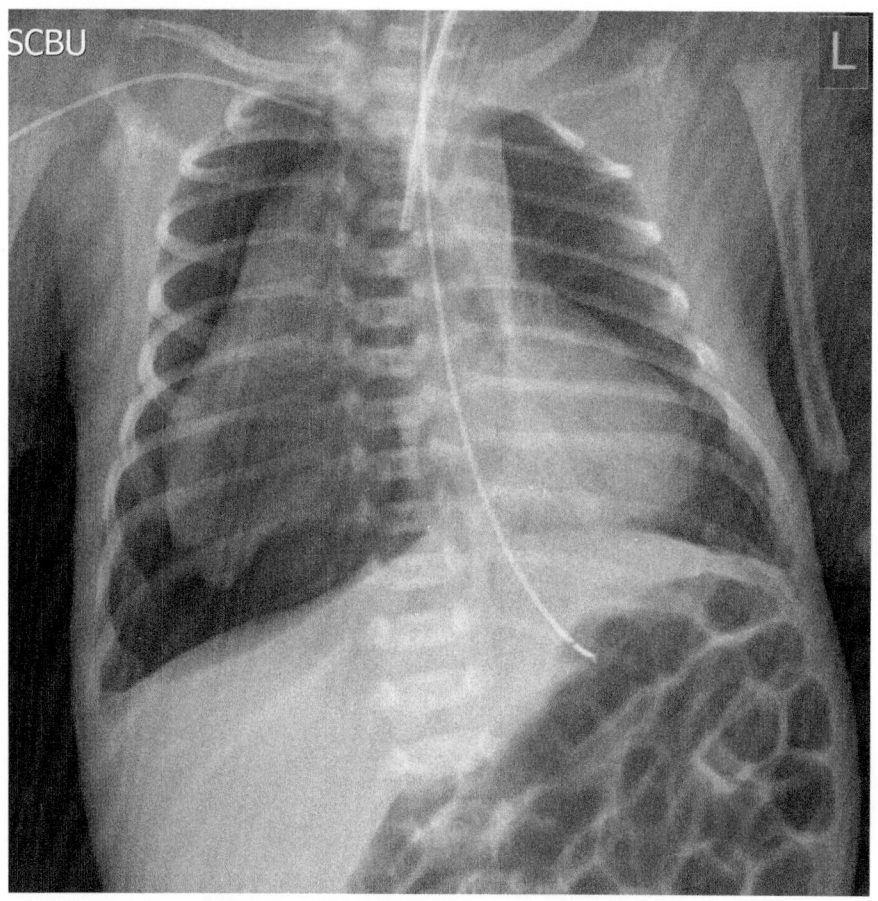

Normal	Abnormal	Diagnosis/Abnormality (only if abnormal)

8.2   Answers

Image	Normal	Abnormal	Diagnosis/abnormality (only if abnormal)
1		✓	Developmental dysplasia right hip
2		✓	Healing bilateral rib #s
3	✓		
4	✓		
5	✓		
6	✓		
7		✓	# right ulna diaphysis
8	✓		
9		✓	Oblique # left second toe proximal phalanx
10		✓	Necrotising enterocolitis
11		✓	Right distal tibial metaphyseal #
12		✓	# left scaphoid
13		✓	# left midshaft femur
14	✓		
15		✓	# (surgical neck) right humerus
16		✓	Proximal bowel obstruction/jejunal atresia
17	✓		
18	✓		
19	✓		
20		✓	Left radial head dislocation
21	✓		
22	✓		
23	✓		
24	✓		
25		✓	Rickets
26	✓		
27		✓	# right scaphoid
28		✓	Pathological # left proximal fibula
29	✓		
30		✓	Right tension pneumothorax

8.3   Explanations

1. **Developmental dysplasia right hip**
   Note the broadening of the right proximal femoral metaphysis with flattening of the right proximal femoral epiphysis. The right acetabulum is sclerotic and irregular, and there is lateral uncovering/subluxation of the proximal femoral epiphysis. See the explanation for Test 2, Image 17.

2. **Healing bilateral rib #s**
   This is the AP chest radiograph from the follow-up skeletal survey for the same child as in Test 2, Image 14 and Test 7, Image 26. This radiograph demonstrates the expanded callus that results from healing rib fractures.
   As previously discussed, acute and/or healing rib fractures may be visualised on chest radiography performed for other indications, which is why vigilance and recognition of these appearances as healing fractures is vital.

7. **# right ulna diaphysis**
   In the presence of an ulnar shaft fracture, a concomitant radial head dislocation should be sought—and vice versa—as part of the Monteggia fracture-dislocation pattern. Formal forearm radiographs should be recommended if they have not yet been obtained. See the explanation for Test 1, Image 28.

9. **Oblique # left second toe proximal phalanx**

10. **Necrotising enterocolitis**
    Necrotising enterocolitis (NEC) is the commonest gastrointestinal condition affecting premature neonates and has an inverse proportional incidence with gestational age—the more premature the infant, the greater the risk of developing NEC. The condition is thought to arise from a number of complex interactions which lead to increased gut wall mucosal permeability to bacteria resulting in inflammation and necrosis.
    Due to the inflammation and subsequent hyperaemia of the immature gut wall, there is bacterial translocation of intestinal flora and formation of gas within the gut wall (i.e. intramural) as a by-product of bacterial metabolism. The overwhelming sepsis that can develop results from a generalised inflammatory response due to the presence of bacteria and toxins entering the blood stream from the breakdown of the gut wall mucosa. The cascade of inflammatory cytokines results in eventual transmural involvement that compromises the microvasculature leading to ischaemia, necrosis, mucosal sloughing, bowel wall thinning, and eventual perforation. The terminal ileum is the commonest affected location.
    Presentation can be non-specific and can mimic neonatal sepsis. Systemic symptoms include 'being unsettled', temperature and blood pressure instability, episodes of bradycardia, desaturation, and apnoeas. Gastrointestinal symptoms may include feed intolerance, vomiting which may be bile-stained,

diarrhoea, blood stained stools, and rectal bleeding. Clinical examination usually reveals a distended abdomen and there may be discolouration of the overlying skin.

This radiograph was obtained in a 6-day-old premature neonate who was 'unsettled' with rectal bleeding. The key radiographic features in this image include:

- Dilated bowel loops: these are often distributed asymmetrically throughout the abdomen and change very little, if at all, on subsequent radiographs.
- Pneumatosis intestinalis: also known as intramural gas, as described above.
- Portal venous gas: can be distinguished from pneumobilia (which is more central) since portal venous gas is peripheral (as in this radiograph).

Another important radiographic feature is pneumoperitoneum, and whilst not present on this radiograph, should be actively sought on every neonatal abdominal radiograph, particularly if there are clinical concerns for NEC. Once the bowel has perforated, the mortality rate increases; thus, prompt recognition of the early radiographic changes of NEC prior to perforation may result in improved morbidity and mortality. However, it is important to note that pneumoperitoneum may not be seen on radiographs in an estimated 50–75% of cases, even in the presence of perforation. A non-exhaustive list of the radiographic signs of pneumoperitoneum includes:

- Rigler sign: free air on both sides of the bowel wall.
- Triangular-shaped lucencies: formed between three overlapping loops of bowel, or two bowel loops and the anterior abdominal wall.
- Continuous diaphragm sign: a large amount of free air which collects under both the left and right hemidiaphragms creating the appearance of uninterrupted lucency underneath the diaphragms creating a 'continuous diaphragm'.
- Football sign: the abdominal cavity and the falciform ligament are outlined by free air and in the case of massive pneumoperitoneum in a supine patient can be thought of as an extension of the continuous diaphragm sign.
- Inverted 'V' sign: free air outlines the lateral umbilical ligaments creating an inverted 'V' shape projected over the pelvis.
- Urachus sign: free air outlines the median umbilical ligament on both sides creating a vertical line between the bladder and the umbilicus projected over the pelvis.

We included this radiograph because of the constellation of radiographic features of NEC present on one radiograph. You may be presented with one or all of these findings on a radiograph in any component of the 2B examination (and in clinical practice), thus awareness and recognition of the radiographic features which support the diagnosis of NEC is paramount. An early paediatric surgical opinion is strongly advised in any neonate about which there is a clinical and/or radiological suspicion of NEC. Also see the explanation for Test 1, Image 19.

11. **Right distal tibial metaphyseal #**

The 'bucket handle' metaphyseal (classic metaphyseal lesion, CML) fracture configuration is better visualised in the magnified image below:

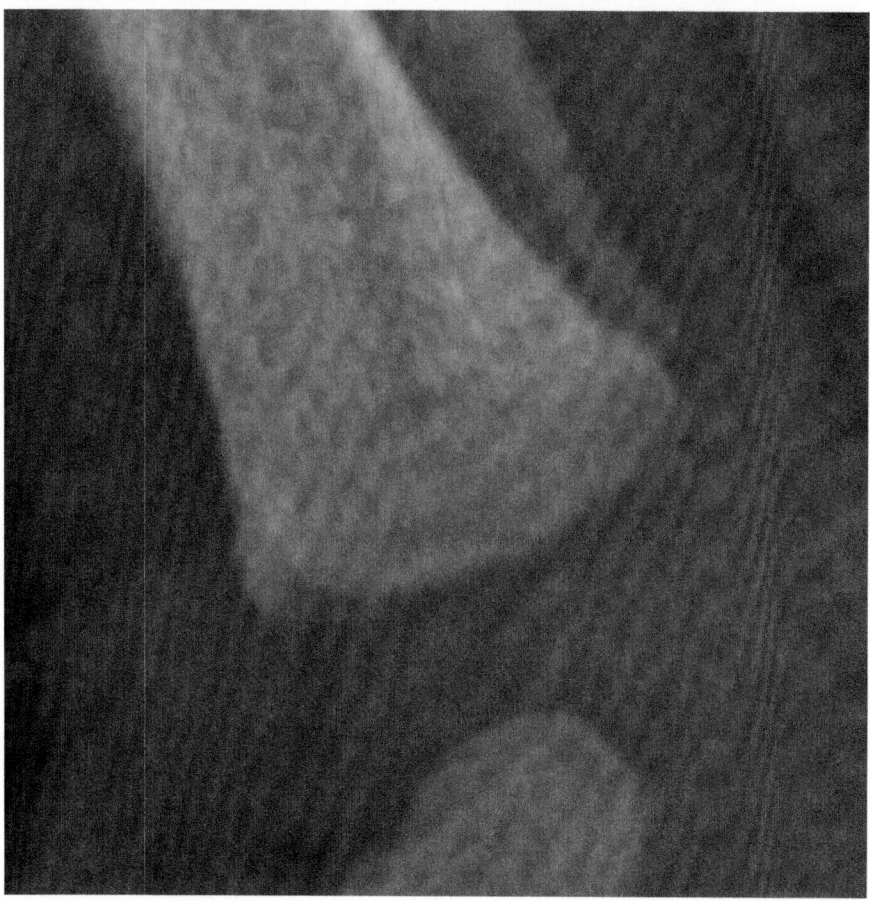

See the explanation for Test 3, Image 2. The fragmented ossification of the tarsal bones is normal.

12. **# left scaphoid**

Carefully tracing the outline of each bone reveals the fracture of the distal pole of the left scaphoid.

Tip for the viva:

- A systematic review published in 2018 demonstrated that there is currently no evidence on which to propose an imaging algorithm for the diagnosis of suspected scaphoid fractures in children. As such, it is recommended that imaging pathways used in adults should be followed until such a time when high quality evidence is available in the paediatric population. You should know your local policy.

13. **# left midshaft femur**

This fracture looks unusual because of the overlapping fracture fragments in the AP plane and the spiral configuration of the fracture.

This 30-month-old child with cerebral palsy was presented to the Emergency Department by his father who heard a 'crack' when he was changing his nappy. Whilst this child is 30-months old, he was not (and may never be) ambulatory because of his cerebral palsy. Those children with a physical developmental problem or disability, and those born premature, are at an increased risk of physical abuse. They are however, also at increased risk of accidental fracture. The initial and follow-up skeletal survey revealed no other acute or healing fracture with normal radiographic bone density and modelling. CT of the head demonstrated no acute intracranial haemorrhage, specifically no subdural haematoma, and long-standing ventriculomegaly with bilateral ventriculoperitoneal shunts. It was felt that the fracture was in keeping with the mechanism proffered by the father. See the explanation for Test 3, Image 23.

The term *inflicted injury* is preferred in these circumstances because it does not necessarily exclude accidental injury and is more accurate in describing the causal mechanism of injury (i.e. an injury that was consequent upon the caregiver's actions) without ascribing a malicious intent to cause harm (i.e. non-accidental injury): it is a subtle but important difference, particularly from a medicolegal perspective.

15. **# (surgical neck) right humerus**

The surgical neck (the 'line' inferior to the greater and lesser tubercles/tuberosities; the start of the proximal humeral diaphysis) is much more commonly fractured than the anatomical neck (the physis in children; the old fused epiphyseal plate in adults) in both adults and children.

16. **Proximal bowel obstruction/jejunal atresia**

The radiographic appearances are in keeping with a proximal (high) bowel obstruction—you can see the distended gas-filled stomach (first bubble), duodenum (second bubble), and the DJ flexure which is visualised in the left upper quadrant with only a short but dilated segment of proximal jejunum (third bubble). There is an abrupt cut-off and an absence of bowel gas distal to this in keeping with the 'triple bubble sign' seen in jejunal atresia. The atresia can be anywhere from the ligament of Treitz (the DJ flexure) to the jejunoileal junction. Additionally, there may be more than one atretic jejunal segment.

Tip for the viva:
- You would be expected to be able to categorise the pattern of obstruction as either proximal (high) or distal (low) and offer an appropriate differential diagnosis depending on the age of the child and the clinical context. See the explanations for Test 1, Image 19 and Test 5, Image 30.

17. **Normal chest radiograph**

This is a normal chest radiograph. The cardiomediastinal contours are well demarcated and the lungs are clear with no confluent consolidation or collapse.

20. **Left radial head dislocation**

See the explanation for Test 1, Image 28.

24. **Normal left elbow radiograph**

This radiograph is normal. All the elbow ossification centres are present in this 11-year-old female (the olecranon ossification centre is not well visualised on AP projections and typically better visualised on contemporaneous lateral projections).

The trochlear may have two or more ossification centres which can often lead to a variable and fragmented appearance during ossification. On the lateral projection, they may also appear as 'fragments' projecting into the joint space, simulating intra-articular loose bodies. It is important to remember that an avulsed medial epicondyle ossification centre may be displaced into the elbow joint space mimicking the normal trochlear officiation centre—a serious finding not to be overlooked. See the explanation for Test 6, Image 9.

It is imperative that when evaluating any paediatric elbow radiograph, you should establish the age of the child and actively consider the expected pattern of ossification centres on **both** orthogonal projections.

Tip for the viva:

• When you are next in work, search for elbow radiographs in children aged 10–14 years of age to familiarise yourself with the normal (and variable) appearances of all the ossification centres, in particular the trochlear ossification centre. Look out for examples of avulsion fractures with which you can compare.

25. **Rickets**

The radiographic appearances are typical for rickets—a condition of bone demineralisation and abnormal growth in children who are vitamin D deficient. The radiographic features include widening and irregularity of the metaphyses with cupping, flaring, and fraying. Splaying of the metaphyses and bowing deformities occur with continued growth in weight-bearing children. The other features can be remembered using the mnemonic, **RICKETS**:

• **R**eaction of the periosteum
• **I**ndistinct cortex
• **C**oarse trabeculation
• **K**nees, wrists, and ankles mainly (the sites of most rapid growth)
• **E**piphyseal plates widened and irregular
• **T**remendous metaphyses
• **S**pur (metaphyseal)

The metaphyses may be fragmented which may sometimes be mistaken for fracture or classic metaphyseal lesions, CMLs (see the explanation for Test 3, Image 2). Whilst the features are obvious in this example, recognition of subtle radiographic features of rickets is imperative so that they are not erroneously reported as suspicious/abusive fractures.

Tips for the viva:
- In the context of unexplained fractures, a low vitamin D level in the *absence* of other biochemical and radiological features of rickets does *not* account for the fractures.
- Do not mistake normal ulnar cupping in infants for the changes of rickets.

27. **# right scaphoid**
There is a fracture of the right scaphoid waist. See the explanation for Image 12 in this test.

28. **Pathological # left proximal fibula**
There is a fracture through the left proximal fibula. There is an underlying lucent, expansile lesion with associated cortical thinning consistent with an aneurysmal bone cyst. Appearances are consistent with a pathological fracture. These fractures are secondary to normal stresses on abnormal bones (in this case, the aneurysmal bone cyst).

30. **Right tension pneumothorax**
Do not forget to assess the positions of all lines and tubes. The tips of the endo-tracheal tube (ETT) and NGT are appropriately sited.

Further Reading

Image 10

Awolaran OT (2015) Radiographic signs of gastrointestinal perforation in children: a pictorial review. Afr J Paediatr Surg 12(3):161–166
Bell DJ, Klaassen K et al (2018) Urachus sign. https://radiopaedia.org/articles/urachus-sign. Accessed June 2018
Bell DJ, Tran T et al (2018) Telltale triangle sign. https://radiopaedia.org/articles/telltale-triangle-sign. Accessed June 2018
Epelman M, Daneman A, Navarro OM et al (2007) Necrotizing enterocolitis: review of state-of-the-art imaging findings with pathologic correlation. Radiographics 27(2):282–305
Sharma R, Jones J et al (2018) Pneumoperitoneum. https://radiopaedia.org/articles/pneumoperito-neum. Accessed June 2018
Sharma R, Khadar O, Thabet MA et al (2018) Inverted "V" sign (pneumoperitoneum). https://radiopaedia.org/articles/inverted-v-sign-pneumoperitoneum. Accessed June 2018
Skandhan AKP, Weerakkody Y et al (2018) Necrotising enterocolitis. https://radiopaedia.org/articles/necrotising-enterocolitis-1. Accessed June 2018

Image 12

Offiah AC, Burke D (2018) The diagnostic accuracy of cross-sectional imaging for detecting acute scaphoid fractures in children: a systematic review. Br J Radiol 91(1086):20170883

Image 15

Torchia M, Taylor B et al (2018) Proximal Humerus Fractures. https://www.orthobullets.com/trauma/1015/proximal-humerus-fractures. Accessed June 2018

Image 16

Glick Y, Bickle I et al (2018) Triple bubble sign. https://radiopaedia.org/articles/triple-bubble-sign. Accessed May 2018
Weerakkody Y, Salam H et al (2018) Jejunal atresia. https://radiopaedia.org/articles/jejunal-atresia. Accessed May 2018

Image 24

Smithuis R (2018) Elbow – fractures in children. http://www.radiologyassistant.nl/en/p58c4d-d5b9219a/elbow-fractures-in-children.html. Accessed June 2018

Image 25

Arundel P, Ahmed SF, Allgrove J et al (2012) British Paediatric and Adolescent Bone Group's position statement on vitamin D deficiency. BMJ 345:e8182

Cheema JI, Grissom LE, Harcke HT (2003) Radiographic characteristics of lower-extremity bowing in children. Radiographics 23(4):871–880

Gaillard F, Sheikh Z et al (2018) Rickets (mnemonic). https://radiopaedia.org/articles/rickets-mnemonic. Accessed June 2018

Kleinman PK, Sarwar ZU, Newton AW et al (2009) Metaphyseal fragmentation with physiologic bowing: a finding not to be confused with the classic metaphyseal lesion. AJR Am J Roentgenol 192(5):1266–1268

Test 9

9

9.1   Images

Image 1

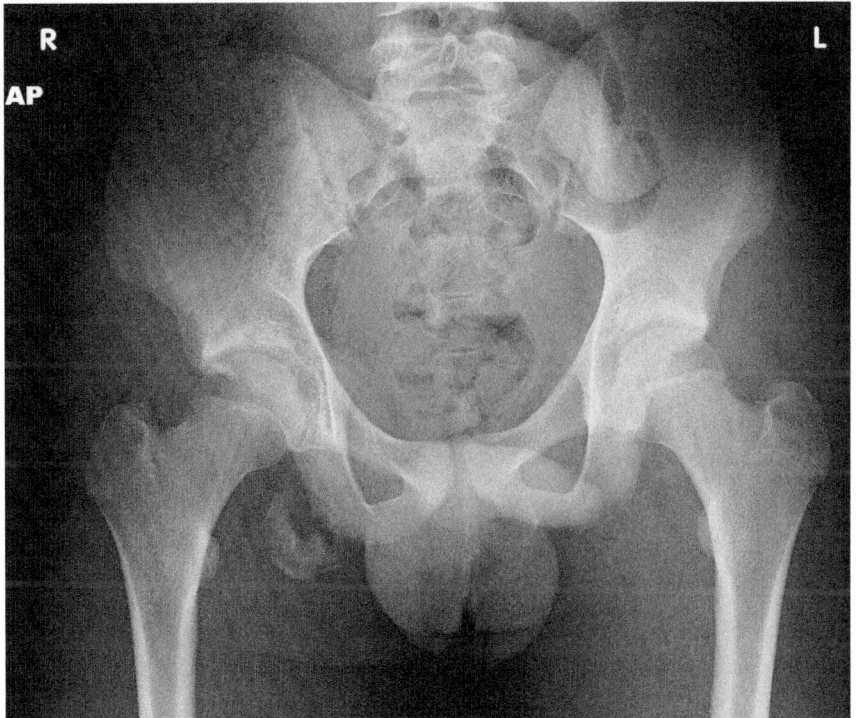

Normal	Abnormal	Diagnosis/Abnormality (only if abnormal)

© Springer Nature Switzerland AG 2019
M. Paddock, A. C. Offiah, *Paediatric Radiology Rapid Reporting for FRCR Part 2B*,
https://doi.org/10.1007/978-3-030-01965-5_9

Image 2

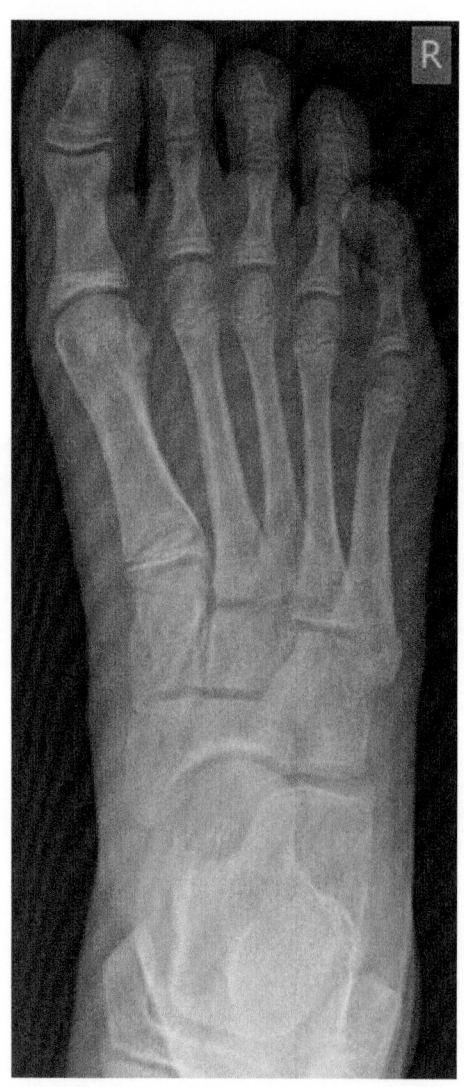

Normal	Abnormal	Diagnosis/Abnormality (only if abnormal)

Image 3

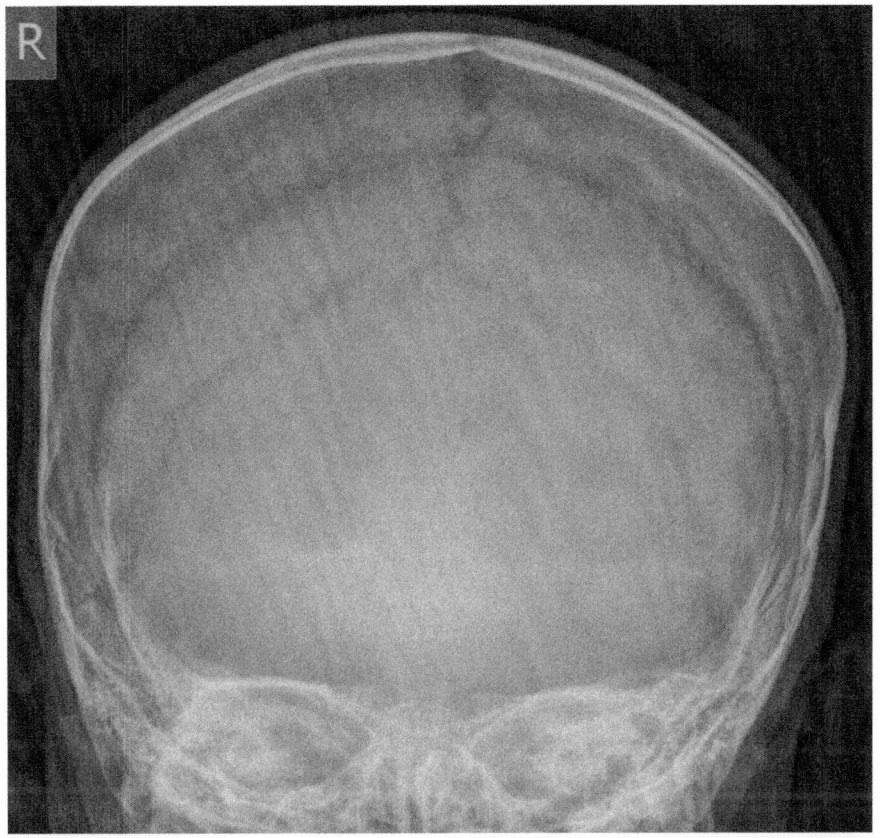

Normal	Abnormal	Diagnosis/Abnormality (only if abnormal)

Image 4

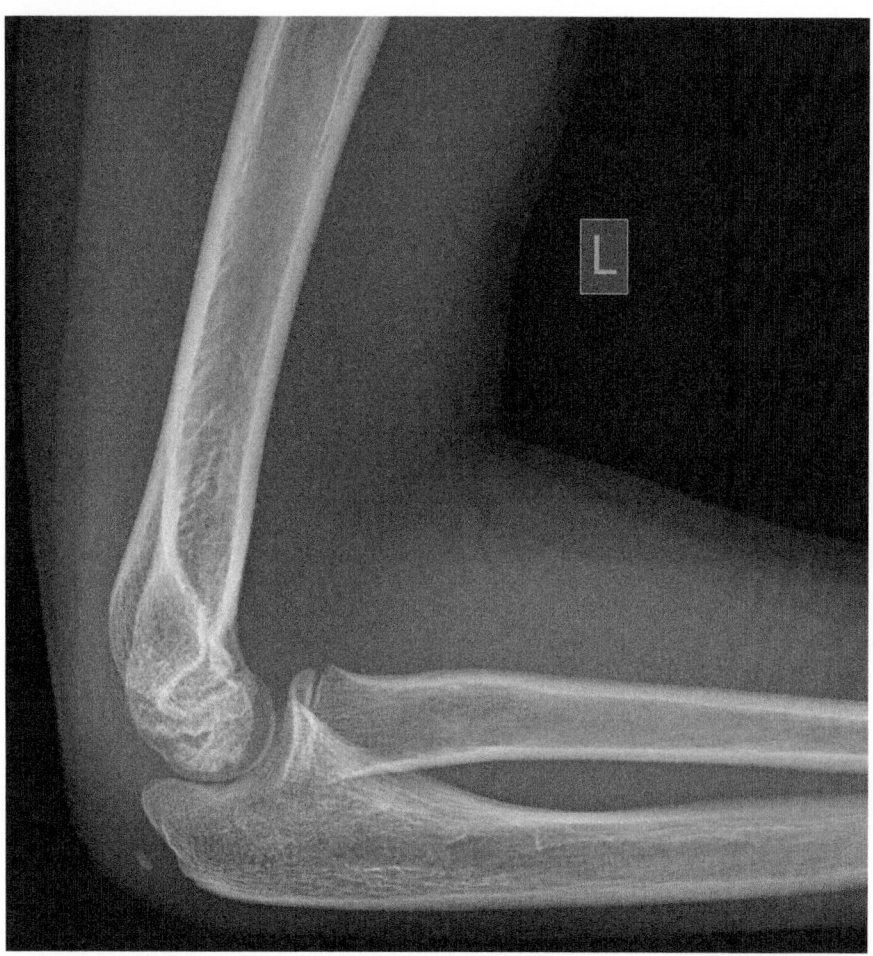

Normal	Abnormal	Diagnosis/Abnormality (only if abnormal)

Image 5

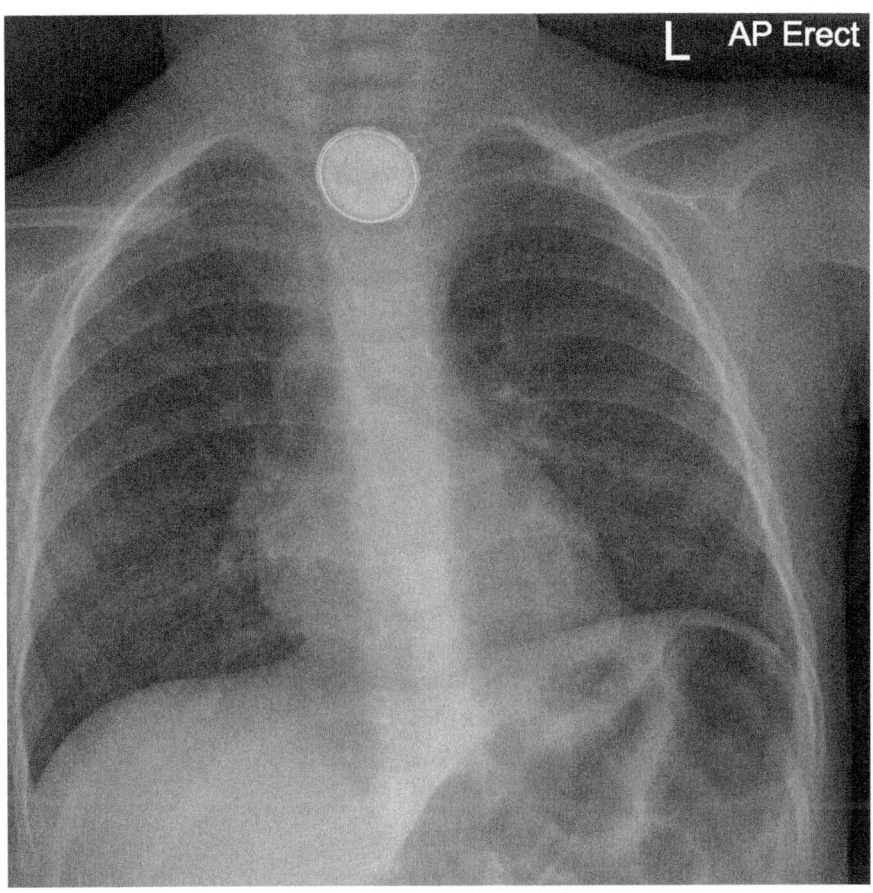

Normal	Abnormal	Diagnosis/Abnormality (only if abnormal)

Image 6

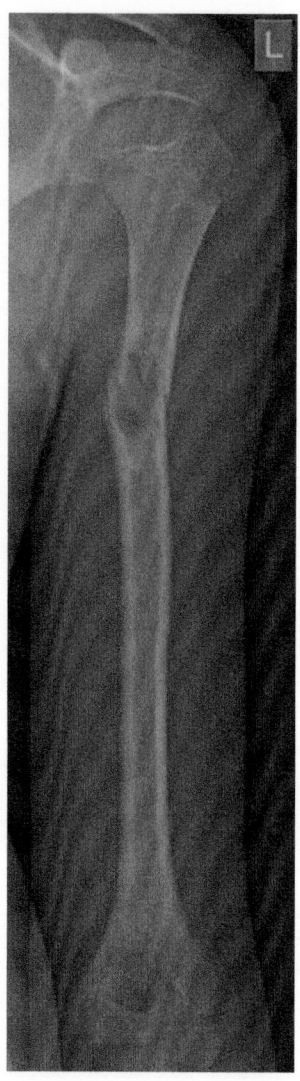

Normal	Abnormal	Diagnosis/Abnormality (only if abnormal)

Image 7

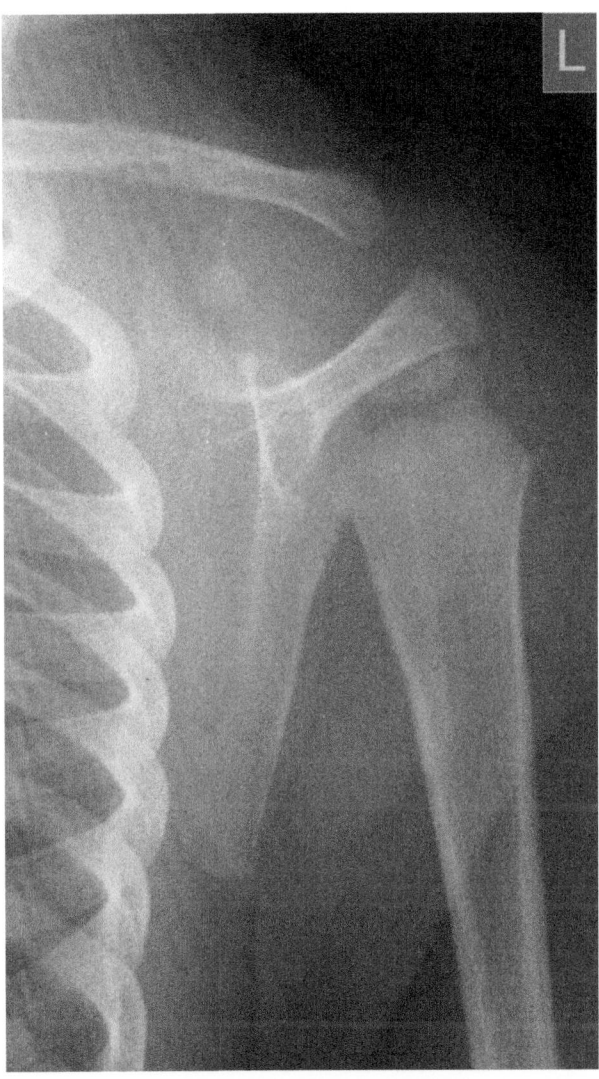

Normal	Abnormal	Diagnosis/Abnormality (only if abnormal)

Image 8

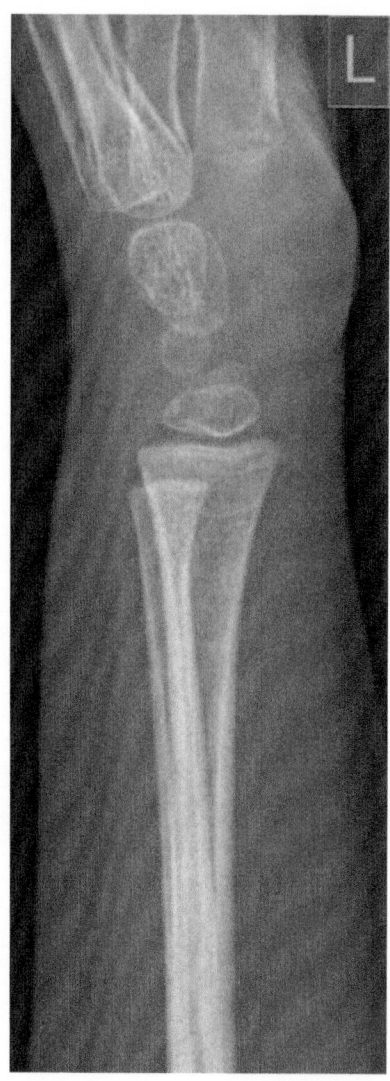

Normal	Abnormal	Diagnosis/Abnormality (only if abnormal)

Image 9

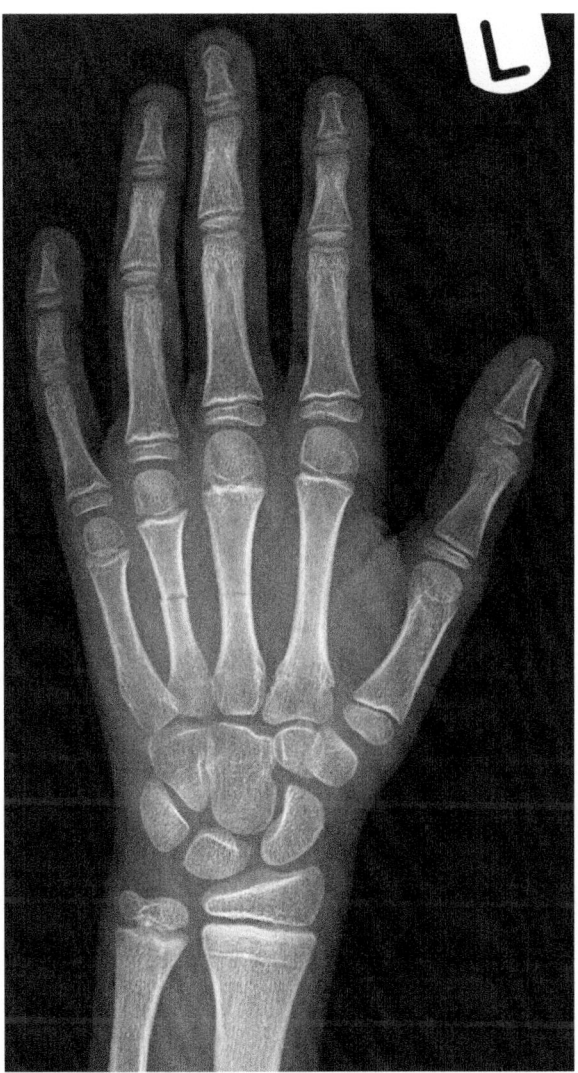

Normal	Abnormal	Diagnosis/Abnormality (only if abnormal)

Image 10

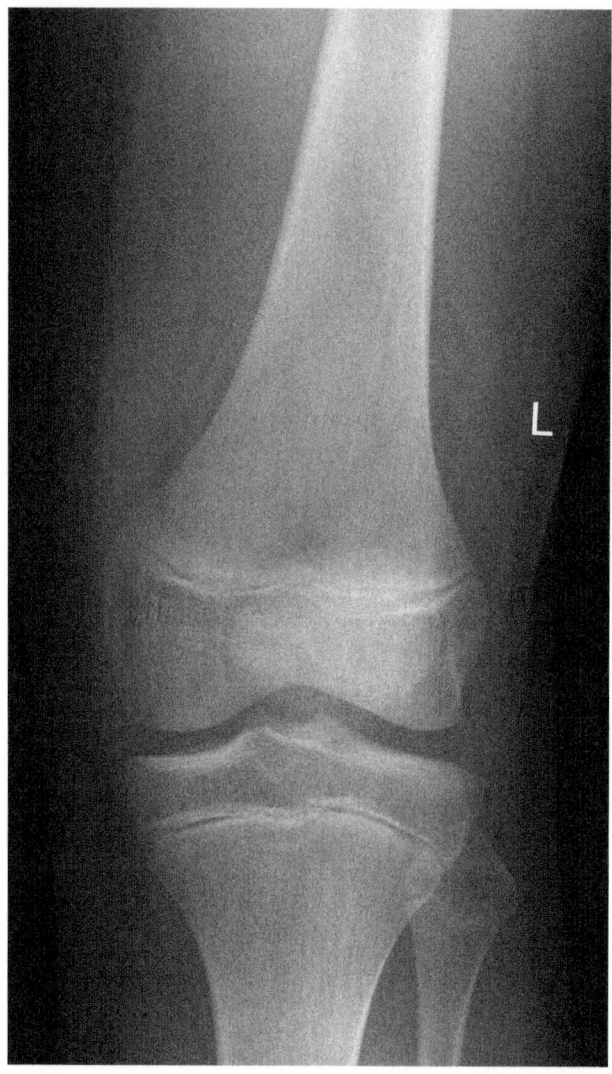

Normal	Abnormal	Diagnosis/Abnormality (only if abnormal)

Image 11

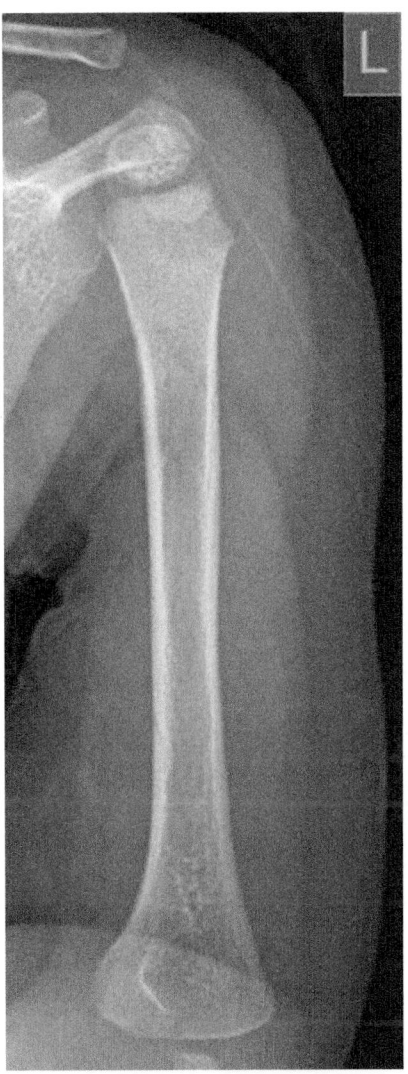

Normal	Abnormal	Diagnosis/Abnormality (only if abnormal)

Image 12

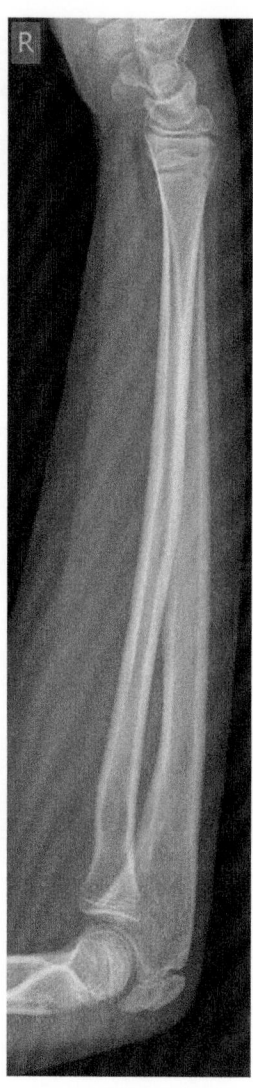

Normal	Abnormal	Diagnosis/Abnormality (only if abnormal)

Image 13

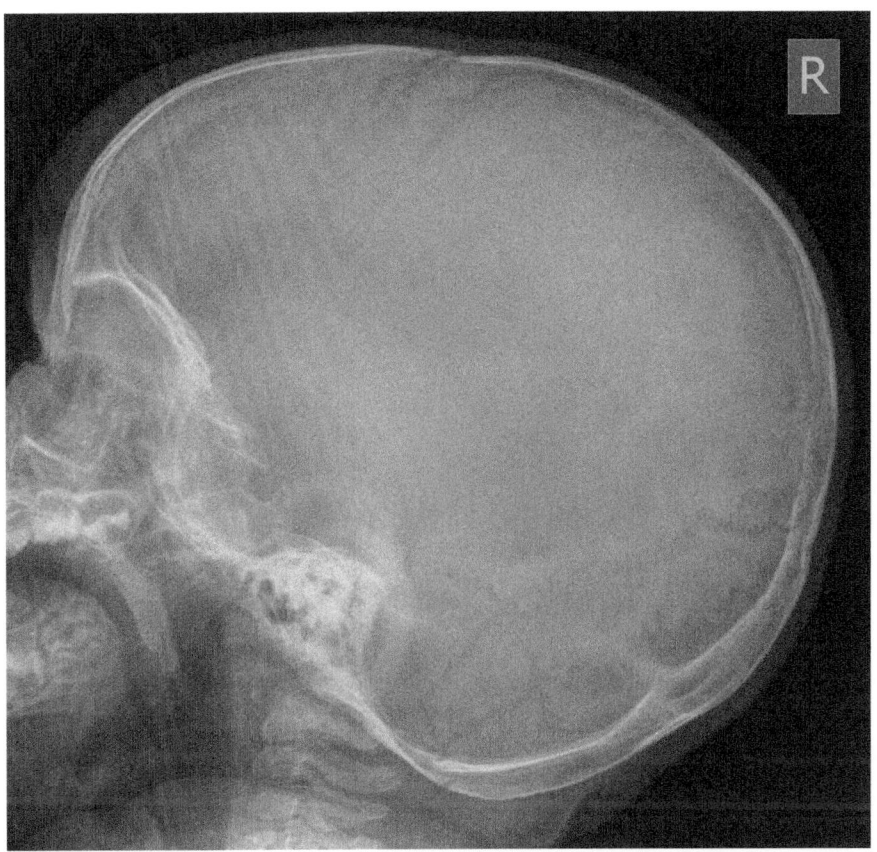

Normal	Abnormal	Diagnosis/Abnormality (only if abnormal)

Image 14

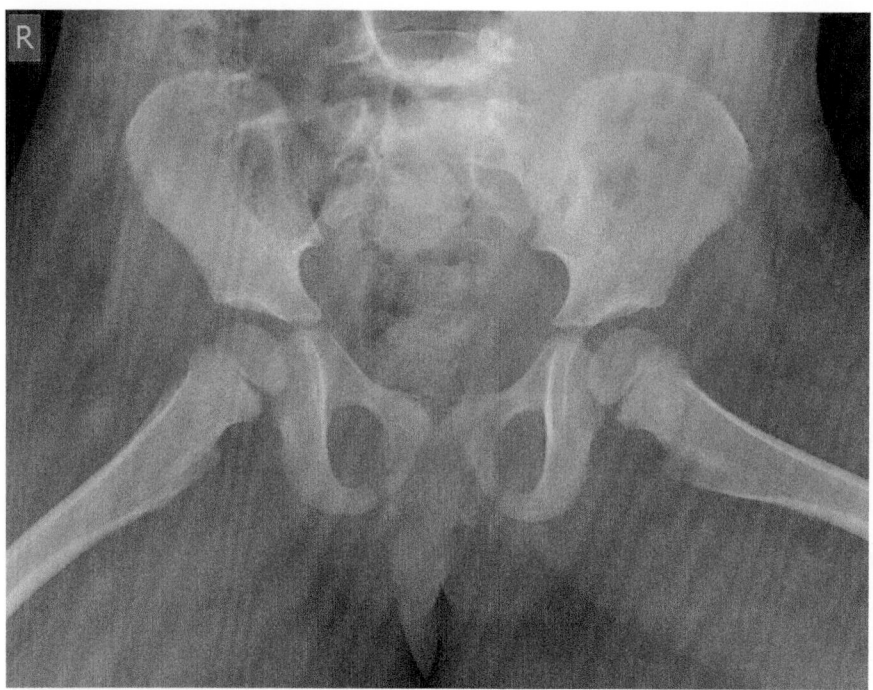

Normal	Abnormal	Diagnosis/Abnormality (only if abnormal)

Image 15

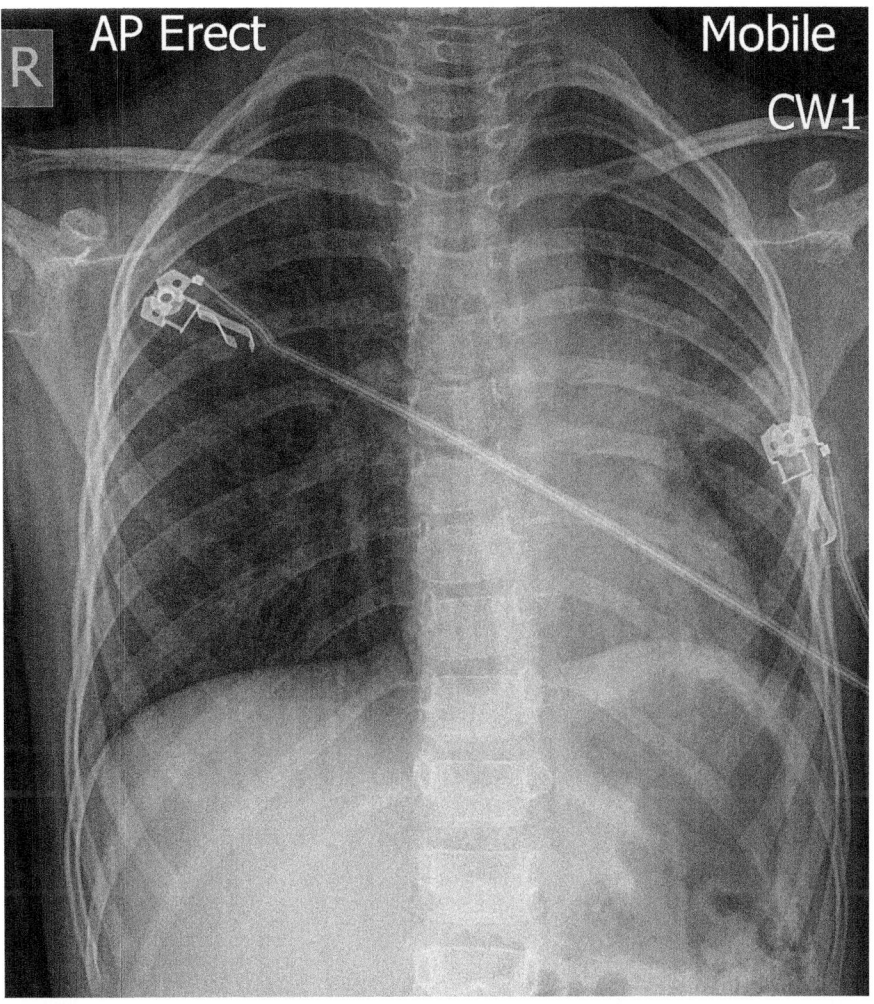

Normal	Abnormal	Diagnosis/Abnormality (only if abnormal)

Image 16

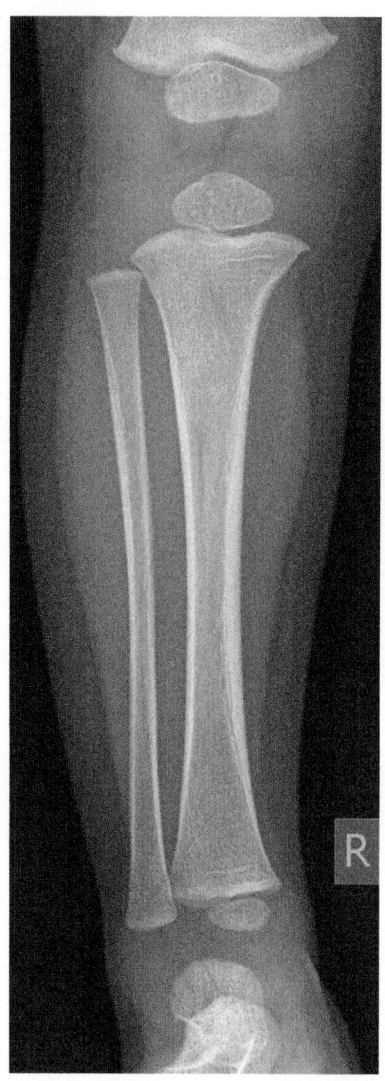

Normal	Abnormal	Diagnosis/Abnormality (only if abnormal)

Image 17

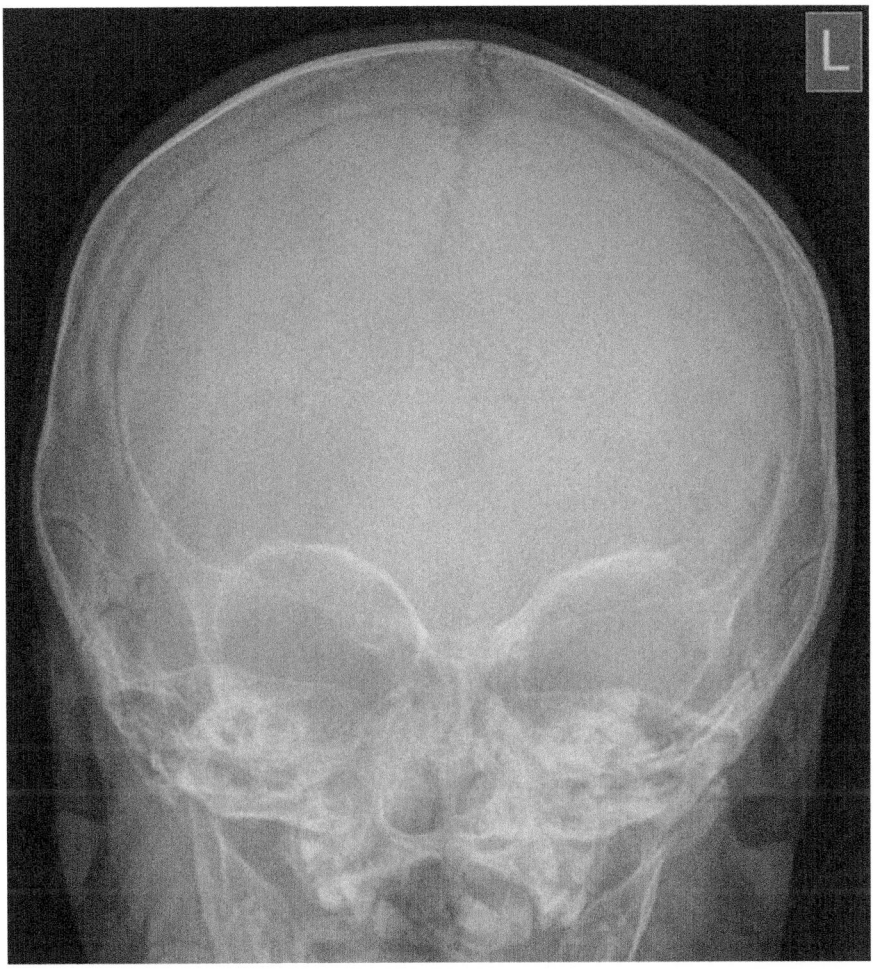

Normal	Abnormal	Diagnosis/Abnormality (only if abnormal)

Image 18

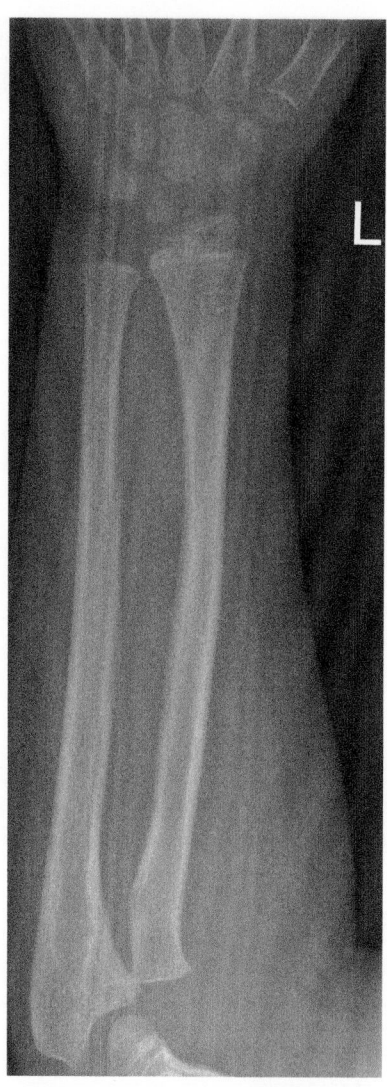

Normal	Abnormal	Diagnosis/Abnormality (only if abnormal)

Image 19

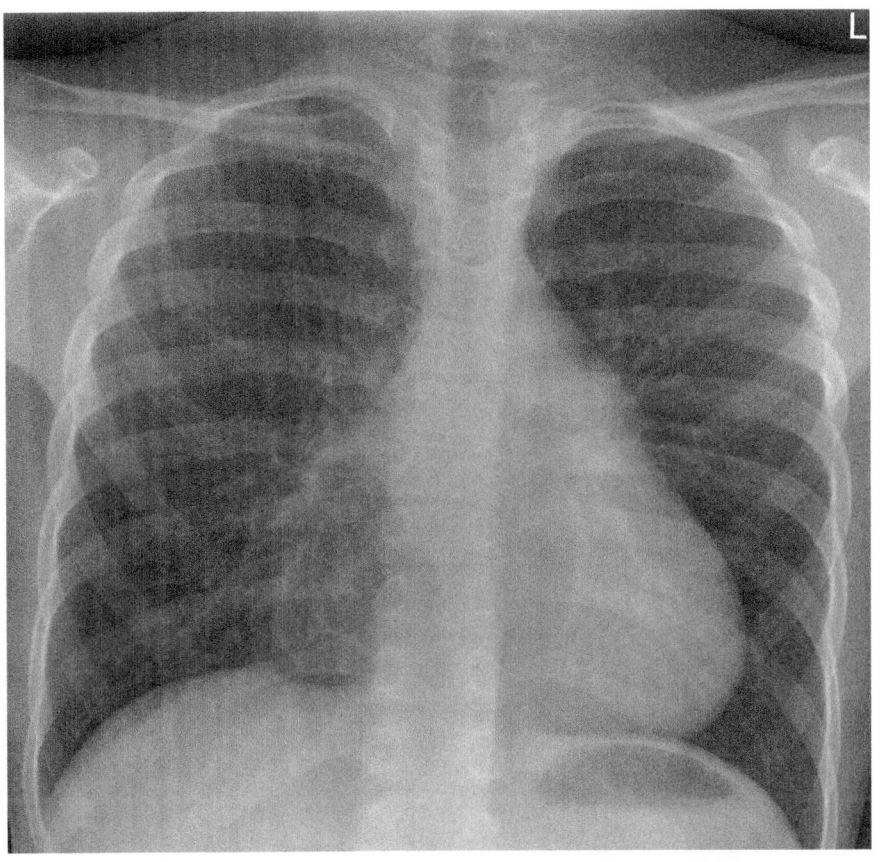

Normal	Abnormal	Diagnosis/Abnormality (only if abnormal)

Image 20

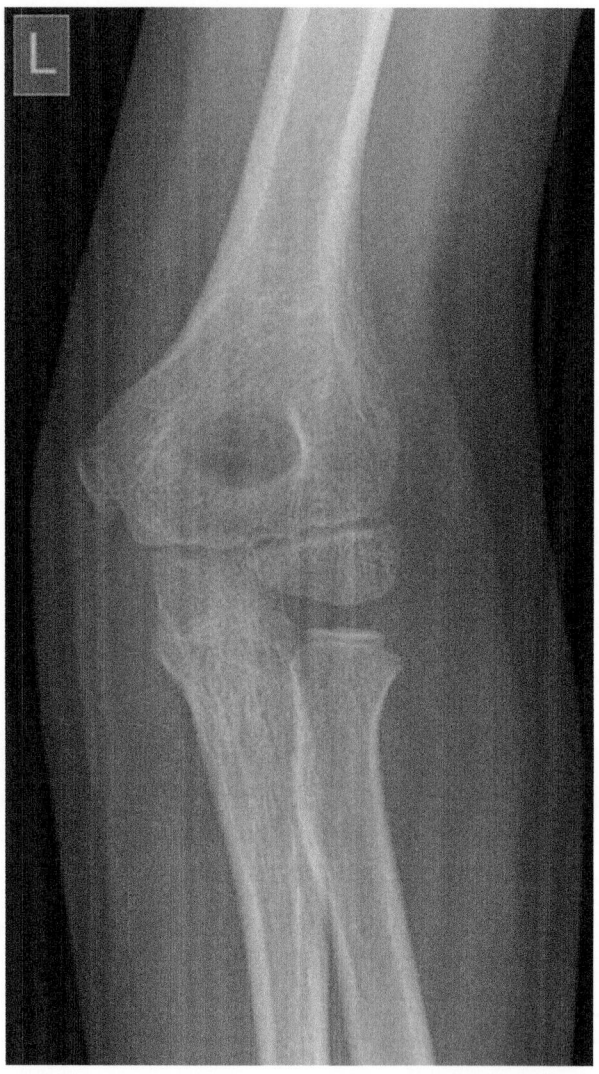

Normal	Abnormal	Diagnosis/Abnormality (only if abnormal)

Image 21

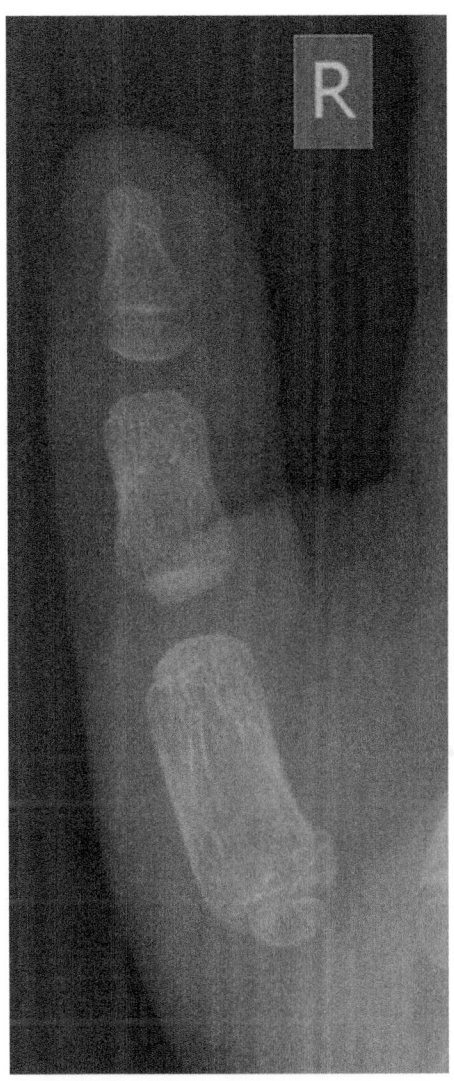

Normal	Abnormal	Diagnosis/Abnormality (only if abnormal)

Image 22

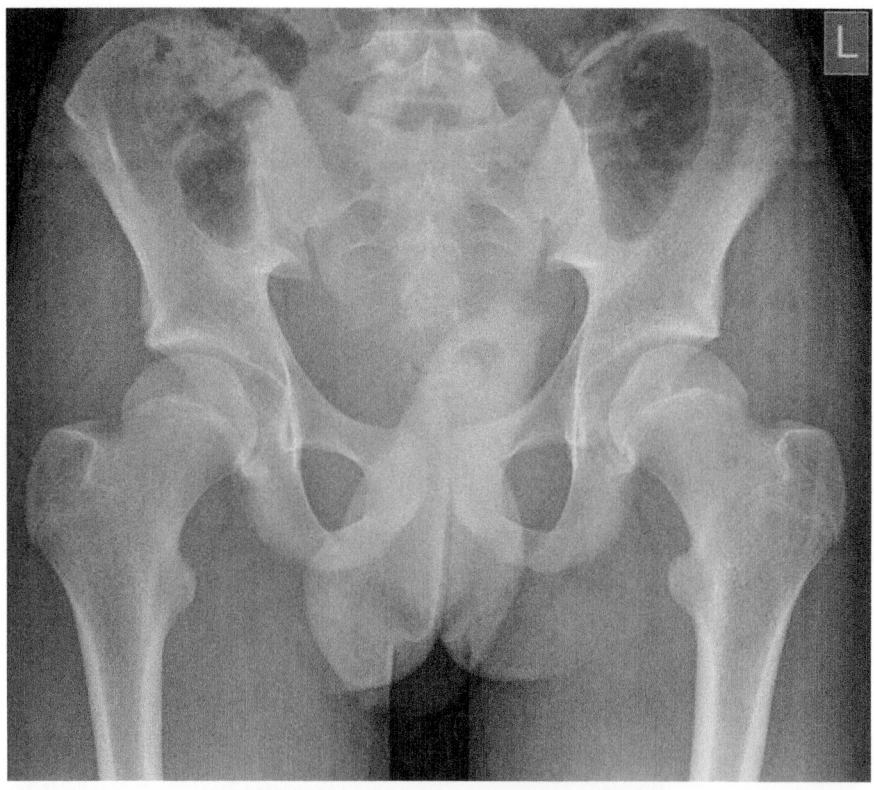

Normal	Abnormal	Diagnosis/Abnormality (only if abnormal)

Image 23

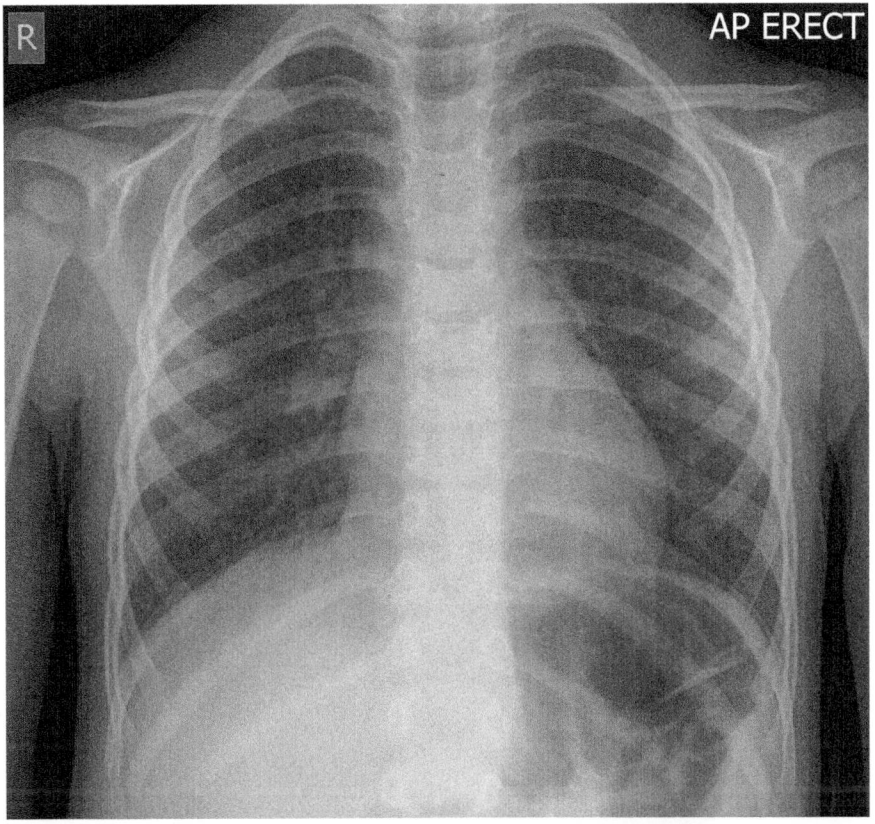

Normal	Abnormal	Diagnosis/Abnormality (only if abnormal)

Image 24

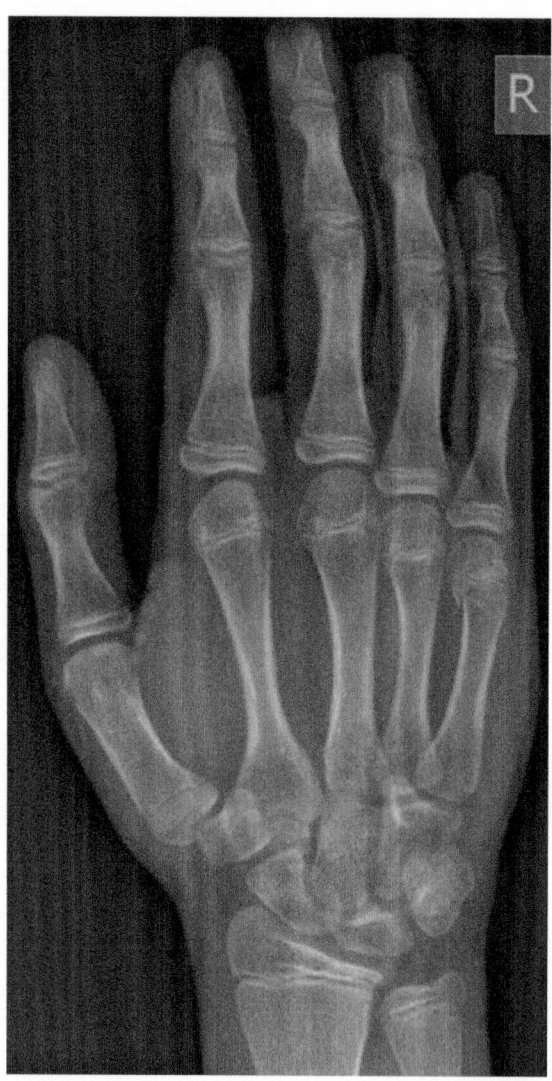

Normal	Abnormal	Diagnosis/Abnormality (only if abnormal)

Image 25

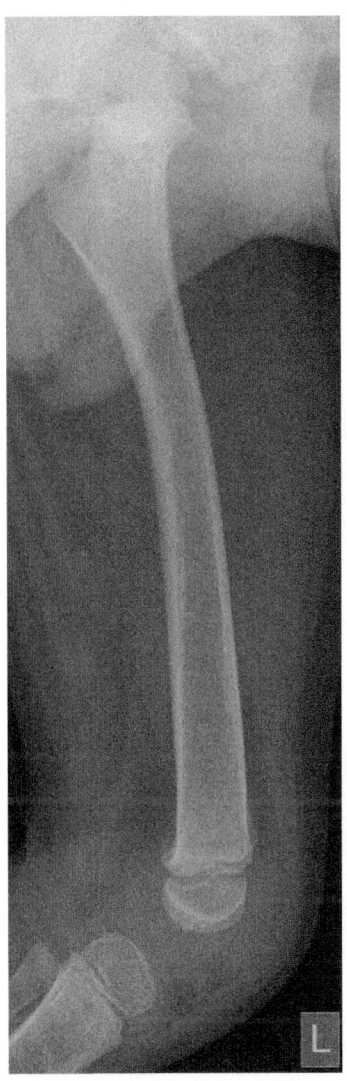

Normal	Abnormal	Diagnosis/Abnormality (only if abnormal)

Image 26

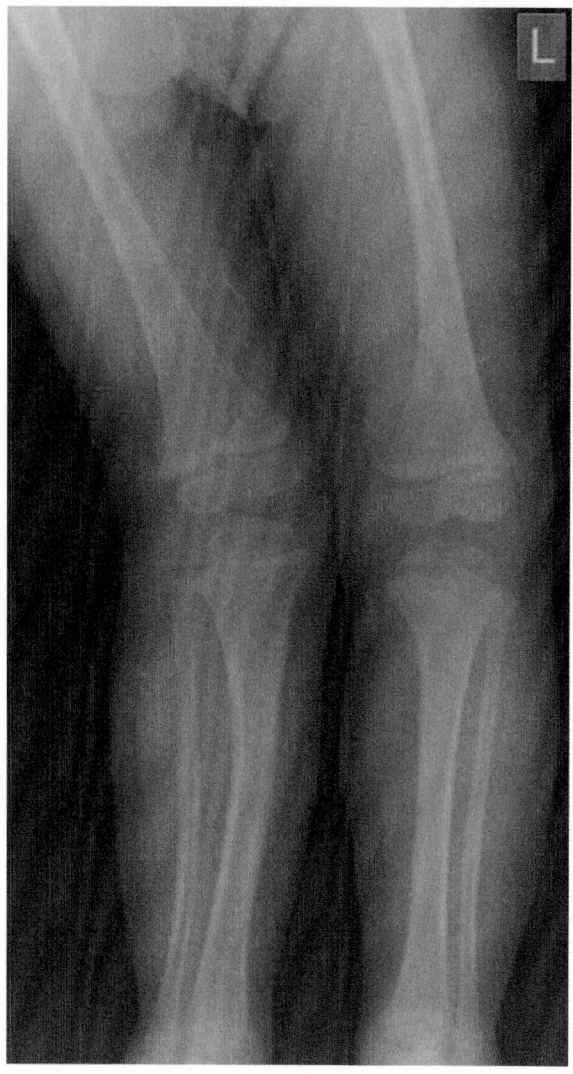

Normal	Abnormal	Diagnosis/Abnormality (only if abnormal)

Image 27

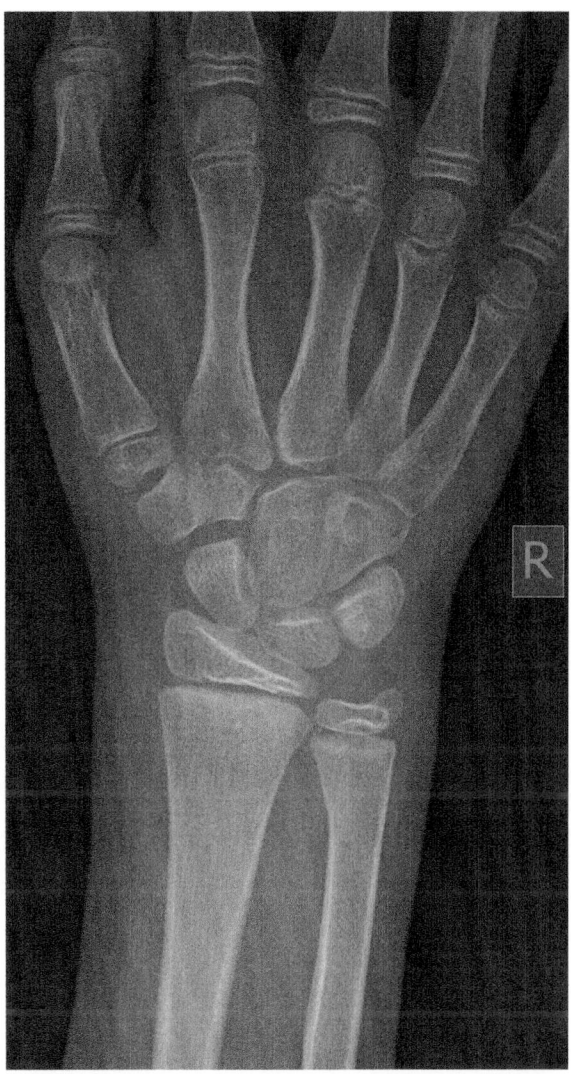

Normal	Abnormal	Diagnosis/Abnormality (only if abnormal)

Image 28

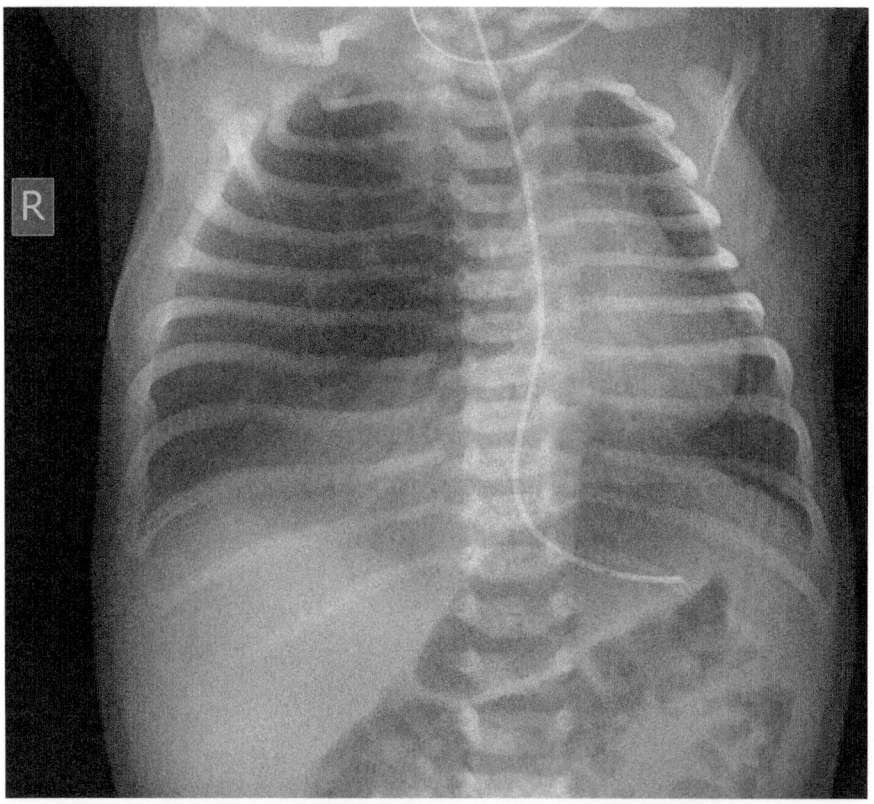

Normal	Abnormal	Diagnosis/Abnormality (only if abnormal)

Image 29

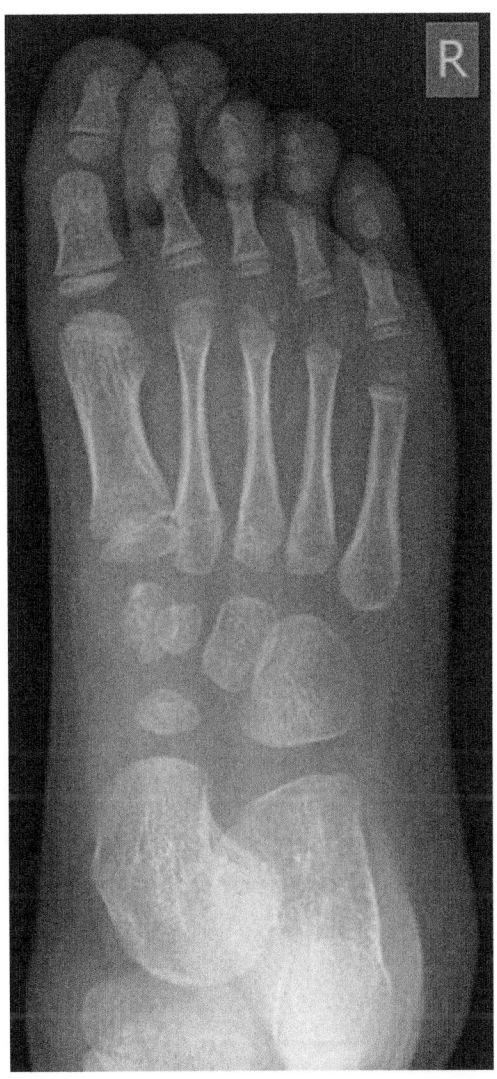

Normal	Abnormal	Diagnosis/Abnormality (only if abnormal)

Image 30

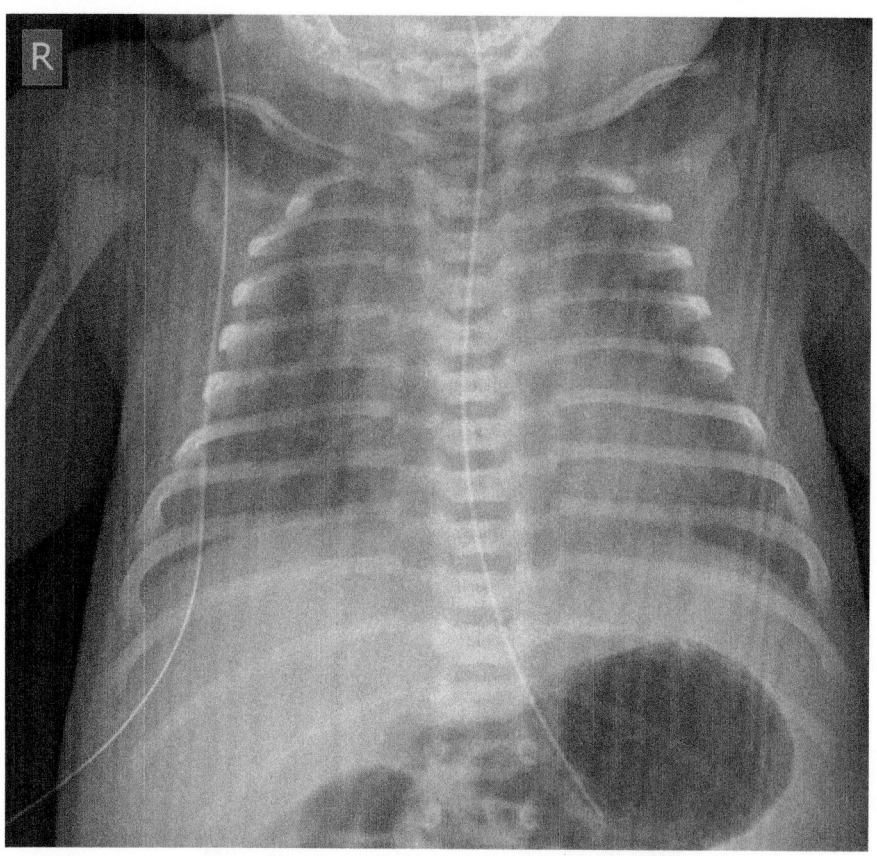

Normal	Abnormal	Diagnosis/Abnormality (only if abnormal)

9.2   **Answers**

Image	Normal	Abnormal	Diagnosis/abnormality (only if abnormal)
1		✓	Healing right ischial tuberosity avulsion # (chronic)
2	✓		
3	✓		
4	✓		
5		✓	Radiopaque foreign body oesophagus
6		✓	Pathological # left humerus
7		✓	# left midshaft clavicle
8	✓		
9		✓	Transverse # left middle and ring finger metacarpals
10	✓		
11	✓		
12	✓		
13	✓		
14	✓		
15		✓	Left upper lobe collapse
16		✓	Buckle # right proximal tibia
17	✓		
18		✓	Left radial head dislocation
19		✓	Pectus excavatum
20	✓		
21		✓	Salter-Harris 2 # base left thumb metacarpal
22	✓		
23		✓	Pneumomediastinum
24		✓	# right little finger metacarpal neck
25	✓		
26		✓	Right genu valgum/Cozen phenomenon
27		✓	Buckle # right distal ulna
28		✓	Right middle lobe congenital lobar overinflation
29		✓	Healing stress # right third metatarsal diaphysis
30	✓		

9.3 Explanations

1. **Healing right ischial tuberosity avulsion # (chronic)**
   See the explanation for Test 4, Image 13. The ischial tuberosity is the insertion for the hamstring tendons. There is displacement and fragmentation of the avulsed fragment.

5. **Radiopaque foreign body oesophagus**
   Whilst the abnormality may be obvious, we have included this radiograph so that you will be able to recognise the foreign body itself: *a button battery*. These have a distinctive radiographic appearance on AP radiographs, often described as a 'double ring', 'double halo', or 'double density'. This is best appreciated on the magnified image below:

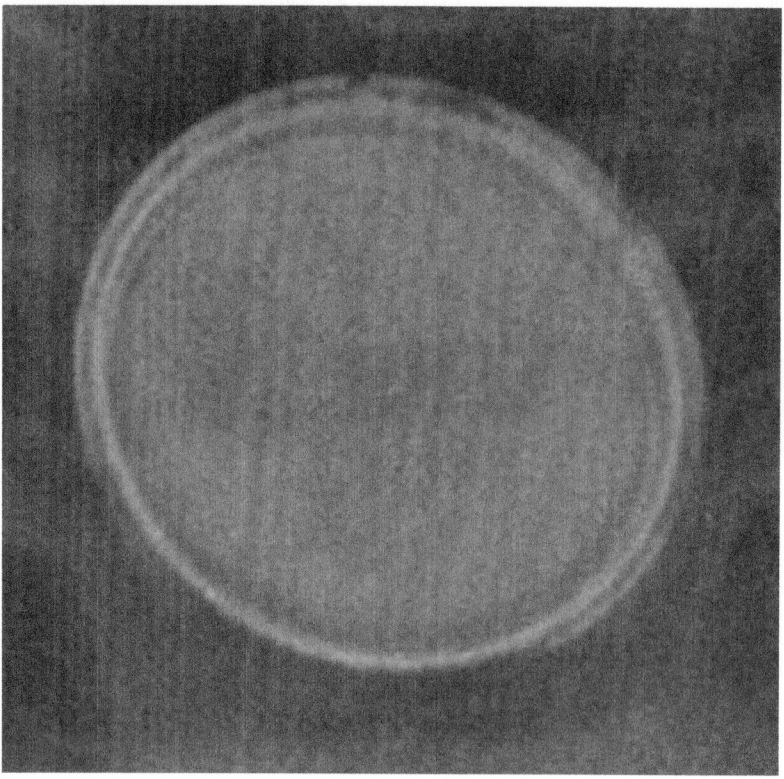

Given its shape, size, and contour, a button battery may be mistaken for a coin. The subsequent significant sequelae that can result from button battery ingestion (BBI), including reported cases of death, necessitates that *any* suspected coin or ingested well-circumscribed radiopaque foreign body be closely scrutinised on radiographs. Given the importance of identifying this radiopaque foreign body, we have also included the corresponding soft tissue neck lateral projection below which may be obtained in the investigation of '*?foreign body*':

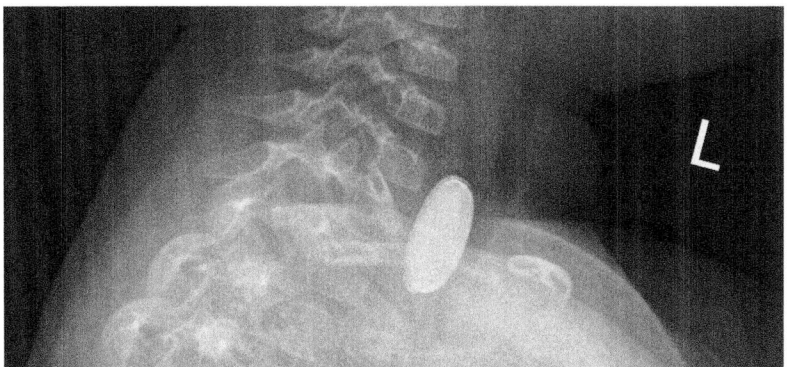

The button battery rests in the oesophagus, posterior to the gas-filled trachea. Note the magnified appearance of the button battery on the lateral projection, below:

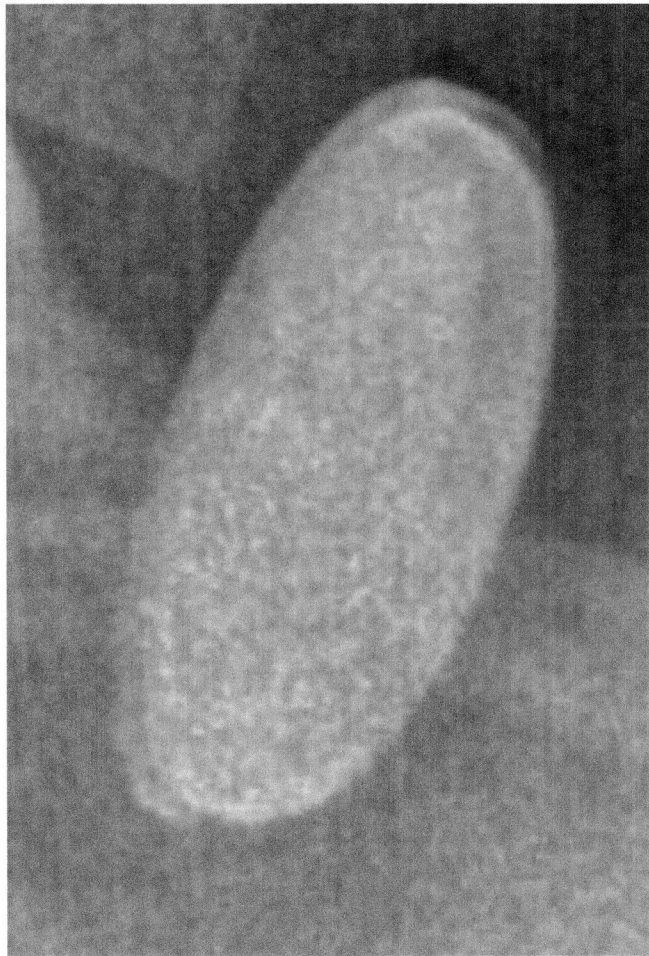

Button batteries account for approximately 2% of all ingested foreign bodies in children with a peak incidence between 6 months and 3 years of age.

Severe tissue damage can result from BBI from as little as 2 h *in situ*. The most important mechanism is that of electrolysis of fluid in local oesophageal tissue which generates a current, and subsequently hydroxide, at the negative pole of the battery. The type of button battery is also important: the ubiquitous lithium button batteries have a higher voltage and capacitance than other types resulting in an increased production of hydroxide and therefore more tissue damage. Other mechanisms include pressure necrosis and leakage of alkaline electrolytes from the battery itself (however, this is supposedly less of a problem with lithium batteries which are said to cause less mucosal irritation). Delayed complications include but are not limited to: oesophageal perforation; oesophageal stricture; tracheo-oesphageal fistula; exsanguination after fistulation into a major blood vessel (e.g. aorto-oesophageal fistula); and vocal cord paralysis.

Urgent surgical opinion should be sought alongside close liaison with ED colleagues. If the battery is located in the stomach or beyond, management (conservative or surgical) is dependent on the age of the child, the size of the battery, and if there is any concern for concurrent oesophageal injury.

6. **Pathological # left humerus**
   This child was presented to the ED with arm pain following a fall at a trampoline park. There is lucency and cortical thinning/scalloping in the left proximal diaphysis consistent with a simple (unicameral) bone cyst through which there is a pathological fracture.

7. **# left midshaft clavicle**
   The fracture is magnified in the image below which shows the acute step in the superior cortex:

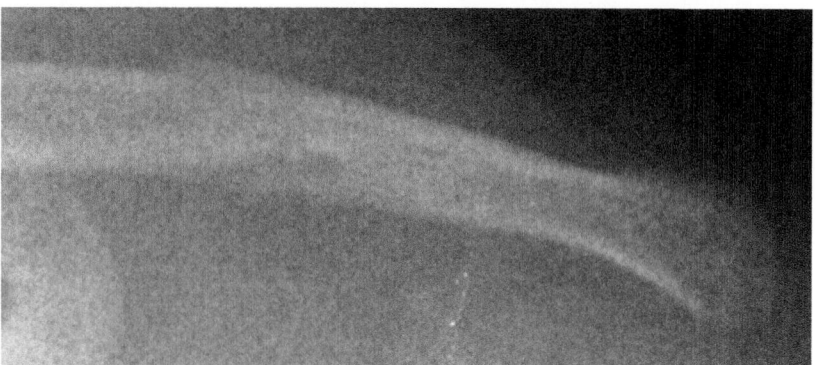

9. **Transverse # left middle and ring finger metacarpals**
    In the examination, there will usually be only one significant diagnosable abnormality per radiograph. However, in those radiographs which demonstrate a well-recognised fracture pattern in which two fractures may occur together, you would be expected to identify and write down both fractures to get the mark.

15. **Left upper lobe collapse**
    This portable chest radiograph demonstrates the distinctive radiographic features of left upper lobe collapse:
    - Veil-like opacity over the left hemithorax: as the left upper lobe collapses, it does so anteriorly, becoming apposed to the anterior chest wall resulting in both volume loss and increased radiographic density of the left hemithorax. Other features of left hemithorax volume loss include:
      - Drawing upwards of the left hilum
      - Elevation of the left hemidiaphragm, which may be 'tented' or 'peaked'
      - Crowding of the left-sided ribs (compare with the right-sided ribs)
      - Mediastinal shift to the left
    - Effacement of the anterior portion of the left heart border reflecting where the collapsed left upper lobe, particularly the lingula, abuts this portion of the left heart border.
    - Luftsichel sign: from the German, literally *air + sickle*, describing the 'air crescent' which can be seen between the aortic arch and the medial border of the collapsed lung. This appearance results from the hyperinflated superior segment of the left lower lobe which interposes itself between the mediastinum and the collapsed left upper lobe.

    A common cause of lobar collapse in children is mucous plugging due to asthma, bronchiolitis (which often results in multifocal areas of atelectasis), or endobronchial infection. A very important cause not to be forgotten is *foreign body inhalation or aspiration*, usually in younger children but also possibly in zealous older children!

    Tip for the viva:
    - This is a classic 'Starter for Ten' viva case, typically in an adult patient with a bronchogenic carcinoma presenting with a left upper lobe collapse on a chest radiograph.

16. **Buckle # right proximal tibia**

See the explanation for Test 6, Image 20. There is a subtle buckle of the lateral cortex of the right proximal tibia, seen in the magnified image below:

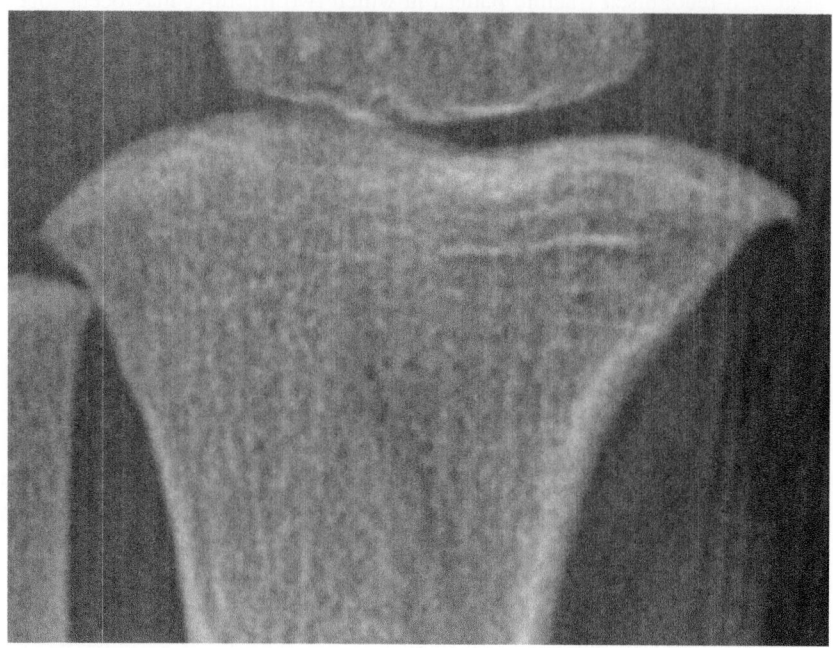

18. **Left radial head dislocation**

Did you spot this at the edge of the image? See the explanation for Test 1, Image 28.

19. **Pectus excavatum**

This image demonstrates the typical radiographic features of pectus excavatum:

- Horizontal posterior ribs with vertical anterior ribs creating the classic '7' configuration of the ribs
- Blurring or obscuration of the right heart border
- Increased density of the right inferomedial lung zone
- Displacement/shift of the heart to the left
- Decreased visualisation/absence of the descending aortic interface

Tip for the viva:

- Pectus excavatum is a common viva case because at a first or quick glance, the radiograph may appear normal. However, it is only on further inspection that the radiographic features of pectus excavatum, as described above, are appreciated.

21. **Salter-Harris 2 # base left thumb metacarpal**

22. **Normal pelvic radiograph**
    Note the normal iliac crest and AIIS apophyses which have not yet fused and are normal.

23. **Pneumomediastinum**
    See the explanation for Test 2, Image 5. This child presented with grunting and respiratory distress. The chest radiograph was obtained for '*?foreign body*'. Whilst this is a subtle finding, it is genuine. Note the subtle lucencies paralleling the upper left heart border and over the right cardiac silhouette, seen in the magnified image below:

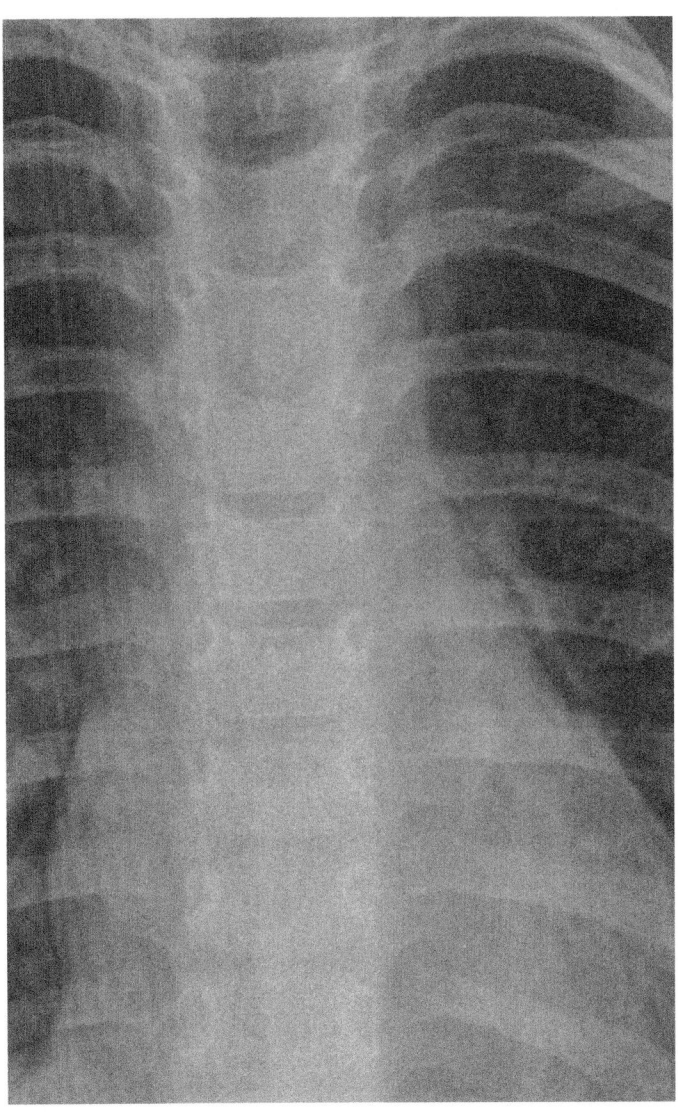

24. **# right little finger metacarpal neck**

26. **Right genu valgum/Cozen phenomenon**
    See the explanation for Test 6, Image 20. This radiograph demonstrates a right genu valgum deformity, or Cozen's phenomenon, following a right proximal tibial fracture 12 months previously.

27. **Buckle # right distal ulna**
    There is angulation of the radial aspect of the right distal ulna—sometimes buckle fractures are subtle, as in this case.

28. **Right middle lobe congenital lobar overinflation**
    Congenital lobar overinflation (CLO), previously known as congenital lobar emphysema (CLE), is a congenital progressive overinflation of a lung lobe(s) with a male predominance. This chest radiograph demonstrates the typical features of an overinflated right middle lobe: hyperlucency with a paucity of blood vessels (pulmonary oligaemia) and resultant mediastinal shift to the left.

    The right horizontal fissure has a tented appearance and has been displaced superiorly between the right second and third rib space medially. The right hemidiaphragm is not depressed and lies slightly higher than the left hemidiaphragm (inferring that the right lower lobe is not overinflated, in which case the right hemidiaphragm would be depressed). Thus, the overinflation can be localised to the right middle lobe.

    Immediate postnatal radiographs may be normal, or the affected lobe may be fluid-filled (with increased lobar opacity representing fetal lung fluid that has yet to clear). Serial radiographs may show progressive distension. Alternatively, as in this case, an initial radiograph taken some days after birth when respiratory distress develops (grunting, increased work of breathing, oxygen requirement) may reveal the lobar inflation and signifies that the normal ipsilateral lobes and contralateral normal lung can no longer compensate for the overinflated lobe.

    Investigation with CT, usually computed tomography pulmonary angiogram (CTPA), will not only delineate the lobe(s) affected but will confirm the CLO and help to differentiate from other pathologies such as congenital pulmonary airway malformation [CPAM], bronchial atresia, and bronchogenic cyst (the differential for this radiographic appearance). Furthermore, this allows the mediastinum and vascular anatomy to be evaluated for an anatomical defect such as an aberrant left pulmonary artery, a known associated abnormality with CLO. Associated cardiac defects include a VSD, PDA, and tetralogy of Fallot for which formal evaluation with echocardiography is advised.

    The right hemithorax is the most commonly affected (right middle and lower lobes affected approximately 30% and 20%, respectively) but there is a greater predilection for the left upper lobe, accounting for approximately 40–45% of cases. Management (which may be conservative or surgical) is determined by the severity of symptoms.

29. **Healing stress # right third metatarsal diaphysis**
    See the explanations for Test 2, Image 10 and Test 4, Image 18. The appearance of the metatarsal epiphyses is normal.

30. **Normal chest radiograph**
    This chest radiograph is normal. The triangular-shaped inferior margin of the right superior mediastinal opacity is the normal thymus—the triangular appearance is known as the 'thymic sail sign'. It can be seen bilaterally but is more commonly seen on the right side, as in this radiograph. Also note the appropriately sited nasogastric tube tip in the gas-filled stomach.

Further Reading

Image 5

Lee JH, Lee JH, Shim JO et al (2016) Foreign body ingestion in children: should button batteries in the stomach be urgently removed? Pediatr Gastroenterol Hepatol Nutr 19(1):20–28

Litovitz T, Whitaker N, Clark L (2010) Preventing battery ingestions: an analysis of 8648 cases. Paediatrics 125(6):1178–1183

Thabet MH, Basha WM, Askar S (2013) Button battery foreign bodies in children: hazards, management and recommendations. Biomed Res Int 2013:846091

Image 15

Do S, Maller VG et al (2018) Luftsichel sign (lungs). https://radiopaedia.org/articles/luftsichel-sign-lungs. Accessed June 2018

Gaillard F et al (2018) Left upper lobe collapse. https://radiopaedia.org/articles/left-upper-lobe-collapse. Accessed June 2018

Image 19

Bickle I, Gaillard F et al (2018) Pectus excavatum. https://radiopaedia.org/articles/pectus-excavatum. Accessed June 2018

Image 28

Chowdhury MM, Chakraborty S (2015) Imaging of congenital lung malformations. Semin Pediatr Surg 24(4):168–175

Daltro P, Fricke BL, Kuroki I, Domingues R, Donnelly LF (2004) CT of congenital lung lesions in pediatric patients. AJR Am J Roentgenol 183(5):1497–1506

Mohammed Abdul Wajid L, Sinha I, Gupta R (2017) An infant with persistent tachypnoea. Arch Dis Child Educ Pract Ed 102(4):222–223

Image 30

Gaillard F, Pradosh KS (2018) Thymic sail sign. https://radiopaedia.org/articles/thymic-sail-sign. Accessed June 2018

10.1 Images

Image 1

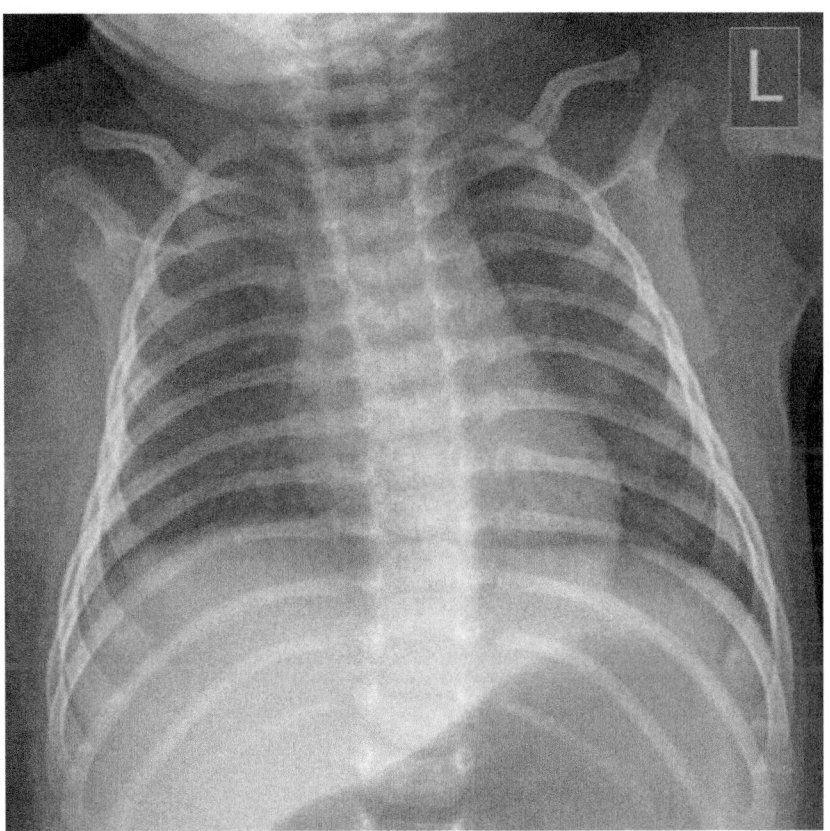

Normal	Abnormal	Diagnosis/Abnormality (only if abnormal)

© Springer Nature Switzerland AG 2019
M. Paddock, A. C. Offiah, *Paediatric Radiology Rapid Reporting for FRCR Part 2B*,
https://doi.org/10.1007/978-3-030-01965-5_10

Image 2

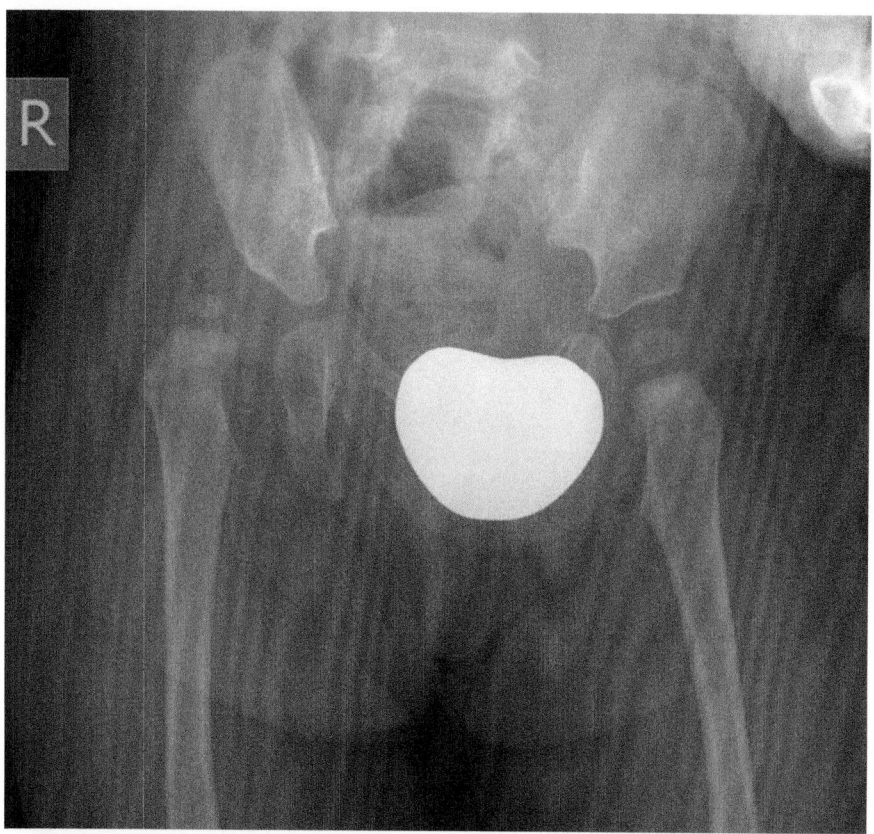

Normal	Abnormal	Diagnosis/Abnormality (only if abnormal)

Image 3

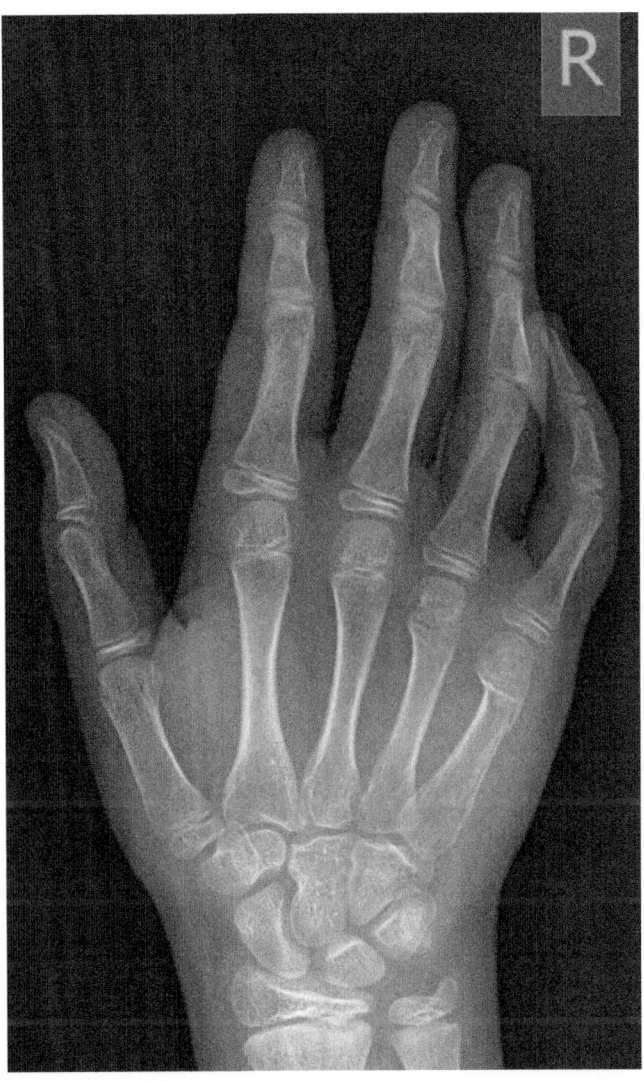

Normal	Abnormal	Diagnosis/Abnormality (only if abnormal)

Image 4

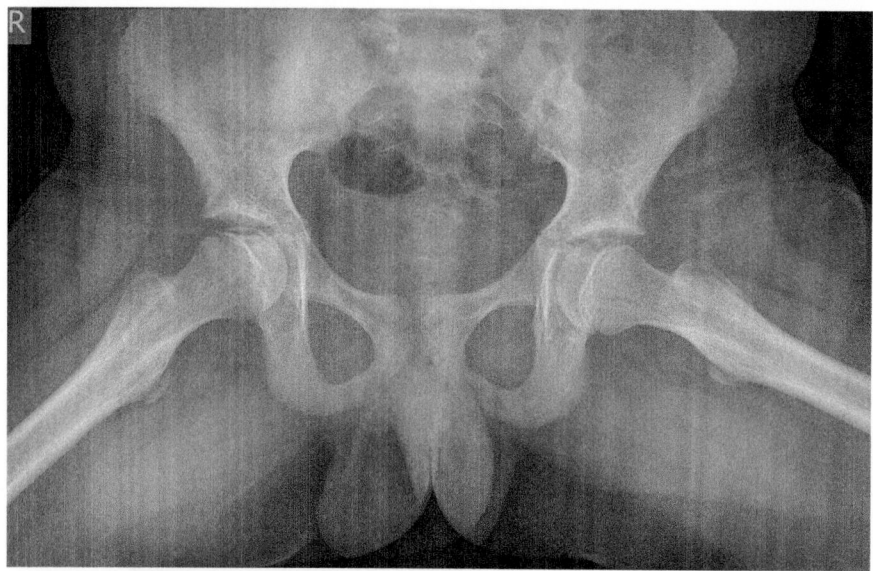

Normal	Abnormal	Diagnosis/Abnormality (only if abnormal)

Image 5

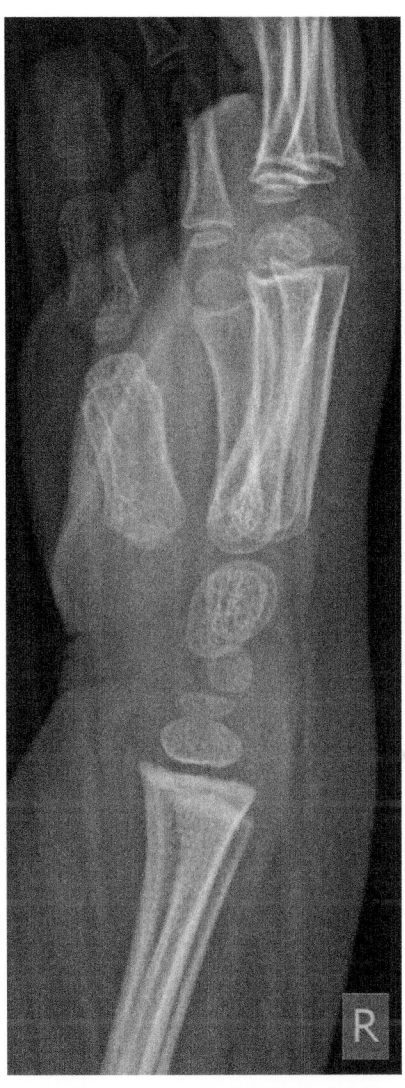

Normal	Abnormal	Diagnosis/Abnormality (only if abnormal)

Image 6

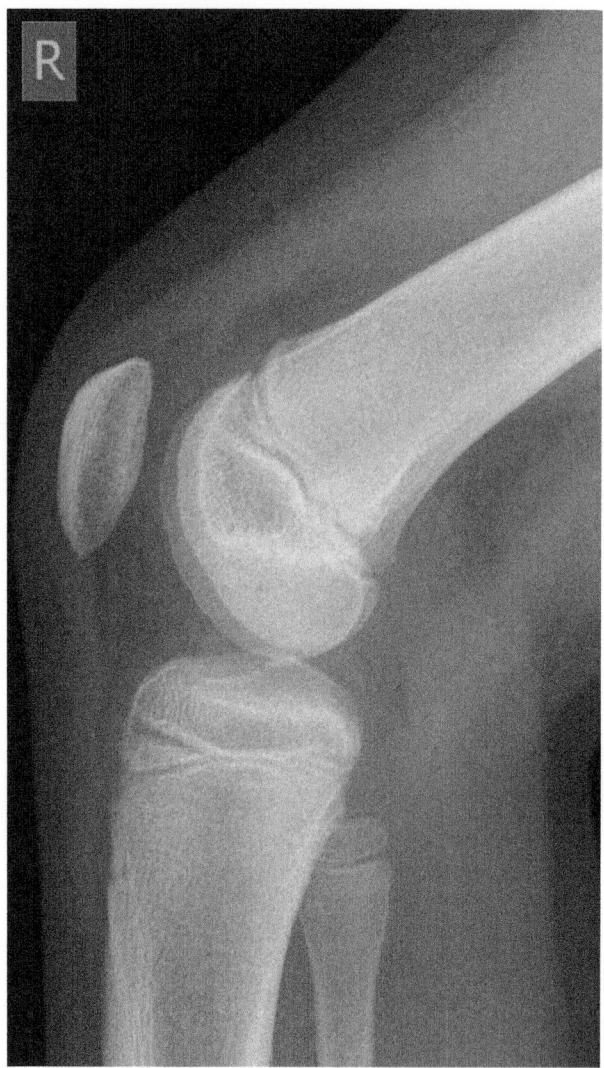

Normal	Abnormal	Diagnosis/Abnormality (only if abnormal)

Image 7

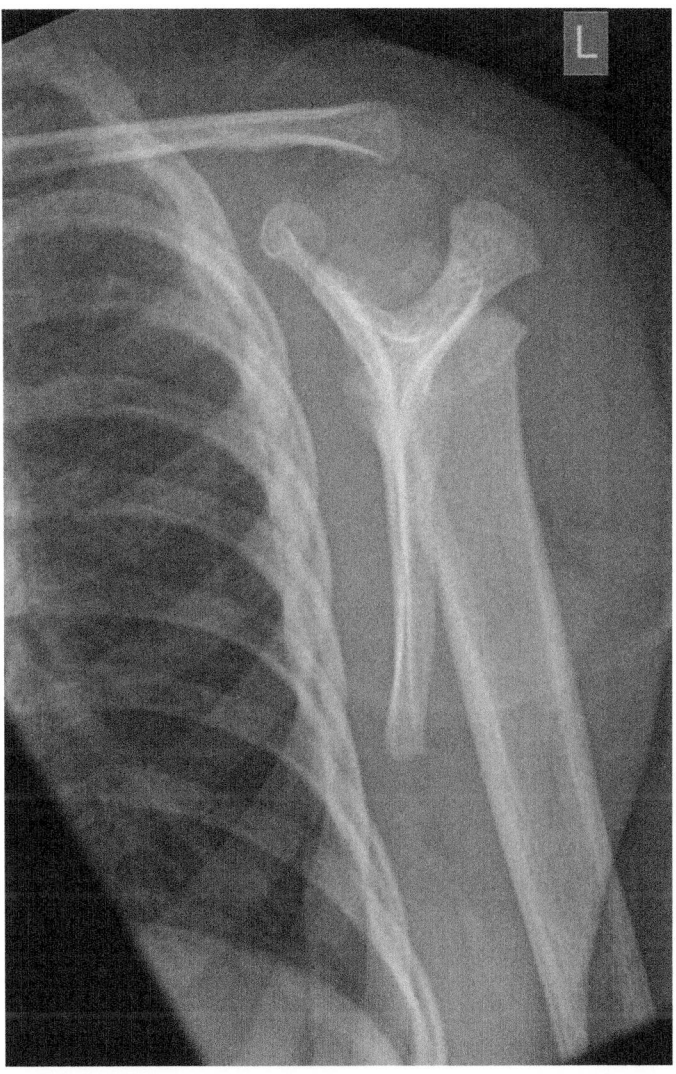

Normal	Abnormal	Diagnosis/Abnormality (only if abnormal)

Image 8

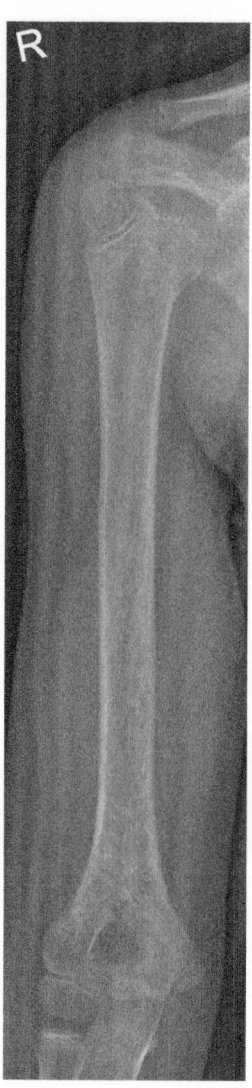

Normal	Abnormal	Diagnosis/Abnormality (only if abnormal)

Image 9

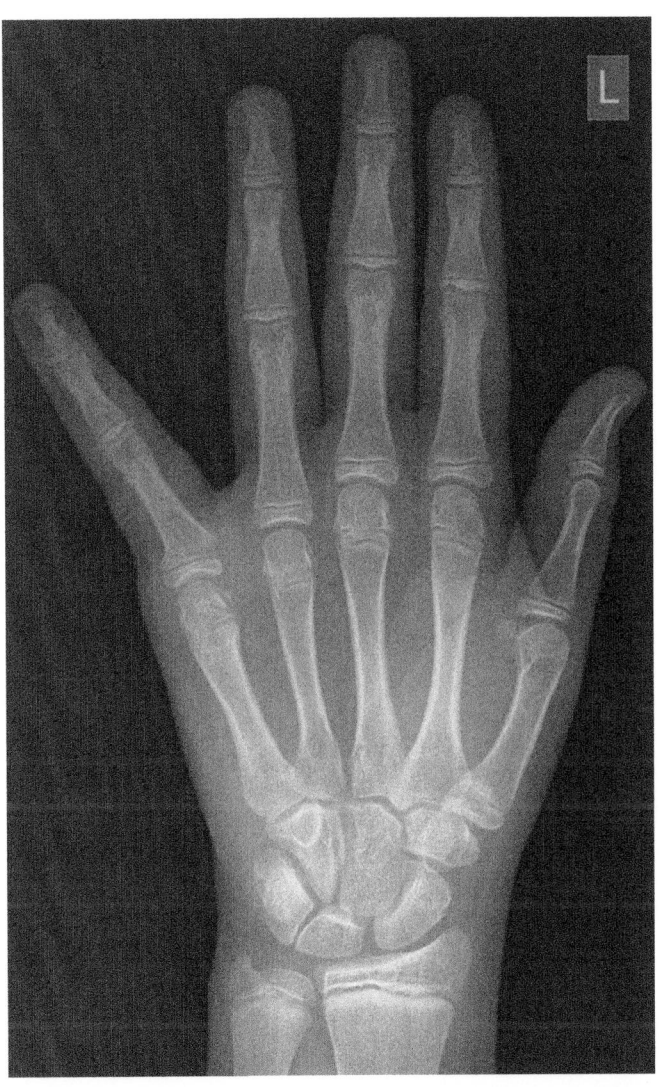

Normal	Abnormal	Diagnosis/Abnormality (only if abnormal)

Image 10

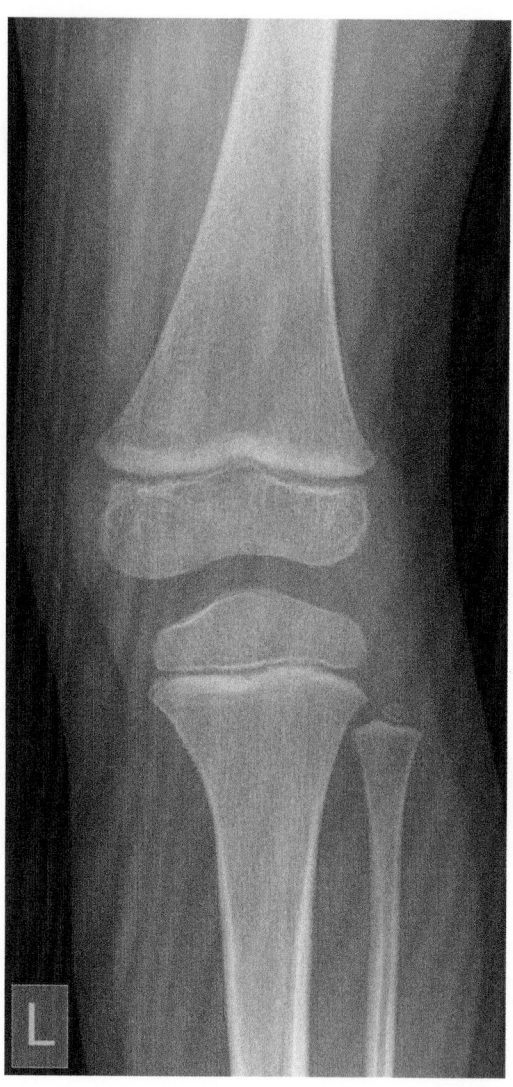

Normal	Abnormal	Diagnosis/Abnormality (only if abnormal)

Image 11

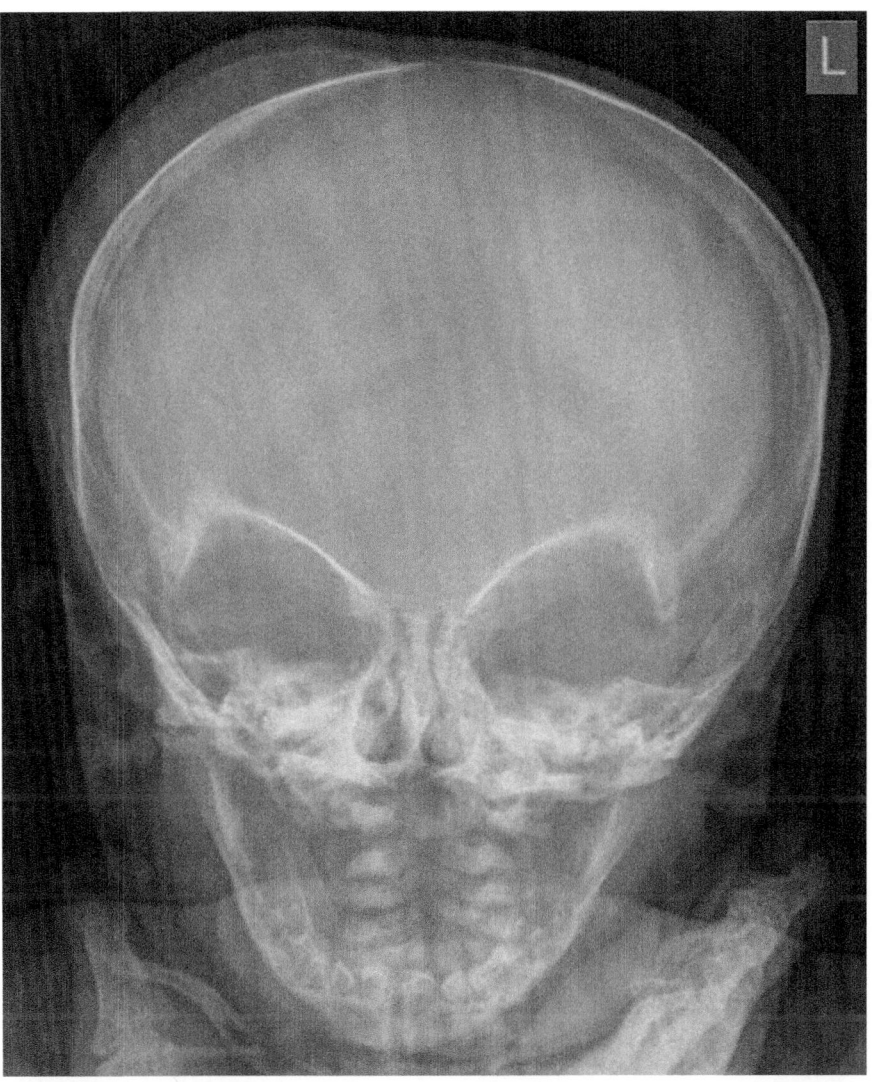

Normal	Abnormal	Diagnosis/Abnormality (only if abnormal)

Image 12

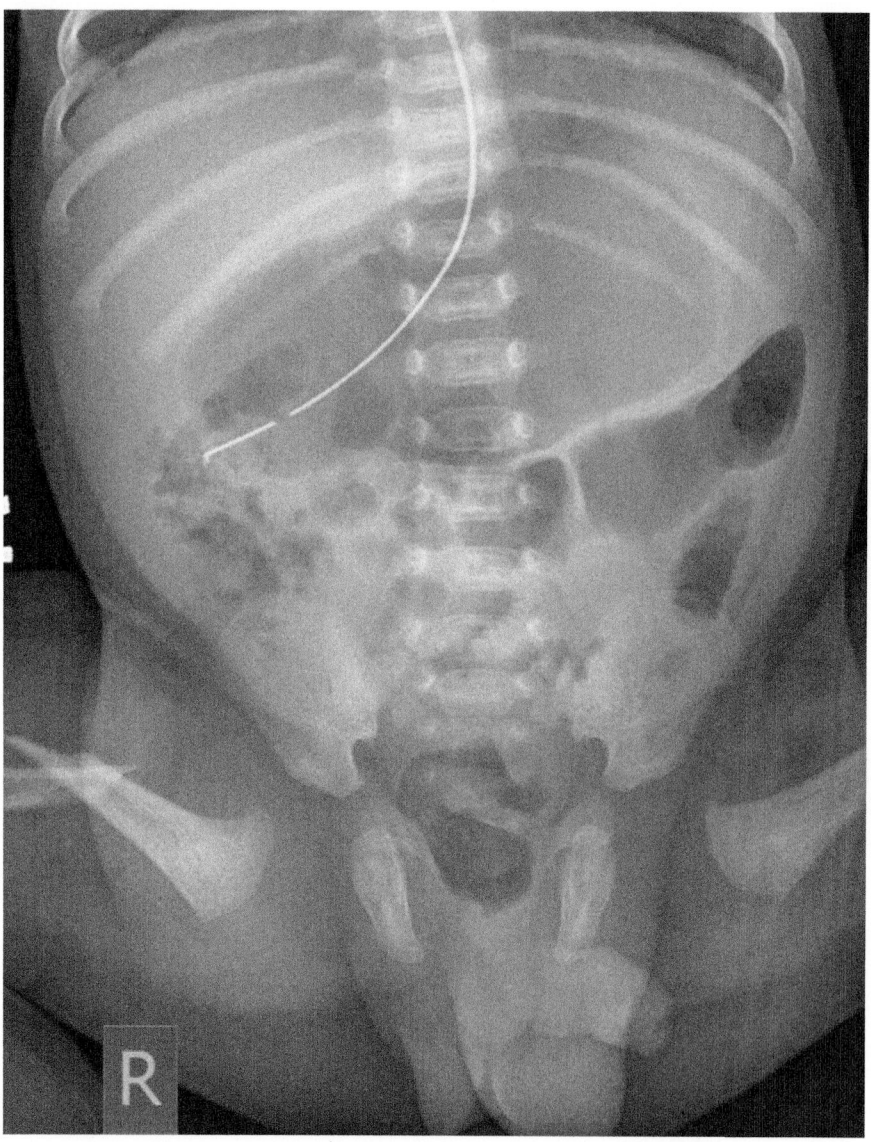

Normal	Abnormal	Diagnosis/Abnormality (only if abnormal)

Image 13

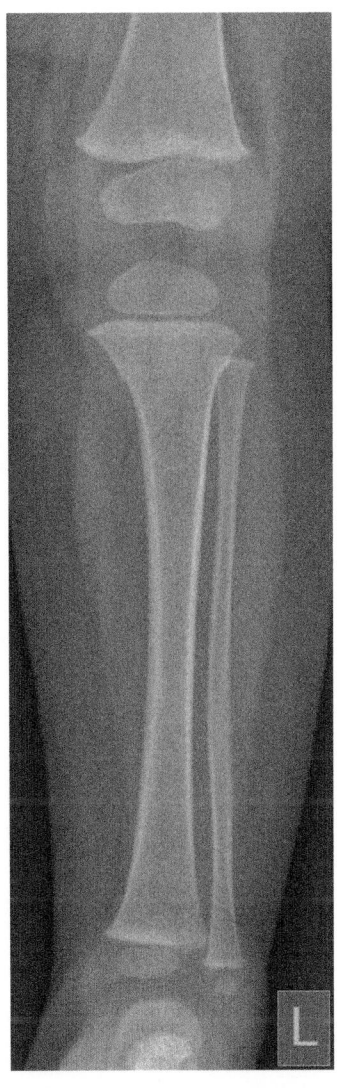

Normal	Abnormal	Diagnosis/Abnormality (only if abnormal)

Image 14

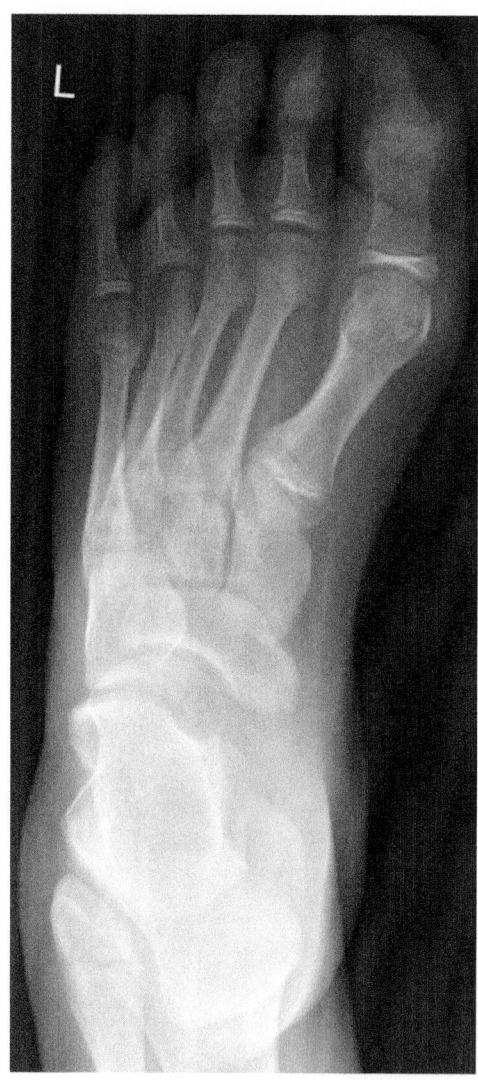

Normal	Abnormal	Diagnosis/Abnormality (only if abnormal)

Image 15

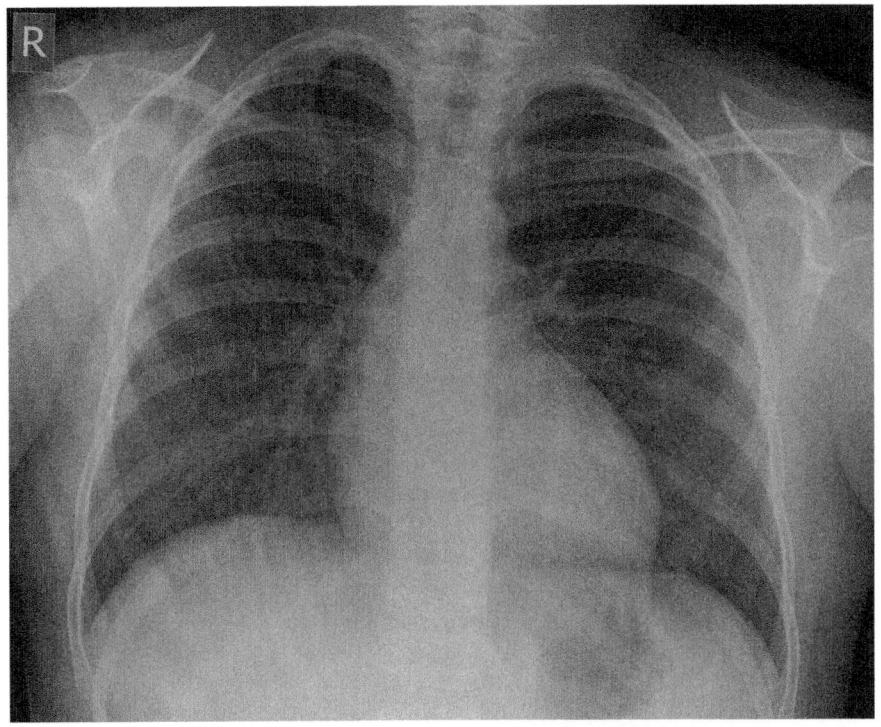

Normal	Abnormal	Diagnosis/Abnormality (only if abnormal)

Image 16

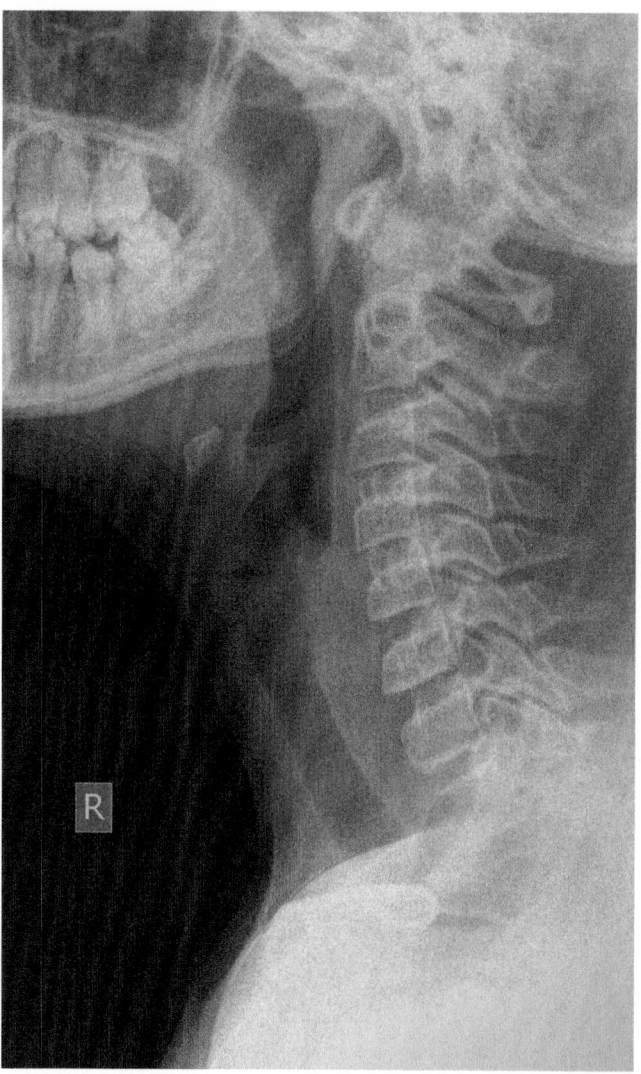

Normal	Abnormal	Diagnosis/Abnormality (only if abnormal)

Image 17

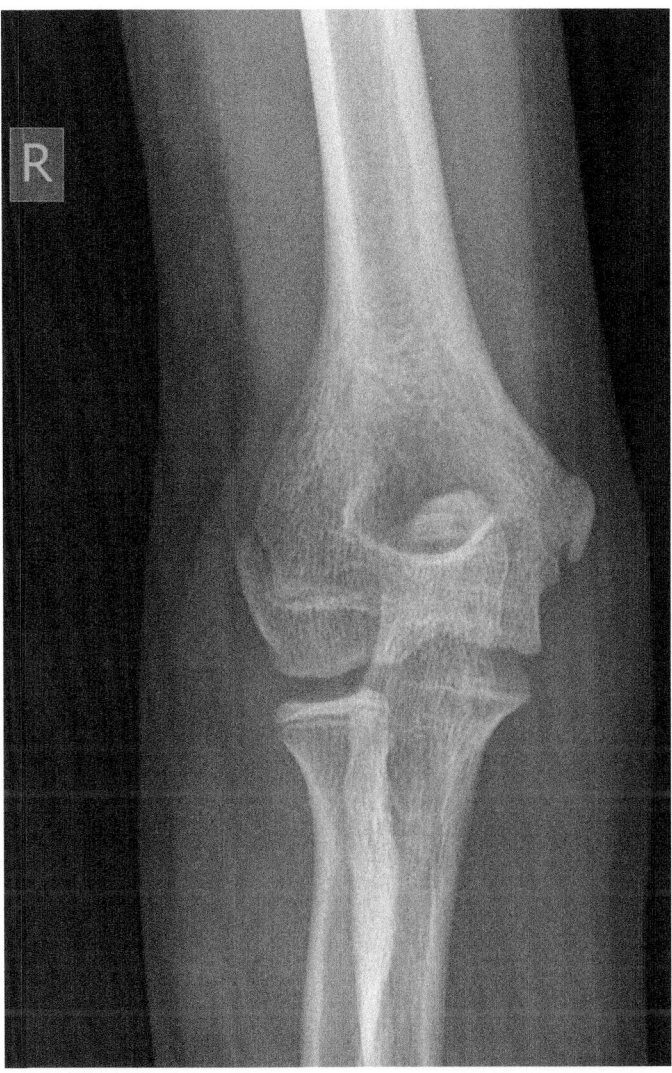

Normal	Abnormal	Diagnosis/Abnormality (only if abnormal)

Image 18

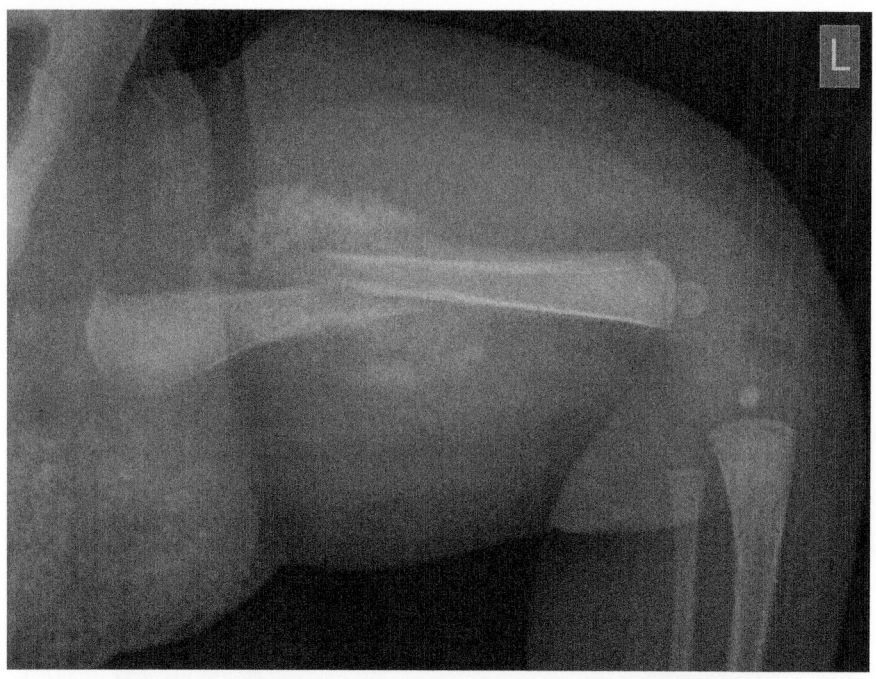

Normal	Abnormal	Diagnosis/Abnormality (only if abnormal)

Image 19

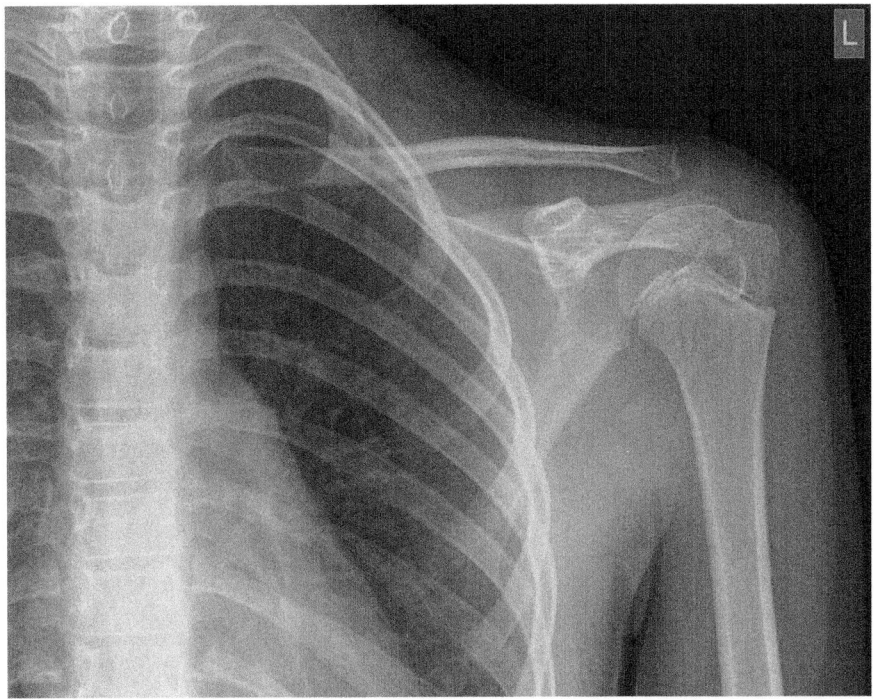

Normal	Abnormal	Diagnosis/Abnormality (only if abnormal)

Image 20

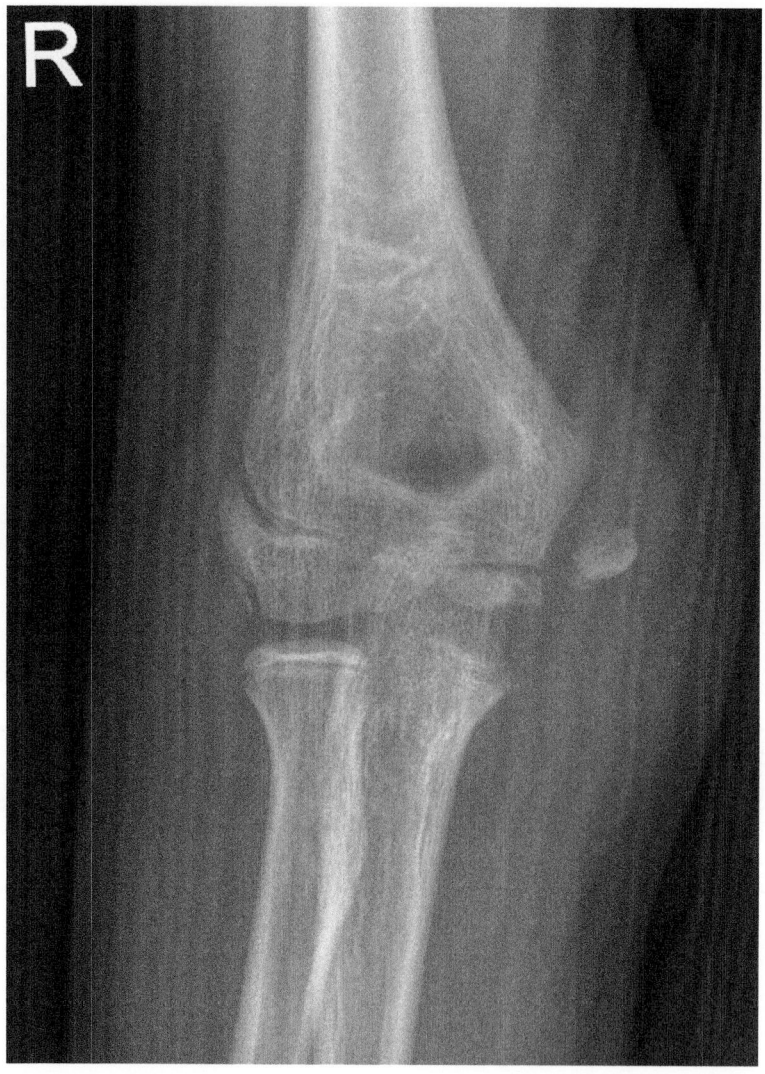

Normal	Abnormal	Diagnosis/Abnormality (only if abnormal)

Image 21

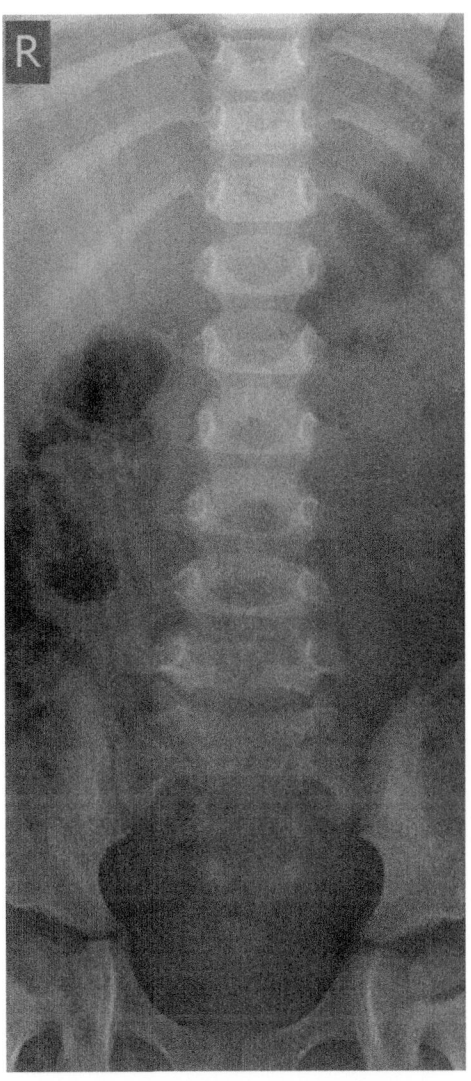

Normal	Abnormal	Diagnosis/Abnormality (only if abnormal)

Image 22

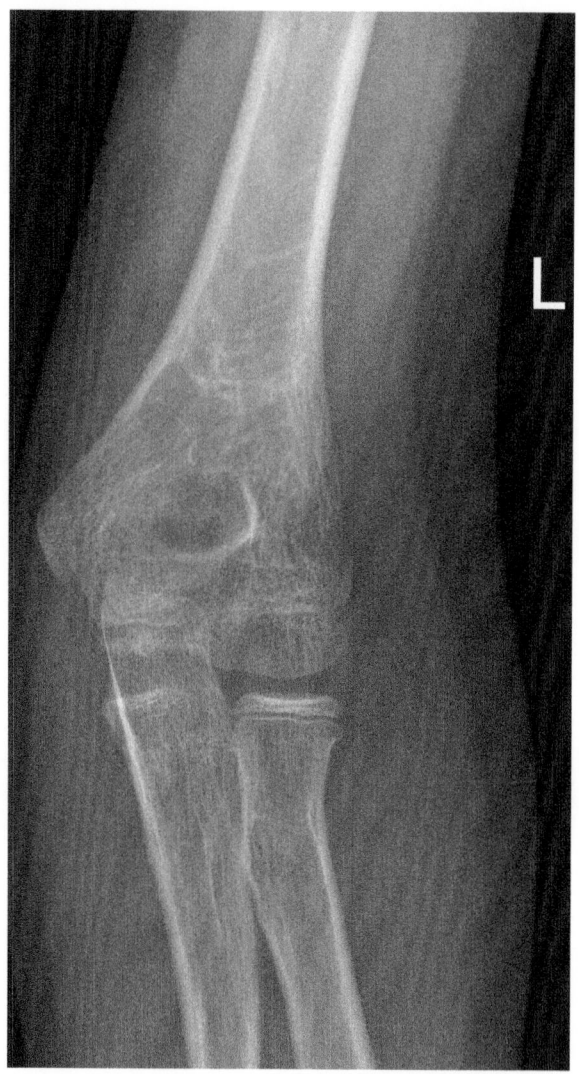

Normal	Abnormal	Diagnosis/Abnormality (only if abnormal)

Image 23

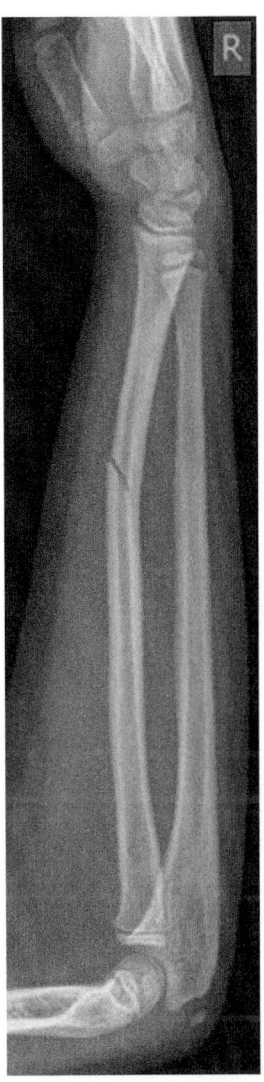

Normal	Abnormal	Diagnosis/Abnormality (only if abnormal)

Image 24

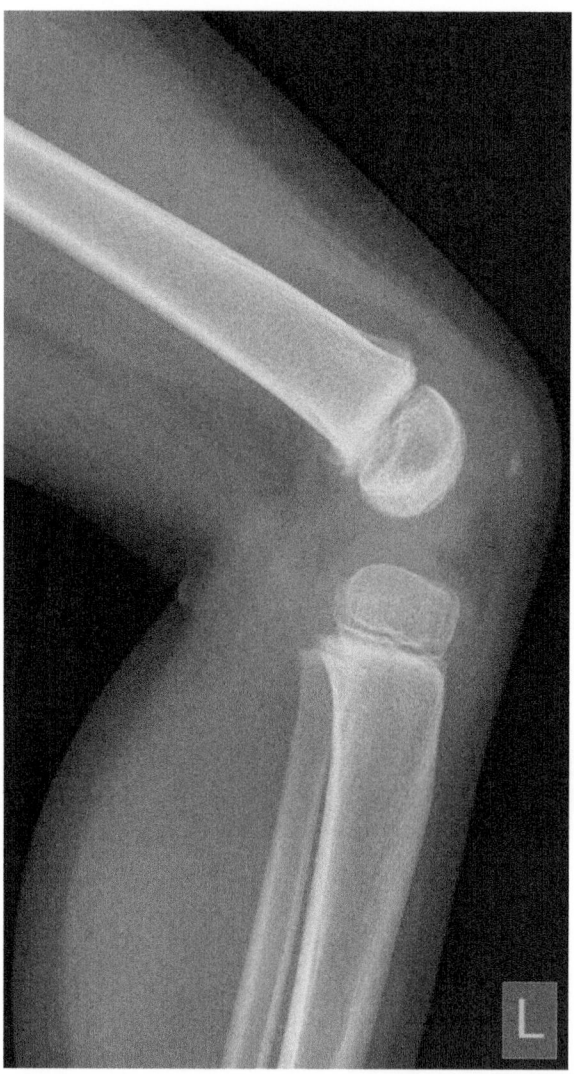

Normal	Abnormal	Diagnosis/Abnormality (only if abnormal)

Image 25

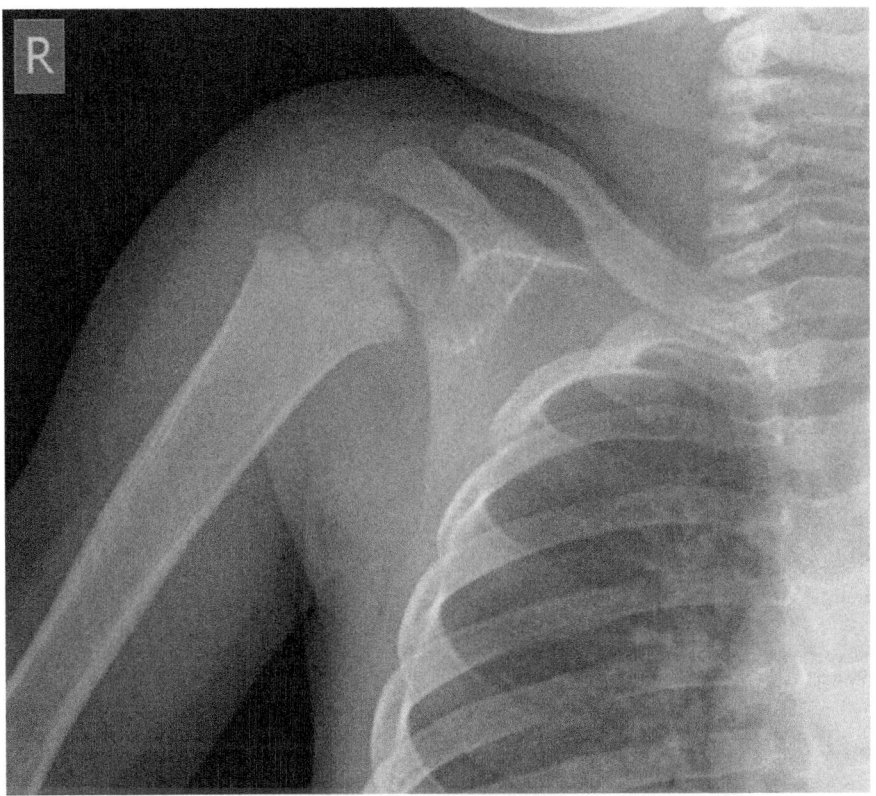

Normal	Abnormal	Diagnosis/Abnormality (only if abnormal)

Image 26

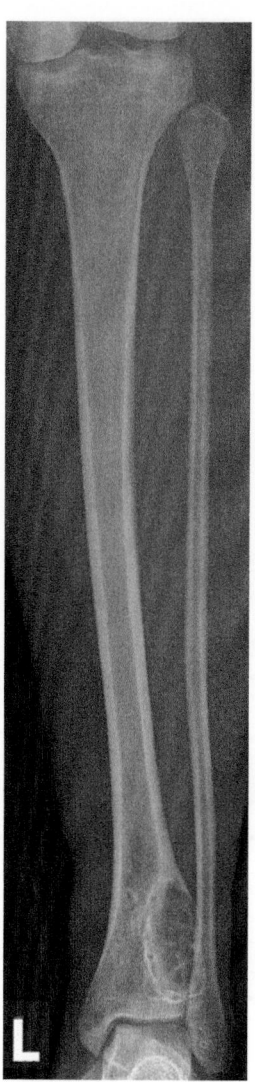

Normal	Abnormal	Diagnosis/Abnormality (only if abnormal)

Image 27

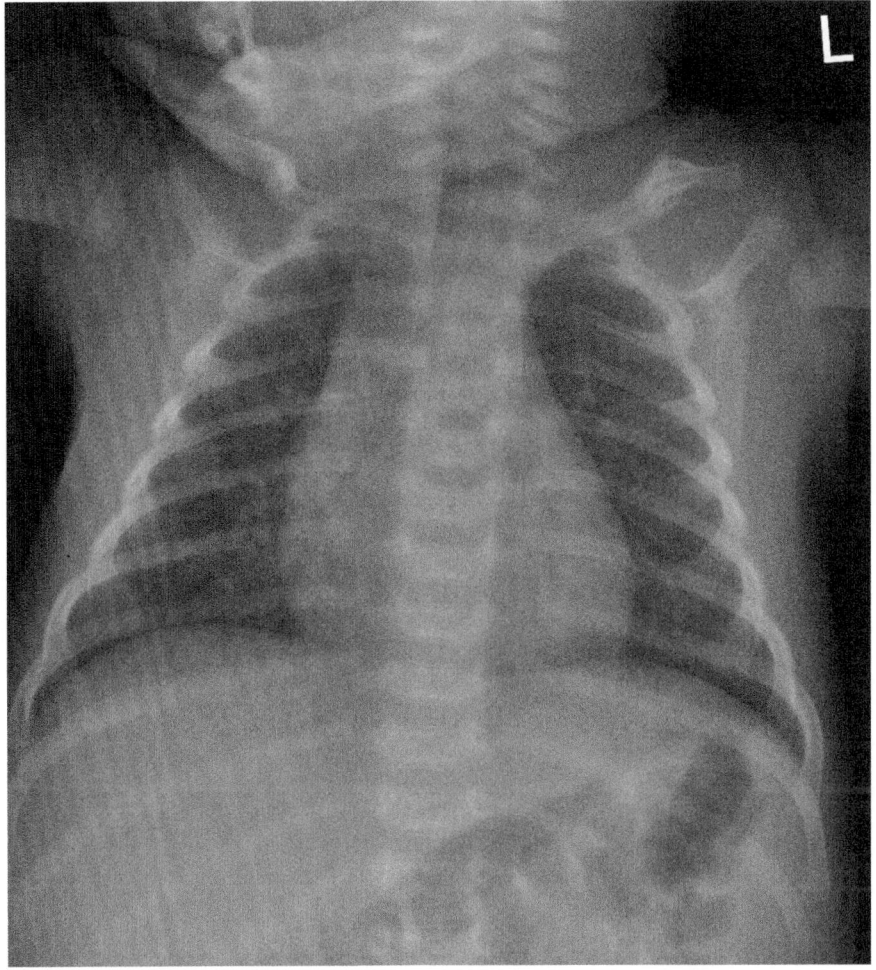

Normal	Abnormal	Diagnosis/Abnormality (only if abnormal)

Image 28

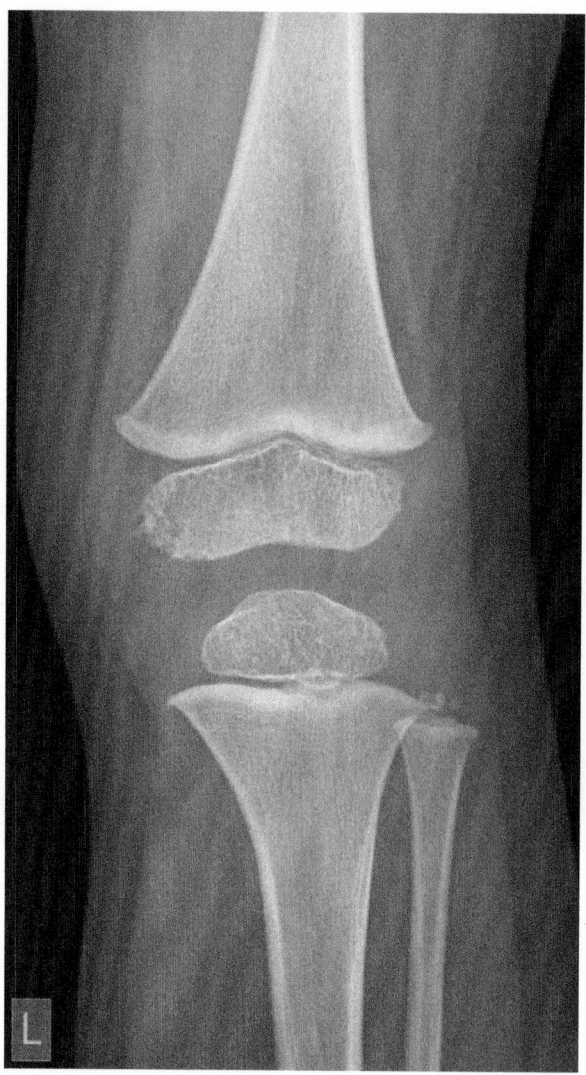

Normal	Abnormal	Diagnosis/Abnormality (only if abnormal)

Image 29

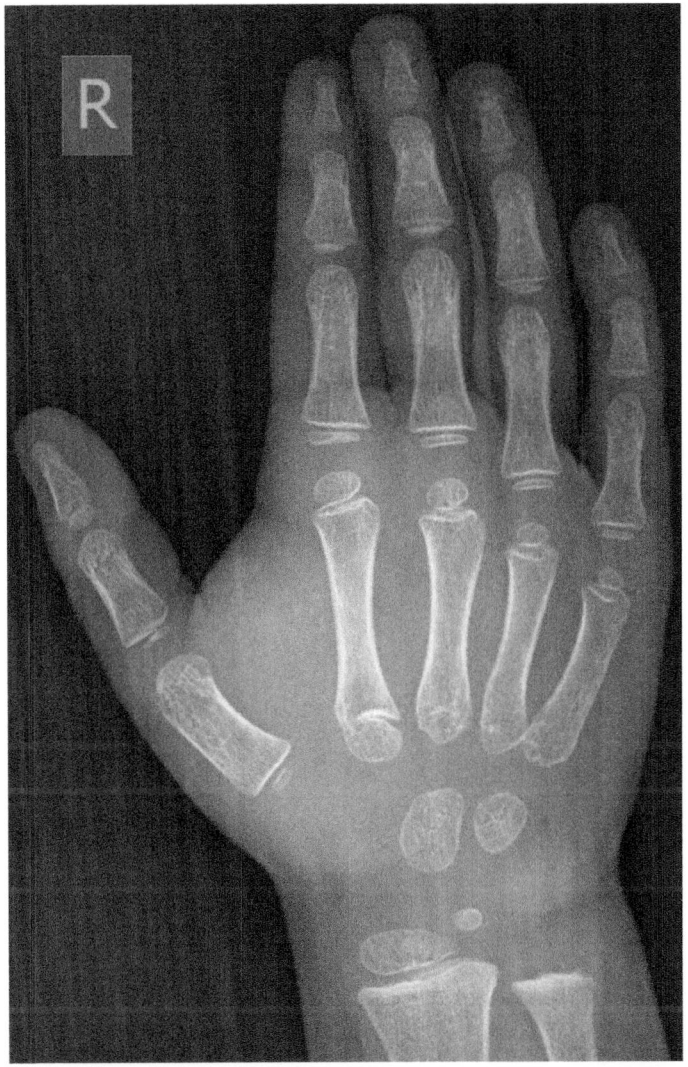

Normal	Abnormal	Diagnosis/Abnormality (only if abnormal)

Image 30

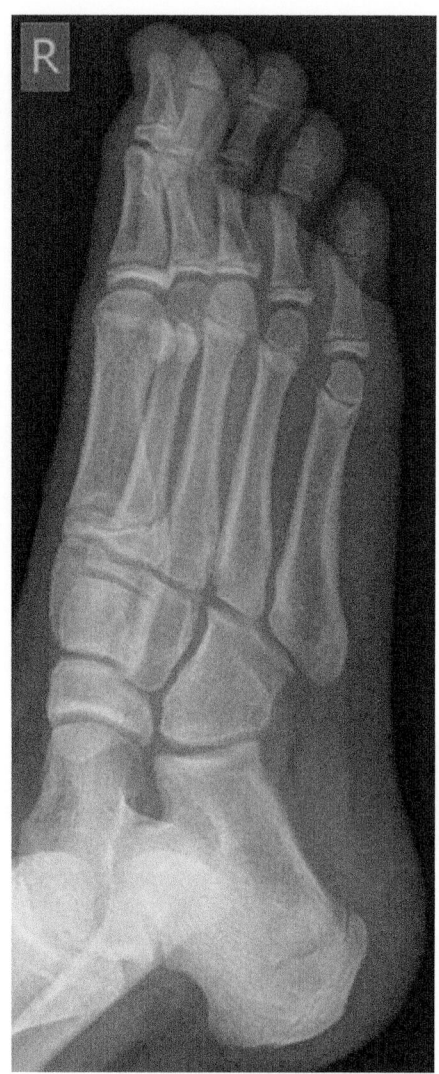

Normal	Abnormal	Diagnosis/Abnormality (only if abnormal)

10.2 Answers

Image	Normal	Abnormal	Diagnosis/abnormality (only if abnormal)
1	✓		
2		✓	Developmental dysplasia right hip
3		✓	# right ring and little finger metacarpal necks
4		✓	Avascular necrosis right proximal femoral epiphysis
5	✓		
6	✓		
7	✓		
8		✓	Aggressive bone lesion right humerus
9		✓	# base left little finger proximal phalanx
10	✓		
11		✓	Right parietal calcified cephalohaematoma
12		✓	Displaced angulated right femoral #
13		✓	Buckle # left proximal tibia
14		✓	# proximal phalanx left hallux
15	✓		
16	✓		
17	✓		
18		✓	Healing left femoral #
19	✓		
20		✓	Avulsion # right medial epicondyle
21	✓		
22		✓	Left radial neck #
23		✓	# right radius at junction of mid and distal thirds
24	✓		
25	✓		
26		✓	Non-ossifying fibroma left distal tibia
27		✓	Healing # left midshaft clavicle
28	✓		
29	✓		
30	✓		

10.3   Explanations

1. **Normal chest radiograph**
   Note the gas-filled stomach in the imaged upper abdomen which is a normal finding in neonates and infants who have been crying before and during image acquisition, causing them to swallow air (aerophagia) which creates this radiographic appearance.

2. **Developmental dysplasia right hip**
   See the explanation for Test 2, Image 17.

3. **# right ring and little finger metacarpal necks**

4. **Avascular necrosis right proximal femoral epiphysis**
   This radiograph demonstrates the 'crescent sign', namely a well-defined subchondral lucency in the lateral aspect of the right proximal femoral epiphysis consistent with AVN. See the explanation for Test 1, Image 1.

7. **Normal left shoulder radiograph**
   This is a normal 'Y-view' projection of the left shoulder. The left first costovertebral recess is normal.

8. **Aggressive bone lesion right humerus**
   There are permeative lucencies throughout the humerus, most notable in the supracondylar region, consistent with an aggressive process. Note the loss of definition of the lateral cortex of the distal humerus. This radiograph was obtained in a 7-year-old female for right arm pain with a known diagnosis of neuroblastoma: the radiographic findings are consistent with metastastic neuroblastoma.

   Tip for the viva:
   • Whilst not present in this case, it is important to look for a pathological fracture in the context of pain with abnormal bone texture.

9. **# base left little finger proximal phalanx**

11. **Right parietal calcified cephalohaematoma**
    This 3-week-old female, born by normal vaginal delivery, was referred to the general paediatricians for a head swelling which had been present from birth but which had not resolved. The radiograph demonstrates a calcified collection overlying the right parietal bone bound by the sagittal suture superiorly and the right squamous suture inferiorly, localising the collection to the subperiosteal

space. Collections in this potential space *cannot* cross suture lines making this a cephalohaematoma and distinguishing it from a subgaleal haematoma which *can* cross suture lines. See the explanation for Test 7, Image 30.

12. **Displaced angulated right femoral #**
A dedicated femoral radiograph was obtained on presentation which demonstrated the displaced and angulated right femoral diaphyseal fracture. This abdominal/pelvic radiograph was taken as part of the initial skeletal survey. See the explanation for Test 3, Image 23.

13. **Buckle # left proximal tibia**
This is another example of a 'trampoline fracture'—see the explanation for Test 6, Image 20 and the longer term complication in Test 9, Image 26. The fracture is magnified in the image below:

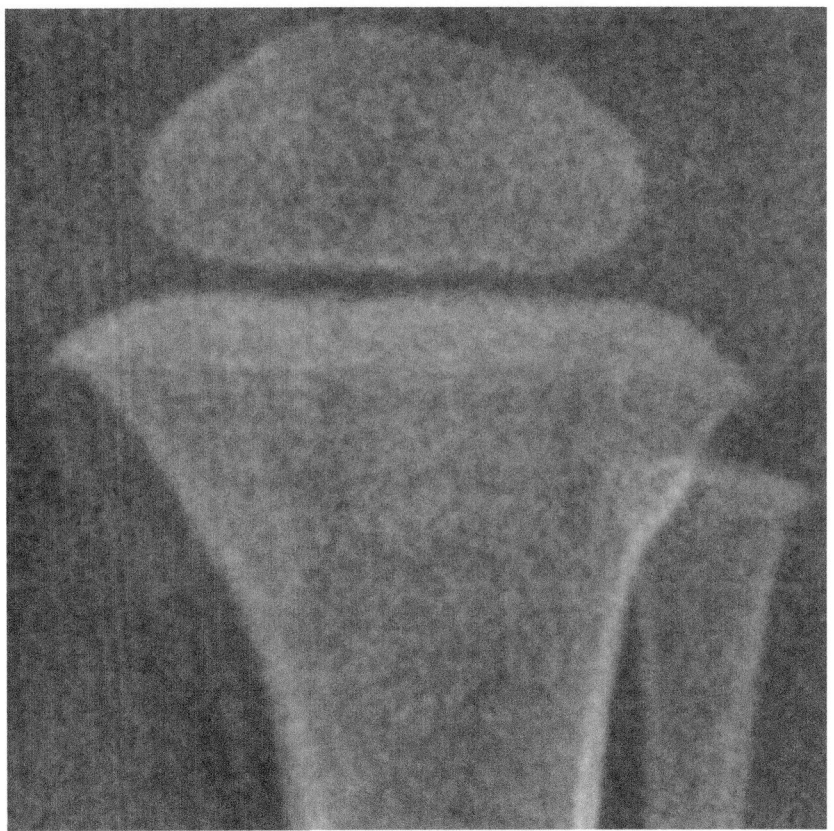

14. **# proximal phalanx left hallux**

This minimally displaced fracture is seen in the magnified image below:

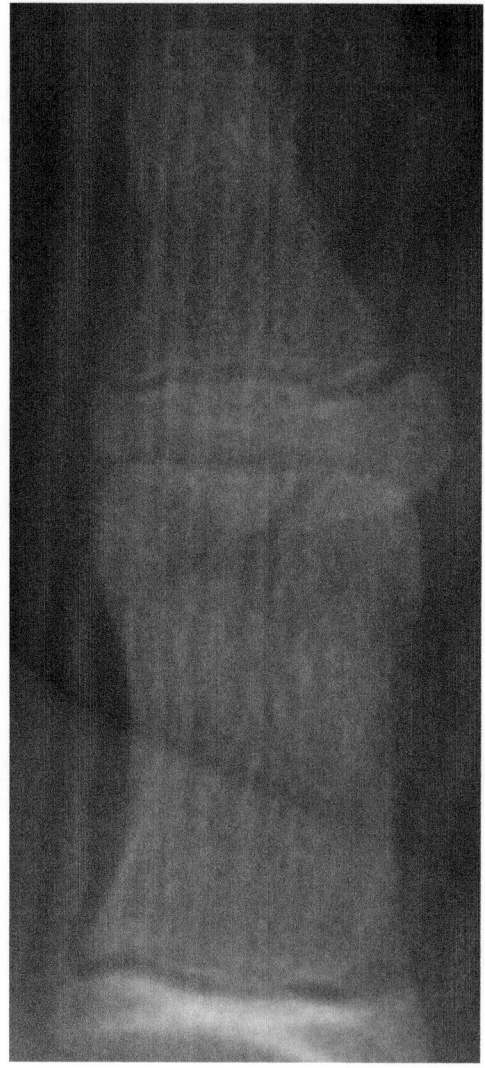

16. **Normal cervical spine radiograph**

    This radiograph is normal. The facet joints are clearly visualised due to the slight obliquity of the projection. There is no subluxation or dislocation and the alignment is normal.

18. **Healing left femoral #**

    This 16-day-old was admitted from the community after a firm swelling of the left thigh was noted on examination. The radiograph reveals a healing fracture of the left femoral mid shaft. Florid periosteal reaction is present and represents calcification (or new bone formation) of the subperiosteal haematoma that occurred at the time of the fracture. Radiographic dating of fractures is complex and subjective. The presence of subperiosteal new bone formation is the most reliable radiographic feature of fracture healing and when present, indicates that the fracture is at least 10 days old. As discussed in the explanation for Test 3, Image 23, depending on the history, a lower limb long bone fracture in a pre-ambulant infant is suspicious of inflicted injury.

    CT of the head showed subdural haemorrhage in the posterior fossa and the right side of the falx; no other brain injury or acute intracranial haemorrhage was demonstrated. Subdural haemorrhages can be found in neonates on imaging following delivery, both normal vaginal and assisted (forceps/ventouse) but are usually 'clinically silent' and when present in asymptomatic infants are usually infratentorial in location and usually resolve by 4 weeks following delivery. This is contrasted with the pattern of subdural haemorrhage found in inflicted injury which is typically supratentorial—bilateral or interhemispheric. The infratentorial haemorrhage in this child had resolved on the MRI performed 2 days later and imaging of the spine was normal. It is imperative that cross-sectional imaging of the neuroaxis (i.e. of the brain *and* spine) is performed in the imaging investigation of suspected physical abuse, as recommended in the national guidance. Investigation with initial and follow-up skeletal survey did not reveal any other acute or healing fractures. It was felt that this fracture, whilst unexplained, alongside the pattern of intracranial haemorrhage, was probably sustained at the time of delivery.

20. **Avulsion # right medial epicondyle**

    The medial epicondyle ossification centre is displaced from its normal position with significant associated soft tissue swelling in keeping with avulsion fracture. See the explanation for Test 6, Image 9. Note the small linear fragmented ossification on the inferolateral aspect of the capitellar ossification centre which is normal.

22. **Left radial neck #**

Note the acute angulation of the lateral aspect of the left radial neck in keeping with fracture, as visualised in the magnified image below:

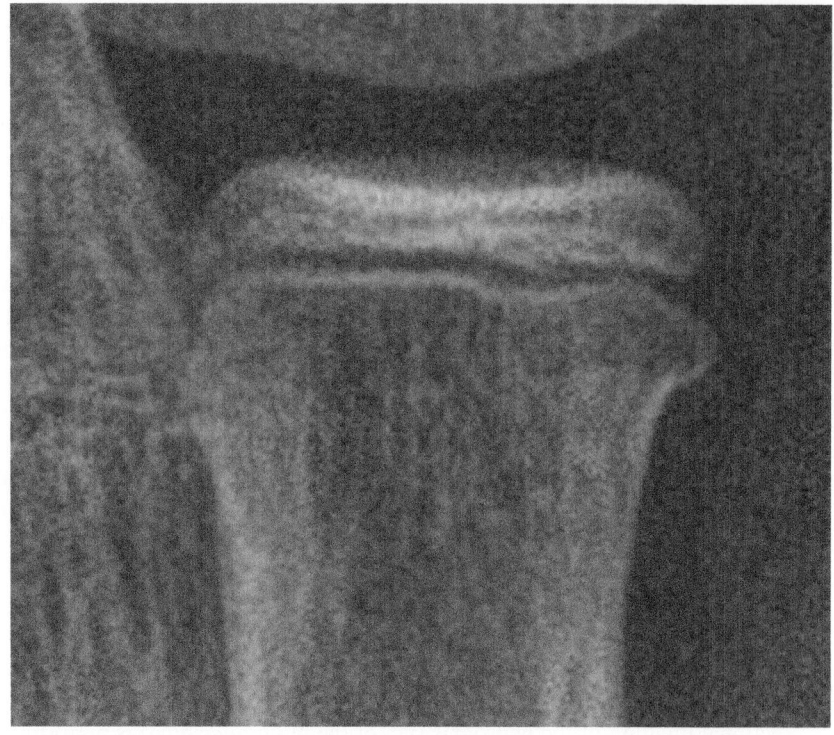

23. **# right radius at junction of mid and distal thirds**

In the context of a distal radial fracture, typically at the junction of the middle and distal thirds (as in this case), one must assess the distal radioulnar joint for dislocation as part of the Galeazzi fracture-dislocation pattern (not present in this case as confirmed on the contemporaneous orthogonal projection). This pattern typically occurs following a FOOSH with the elbow in flexion.

See Test 1, Image 28 and Test 8, Image 7 for a discussion regarding the Monteggia fracture-dislocation pattern (ulnar shaft fracture + concomitant radial head dislocation).

Tip for the viva:

- Formal forearm radiographs should be recommended if they have not yet been obtained: ensure that the wrist and elbow joints have *both* been imaged.

26. **Non-ossifying fibroma left distal tibia**

See the explanation for Test 5, Image 5.

27. **Healing # left midshaft clavicle**

The chest radiograph demonstrates a healing fracture of the left clavicle with callus formation and remodelling. It was obtained in a 6-week-old male following presentation to the ED following a brief resolved unexplained event (BRUE), previously termed an apparent life-threatening event (ALTE). These events are typified by a combination of apnoea, colour change, change in muscle tone (often hypotonia or 'floppy baby'), and choking and gagging. Mean age of presentation is 1–3 months of age. These events are frightening for parents/caregivers who observe and report this presentation to clinicians.

Aetiologies include: gastrointestinal (typically gastro-oesophageal reflux); neurological (seizure is the most common disorder associated with BRUE/ALTE); respiratory (infection, such as bronchiolitis, or lung disease of prematurity); cardiovascular (structural heart disease); and metabolic and endocrine (hypoglycaemia or inborn errors of metabolism).

Whilst less than 3% are reported to result from physical child abuse, this aetiology must be ever present in the mind of all clinicians who assess infants presenting with BRUE/ALTE. Similarly, as clinical radiologists, when reporting any imaging performed for 'BRUE/ALTE', 'blue episode', 'collapse', or 'apnoea', physical child abuse should always be suspected particularly if there is evidence of acute or healing bony injury (as in this case). Close liaison with paediatric colleagues is advised, particularly given that the recently published guidance recommends that chest radiography should not be performed for this indication—please see the references.

The initial and follow-up skeletal survey did not reveal any further acute or healing fractures. There was normal radiographic bone modelling and density (i.e. no radiographic evidence of a skeletal dysplasia). CT imaging of the brain was normal.

Whilst the healing fracture was unexplained, it was felt that the fracture was likely sustained at the time of delivery (normal vaginal delivery). Any birth injury should have healed completely by the age of 3 months.

Further Reading

Image 12

Hui C, Joughin E, Goldstein S et al (2008) Femoral fractures in children younger than three years: the role of nonaccidental injury. J Pediatr Orthop 28:297–302

Kemp AM, Dunstan F, Harrison S et al (2008) Patterns of skeletal fractures in child abuse: systematic review. BMJ 337:a1518

Schwend RM, Werth C, Johnston A (2000) Femur shaft fractures in toddlers and young children: rarely from child abuse. J Pediatr Orthop 20:475–481

Thomas SA, Rosenfield NS, Leventhal JM et al (1991) Long-bone fractures in young children: distinguishing accidental injuries from child abuse. Pediatrics 88:471–476

Image 18

Whitby EH, Griffiths PD, Rutter S et al (2004) Frequency and natural history of subdural haemorrhages in babies and relation to obstetric factors. Lancet 363(9412):846–851

Image 23

Luijkx T, Gaillard F et al (2018) Galeazzi fracture-dislocation. https://radiopaedia.org/articles/galeazzi-fracture-dislocation. Accessed August 2018

Image 27

Choi HJ, Kim YH (2016) Apparent life-threatening event in infancy. Korean J Pediatr 59(9):347–354

Jobe AH (2008) What is ALTE? J Pediatr 152(3):A2

Tate C, Sunley R (2018) Brief resolved unexplained events (formerly apparent life-threatening events) and evaluation of lower-risk infants. Arch Dis Child Educ Pract Ed 103(2):95–98

CPI Antony Rowe
Eastbourne, UK
January 28, 2020